Tissue Engineering and Regeneration in Dentistry

Tissue Engineering and Regeneration in Dentistry

Current Strategies

EDITED BY

Rachel J. Waddington, PhD

School of Dentistry, Cardiff Institute of Tissue Engineering and Repair, Cardiff University, Cardiff, UK

Alastair J. Sloan, PhD

School of Dentistry, Cardiff Institute of Tissue Engineering and Repair, Cardiff University, Cardiff, UK

WILEY Blackwell

This edition first published 2017 © 2017 John Wiley & Sons, Ltd

Registered Office
John Wiley & Sons, Ltd, The Atrium, Southern Gate, Chichester, West Sussex, PO19 8SQ, UK

Editorial Offices
9600 Garsington Road, Oxford, OX4 2DQ, UK
The Atrium, Southern Gate, Chichester, West Sussex, PO19 8SQ, UK
1606 Golden Aspen Drive, Suites 103 and 104, Ames, Iowa 50010, USA

For details of our global editorial offices, for customer services and for information about how to apply for permission to reuse the copyright material in this book please see our website at www.wiley.com/wiley-blackwell.

Library of Congress Cataloging-in-Publication Data

Names: Waddington, Rachel (Rachel J.), editor. | Sloan, Alistair J., editor.
Title: Tissue engineering and regeneration in dentistry : current strategies / edited by Rachel J Waddington and Alistair J Sloan.
Description: Chichester, West Sussex, UK ; Ames, Iowa : John Wiley & Sons Inc., 2017. | Includes bibliographical references and index.
Identifiers: LCCN 2016022478 | ISBN 9781118741108 (pbk.) | ISBN 9781118741047 (Adobe PDF) | ISBN 9781118741078 (epub)
Subjects: | MESH: Tissue Engineering–methods | Dentistry–methods | Guided Tissue Regeneration–methods | Stomatognathic Diseases–therapy
Classification: LCC RK320.T47 | NLM WU 100 | DDC 617.6/340592–dc23
LC record available at https://lccn.loc.gov/2016022478

A catalogue record for this book is available from the British Library.

Wiley also publishes its books in a variety of electronic formats. Some content that appears in print may not be available in electronic books.

Cover image: © Andrew Brookes/Gettyimages

Set in 8.5/12pt Meridien by SPi Global, Pondicherry, India

Printed and bound in Singapore by Markono Print Media Pte Ltd

1   2017

Contents

List of contributors

Wayne Nishio Ayre
School of Dentistry
Cardiff Institute of Tissue Engineering and Repair
Cardiff University
Cardiff, UK

P. Mark Bartold
Colgate Australian Dental Research Centre
Dental School
University of Adelaide
Adelaide, SA, Australia

Vanessa Chrepa
School of Dentistry
University of Texas Health Science Center
San Antonio, TX, USA

John Colombo
School of Dentistry
University of Utah
Salt Lake City, UT, USA

Lindsay C. Davies
Centre for Hematology and Regenerative Medicine
Karolinska Institutet
Stockholm, Sweden;
School of Dentistry
Cardiff University
Heath Park
Cardiff, UK

David de Silva Thompson
University College London
London, UK

Anibal Diogenes
School of Dentistry
University of Texas Health Science Center
San Antonio, TX, USA

Ikbale El Ayachi
Department of Bioscience Research
College of Dentistry
University of Tennessee Health Science Center
Memphis, TN, USA

Stan Gronthos
School of Medical Sciences
Faculty of Health Sciences
University of Adelaide
Adelaide, SA, Australia
South Australian Health and Medical Research Institute
Adelaide, SA, Australia

George T.-J. Huang
Department of Bioscience Research
College of Dentistry
University of Tennessee Health Science Center
Memphis, TN, USA

Dietmar W. Hutmacher
Institute of Health and Biomedical Innovation
Queensland University of Technology
Brisbane, Queensland, Australia

Saso Ivanovski
Menzies Health Institute Queensland
School of Dentistry and Oral Health
Griffith University
Gold Coast, Queensland, Australia

S. Quentin Jones
School of Dentistry
Cardiff Institute of Tissue Engineering and Repair
Cardiff University
Cardiff, UK

Katarina Le Blanc
Centre for Hematology and Regenerative Medicine
Karolinska Institutet
Stockholm, Sweden

Ryan Moseley
School of Dentistry
Cardiff Institute of Tissue Engineering and Repair
Cardiff University
Cardiff, UK

Roman Perez
Institute of Tissue Regeneration Engineering (ITREN)
Dankook University
Cheonan, Republic of Korea

Carlotta Peticone
University College London
London, UK

Jessica Roberts
North Wales Centre for Primary Care Research
Bangor University
Wrexham, UK

Nikita B. Ruparel
School of Dentistry
University of Texas Health Science Center
San Antonio, TX, USA

Alastair J. Sloan
School of Dentistry
Cardiff Institute of Tissue Engineering and Repair
Cardiff University
Cardiff, UK

Rachel J. Waddington
School of Dentistry
Cardiff Institute of Tissue Engineering and Repair
Cardiff University
Cardiff, UK

Ivan Wall
University College London
London, UK;
Institute of Tissue Regeneration Engineering (ITREN)
Dankook University
Cheonan, Republic of Korea

Xiao-Ying Zou
Department of Cariology, Endodontology and Operative
Dentistry
Peking University School and Hospital of Stomatology
Beijing, China

Preface

Over the past twenty years there has been an explosion in published research studies characterising and investigating the behaviour of adult stem cells from the dental and oral tissues, and much excitement has been anticipated in their ability to regenerate a variety of connective tissues. Research in this field is rapidly expanding, facilitated by the many interdisciplinary collaborative opportunities for the repair of dental and craniofacial tissues. Their use has been championed for much wider translational opportunities, from large tissue volume regeneration of the musculoskeletal system to repair of ischaemic heart and liver tissue injury, replacement of misfunctioning cells such as pancreatic islet cells, and regeneration of neuronal networks and spinal cord injury. However, when entering the expansive literature, it is clear that many different experimental protocols have been utilised that examine heterogeneous stem cells, subpopulations, and clonally established cell lines where consideration of the environmental conditions are a critical for interpreting biological response. It is now very clear that adult stem cells represent a heterogeneous family of mesenchymal stem cells, where biological responses and translational applications are clearly going to be affected by the age and tissue source, with isolation and culture procedures affecting their peri-cellular and niche environment. In addition, the clinical use of such cells requires consideration of a number of practical limitations that need to be overcome, such as scale up and delivery. As the field of stem cell biology develops, characterisation of the cell populations is becoming ever more complex, although it should remain an important research element in assessing the therapeutic potential of stem cells. Indeed, exciting opportunities exist for reprogramming these cells, which may hold promise for expanding therapeutic potential. It is evident that much research in the area is needed to further our understanding.

In compiling this book, our aim was to highlight the varied breadth and considerations of the current research and the plethora of published literature to display key findings and current hypotheses. However, rather than simply produce a review of the current "state of the literature" we also aim to help active researchers in the field, both scientists and clinicians, through the provision of invaluable tools and methodologies utilised in undertaking research in this field, and to highlight important biological and practical considerations to facilitate successful migration of research from bench to clinic. As such, the chapters contained within this book not only provide a comprehensive overview of the published literature, but they highlight considerations that must be made for current data, indicate areas for development, and also provide clear protocols, methods, or "case studies" for aspects of research that can be used by other researchers in the field. With the help of leading experts in craniofacial and dental stem cell research and tissue engineering, we wanted to produce a textbook that becomes a valuable reference handbook and a practical guide that comes to be an invaluable lab text.

Professor Rachel J. Waddington
Professor Alastair J. Sloan

CHAPTER 1

Induced pluripotent stem cell technologies for tissue engineering

George T.-J. Huang[1], Ikbale El Ayachi[1], and Xiao-Ying Zou[2]

[1] Department of Bioscience Research, College of Dentistry, University of Tennessee Health Science Center, Memphis, TN, USA

[2] Department of Cariology, Endodontology and Operative Dentistry, Peking University School and Hospital of Stomatology, Beijing, China

Induced pluripotent stem cells (iPSCs) were first established by delivering the four factors c-Myc/Klf4/Oct4/Sox2 or Lin28/Nanog/Oct4/Sox2 into dermal fibroblasts via a viral vector-based approach (Takahashi et al., 2007; Takahashi and Yamanaka, 2006; Yu et al., 2007). To avoid permanent integration of these introduced exogenous genes, plus the vector that carries them, significant efforts have been put into removing the transgenes and vectors from cells after they have been reprogrammed into iPSCs (Gonzalez et al., 2009; Kaji et al., 2009; Soldner et al., 2009; Woltjen et al., 2009; Yu et al., 2009a). Because of the reactivation of endogenous pluripotent genes that function to maintain the pluripotent state after reprogramming, these exogenous transgenes can be removed without affecting the reprogrammed status. In fact, removing these exogenous transgenes renders iPSCs more similar to human embryonic stem cells (hESCs) (Soldner et al., 2009). Besides using viral vector systems to reprogram cells, other methods that can completely circumvent the use of vectors have been utilised, including delivery of recombinant protein-based or synthetic mRNAs of the four factors to generate iPSCs (reviewed by Rao and Malik, 2012). There are many applications that iPSCs can contribute to; among others, this chapter focuses on (1) cell-based tissue regeneration and (2) generation of patient-specific iPSCs to study disease mechanisms.

With respect to the source of cells for human iPSC generation, various cell types are capable of converting into iPSCs, although dermal fibroblasts are most commonly used due to their relative ease of access and availability (Aasen et al., 2008; Giorgetti et al., 2009; Giorgetti et al., 2010; Li et al., 2009; Loh et al., 2009; Miyoshi et al., 2010a; Nakagawa et al., 2008; Park et al., 2008b; Sun et al., 2009; Takahashi et al., 2007; Yan et al., 2010). In general it is easier to reprogram more immature cells than more differentiated cells. From the perspective of clinical applications, cells that are not easily accessible, such as neural stem cells, are not a suitable cell source for iPSC generation. The oral cavity harbours a rich source of mesenchymal stem cells (MSCs), including those from various dental tissues, gingival/mucosal tissues, and alveolar bone (Huang et al., 2009; Morsczeck et al., 2013). Extracted teeth are considered biomedical waste and gingival/mucosal tissues are easily accessible and available. Oral MSCs are also relatively robust in respect to cell proliferation and population doubling (Huang et al., 2009); therefore, these cells may be one of the best sources for generating iPSCs.

While many aspects of iPSCs require investigation concerning their clinical safety, utilising iPSCs for cell therapy is anticipated to take place in the future. Studies focusing on guiding iPSCs to differentiate into various cell types for regeneration purposes have been rigorously undertaken. This chapter will overview current progress in this area, particularly emphasising neurogenesis. Additionally, utilising iPSCs as a tool for studying genetics and disease mechanisms will also be reviewed.

Overview of iPSCs

iPSC derivation

While various approaches or conditions may lead to the derivation of pluripotent stem cells in mammals (Cowan et al., 2005; Gómez et al., 2006; Miyashita et al., 2002;

Tissue Engineering and Regeneration in Dentistry: Current Strategies, First Edition. Edited by Rachel J. Waddington and Alastair J. Sloan.
© 2017 John Wiley & Sons, Ltd. Published 2017 by John Wiley & Sons, Ltd.

Oh et al., 2009; Thuan et al., 2010; Wilmut et al., 1997; Yu et al., 2006), attempts to generate human (h) ESCs by somatic cell nuclear transfer continues to be unsuccessful. Human triploid blastocysts have been generated and are capable of giving rise to ESCs (Noggle et al., 2011); however, triploid hESCs are an unlikely or favorable cell source for clinical applications. Cells that have potential clinical value are hESCs derived from the parthenogenetic approach (Revazova et al., 2007; Revazova et al., 2008). Nonetheless, such a technology is inconvenient and difficult to perform. Yamanaka and his team utilised a $Fbx15^{\beta geo/\beta geo}$ mouse model and found that by introducing 4 factors, c-Myc, Klf4, Oct4 and Sox2 were sufficient to reverse fibroblasts to ES-like cells, termed "induced pluripotent cells (iPSCs)" (Takahashi and Yamanaka, 2006). These mouse (m) iPSCs demonstrate the features resembling ES cells. These include similar morphology in cultures, growth rate, key pluripotent genes, global gene profiles, epigenetic profiles, and capability of embryoid body (EB) formation. In addition, differentiation into cells of all germ layers is observed in EBs *in vitro*, as well as formation of teratomas *in vivo* containing tissues of all germ layers, and above all, the formation of chimeras after iPSCs were injected into blastocysts in an animal system. Subsequently, Yamanaka's group further demonstrated that the same four factors c-Myc, Klf4, Oct4 and Sox2 were also effective in humans in reprogramming fibroblasts into iPSCs, exhibiting similar features mentioned above for miPSCs, except the formation of chimeras which cannot be tested for the human system (Takahashi et al., 2007). Thomson's group independently identified a core set of 4 genes, Oct4, Sox2, Nanog and Lin28 that were also able to reprogram human fibroblasts into iPSCs (Yu et al., 2007).

The successful rate of iPS generation is generally low; the highest was at 0.1% in a mouse system using embryonic fibroblasts as the cell source (Smith et al., 2009). With a single lentiviral vector expressing all four Yamanka's factors, Sommer et al. (2009) were able to demonstrate a reprogramming efficiency of 0.5% using mouse tail-tip fibroblasts. In human systems, adipose tissue stem cells can reach a successful reprogramming rate of 0.2% (Sun et al., 2009). In general, it is difficult to assess the absolute efficiency as different laboratories are using various vector systems and the viral activities can vary widely as well. Compared to other means of deriving human pluripotent stem cells, iPSCs appear to be the desired method for potential clinical utilisation.

Characteristics of iPSCs

One critically important hallmark of ESCs as pluripotent stem cells is the capability to form embryos and be born into live animals via a tetraploid-complementation procedure. Using a mouse system, such cell characteristics can be demonstrated and the generation of live pups by iPSCs, some of which lived to adulthood, has been demonstrated (Boland et al., 2009; Kang et al., 2009; Zhao et al., 2009). The successful rate of giving rise to tetraploid complementation by iPSCs is similar to that by ESCs; however, there are variables in iPSC lines. Some iPSC lines showed early termination of fetal development at the embryonic stage (Zhao et al., 2009). Generally, iPSCs are functionally similar if not identical to ESCs. One drawback is the variability among different iPSC clones. hiPSCs cannot be tested by such methodologies; therefore, characterisation at genetic and epigenetic levels should be carried out to establish the molecular basis of the reprogrammed hiPSC clones.

In the human system, the global gene-expression patterns and epigenetic profiles between iPS and ES cells were shown to be similar (Takahashi et al., 2007; Yu et al., 2007). Regarding the telomere regaining length in iPSCs, this was addressed in the reprogramming of cells from patients with Dyskeratosis congenita (DC), a disorder of telomere maintenance (Agarwal et al., 2010). Reprogramming can restore telomere elongation in DC cells despite genetic lesions affecting telomerase (Agarwal et al., 2010).

Examining the whole-genome profiles of DNA methylation at single-base resolution of hiPSC lines revealed that there is reprogramming variability, including somatic memory and aberrant reprogramming of DNA methylation (Lister et al., 2011). iPSCs are thought to harbor a residual DNA methylation signature related to their cell of origin, termed "epigenetic memory". This predisposes them toward differentiation along lineages related to that cell type and restricts differentiation to alternative cell fates (Kim et al., 2010; Polo et al., 2010). Epigenetic memory can also be correlated with a residual transcriptional profile in iPSCs that is related to the cell from which it was originally reprogrammed (Ghosh et al., 2010). Epigenetic analysis of the iPSC clones may be needed to provide a critical baseline for studying cellular changes occurring during the controlled *in vitro* differentiation concerning the utility of these cells for future therapies. There are also reprogramming-associated mutations that occur during or after reprogramming. It is suggested that extensive genetic screening should become a standard procedure to ensure hiPSC safety before clinical use (Gore et al., 2011). Despite these caveats, efforts have been made to produce pure, stable, and good manufacturing practice (GMP)–grade hiPSCs potentially suited for clinical purposes (Durruthy-Durruthy et al., 2014).

While mutations may occur during reprogramming, whether hiPSCs cause tumors has yet to be fully investigated. Neural precursor cells derived from miPSCs have been shown to form teratomas after *in utero* transplantation into the brain of mouse embryos. This may be avoided by FACS (fluorescent activated cell sorting) depletion of the SSEA1-positive cell fraction prior to transplantation (Wernig et al., 2008a). Although there is concern of the genomic instability in pluripotent stem cells such as ESCs, it is not known whether genomic instability in hPSCs increases the likelihood of tumorigenesis. It has been proposed that high-resolution methods such as single nucleotide polymorphism genotyping be performed before any hPSCs are used for clinical transplantation (Peterson and Loring, 2014).

Feasible cell types for iPSC generation

Dermal fibroblasts have been the popular cell type of choice to generate iPSCs because they are ubiquitous and easily acquired in the skin. However, another source of cells, which is possibly more feasible and accessible, is the oral cavity. Fibroblasts from the oral mucosa can be reprogrammed into iPSCs, and acquiring a small amount of oral mucosa tissue leaves behind no scar (Miyoshi et al., 2010a), while it harbours a robust mesenchymal stem cell population (Morszczeck et al., 2013). MSCs in the jawbone can also be easily accessed. Acquiring alveolar bone in the jaw may be slightly more invasive; if needed, its acquisition protocol to isolate MSCs has been well established (Mason et al., 2014), and no report associates significant postoperative pain with this procedure. Blood cells are another easily obtainable cell type for iPSC generation; however, it requires subpopulation isolation and growth factor stimulation before reprogramming. This tedious process makes them makes them less attractive as a feasible cell source for reprogramming (Loh et al., 2009; Staerk et al., 2010; Su et al., 2013).

Discarded extra-embryonic tissues such as umbilical cord are a good cell source to generate iPSCs, as they are immature cells, highly suitable for such a purpose (Jiang et al., 2014; Song et al., 2014). Extracted teeth contain mesenchymal-like stem/progenitor cells including dental pulp stem cells (DPSCs), stem cells from exfoliated deciduous teeth (SHED), stem cells from apical papilla (SCAP), and periodontal ligament stem cells (PDLSCs) that are also a good cell source to derive iPSCs (Tamaoki et al., 2010; Wada et al., 2011; Yan et al., 2010). These stem cells are normally from children or young adults—SHED are from children around ages 6–12; SCAP, DPSCs, and PDLSCs from third molars are from those ages 16–22. These age groups contain more immature stem cells suitable for generating iPSCs. As summarised in Figure 1.1, a number of cell sources may be used for transgene-/vector-free iPSC generation and their subsequent medical applications.

Applications for iPSCs in cell-based therapy

While adult stem cells are multipotent and some are near pluripotent, their acquisition is nonetheless often inconvenient, and they have a limited life span in cultures (Kim et al., 2007; Kolf et al., 2007). Partial reprogramming by directing fibroblasts into specific lineages appears to be a good option for cell-based therapy; however, the key issue is still the limitation of cell source and their life span *in vitro*. With respect to their capacity for tissue regeneration, the pluripotency of ESCs, which can generate all cell types, is unparalleled by adult stem cells. The main concern of using hESCs is their safety, as ESCs may form teratomas *in vivo* if they fail to differentiate. One report of two clinical cases and phase I/II studies of 18 patients using hESCs for restoring eyesight of patients showed no adverse effects after a median of 22 months of follow-ups (Schwartz et al., 2012; Schwartz et al., 2015). Teratoma formation normally occurs within 8 weeks, suggesting that these clinical cases are unlikely to develop any tumor formation in the future. Currently, there are a number of clinical trials mainly using hESC-derived retina pigmented epithelial cells for transplantation to treat retinal degenerative diseases, and none have shown development of tumors (Peterson and Loring, 2014). The clinical trials operated by Geron for treating spinal cord injury using hESCs have, unfortunately, been discontinued due to financial reasons. If proven that hESCs are clinically safe, it is possible that iPSCs are also safe, and the

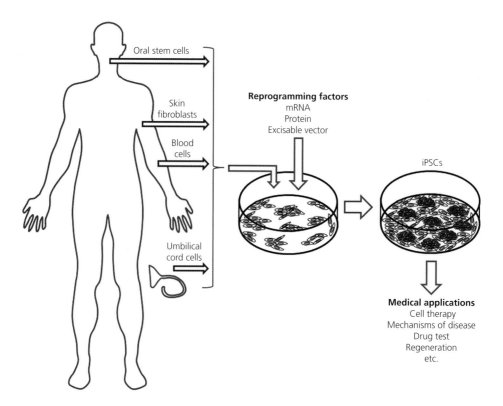

Figure 1.1 Feasible source of cells or stem cells for transgene-free iPSC generation and subsequent medical applications. Oral stem cells are the most accessible and easiest cells for the reprogramming process. Use of mRNA, protein, or an excisable vector approach allows generation of transgene-free iPSCs. Note: Although blood cells appear to be the easiest cell type to obtain, multiple steps are involved in their processing before they are ready for reprogramming, which is very inconvenient.

ongoing clinical trials with iPSCs will verify this possibility (Cyranoski, 2013). Recently it has been shown that transplantation of hiPSC-derived neural stem cells (NSCs) enhanced axonal sparing, regrowth and angiogenesis, prevented demyelination after spinal cord injury, and promoted functional recovery in the common marmoset animal model without tumor formation (Kobayashi et al., 2012).

Guiding hESCs towards differentiation into various tissue specific cells *in vitro* has been rigorously tested, and various protocols have been established. These protocols are being utilised for iPSC differentiation. Various differentiation pathways have been tested for guiding iPSCs into specific lineages representing all of the three germ layers (Efthymiou et al., 2014). Examples are ectodermal-related neural cells (Cai et al., 2010; Hu et al., 2010), mesodermal-related haematopoietic and endothelial cells (Choi et al., 2009; Feng et al., 2010) and skeletal muscle cells (Mizuno et al., 2010), and

endodermal-related hepatocytes (Gallicano and Mishra, 2010; Si-Tayeb et al., 2010; Sullivan et al., 2010). Studies are being continuously undertaken to refine the differentiation protocols of guiding ESCs or iPSCs into specific cell types, and to understand the extent of variation in differentiation potential among different cell lines and clones that is related to the effects of cell origin or reprogramming methods. Most importantly, iPSC-derived differentiated cells must have equivalent functions to the naturally formed tissue cells (Efthymiou et al., 2014).

iPSCs for tissue engineering and regeneration

iPSCs for tissue regeneration in general
Cell-based therapy to regenerate tissues may be the best and the only option when defect size reaches a point where non-cell-based approaches cannot work. iPSCs,

similar to ESCs, undergo continuous self-renewal in cultures and may provide unlimited cell source for tissue regeneration (Efthymiou et al., 2014; Hirschi et al., 2014; Lengner, 2010). With regard to human systems, a number of different cell types may be differentiated from hiPSCs for regenerative medicine. The following listed are a few examples.

(a) Cardiac regeneration with iPSCs

hiPSCs can differentiate into functional cardiomyocytes (Germanguz et al., 2011; Seki et al., 2014; Zhang et al., 2009; Zwi et al., 2009). Successful differentiation of hiPSCs into cardiomyocytes was first reported in 2009 (Zhang et al., 2009). Electrophysiology studies indicated that iPSCs differentiate into nodal-, atrial-, and ventricular-like phenotypes and exhibit responsiveness to beta-adrenergic stimulation. Overall, cardiomyocytes obtained from iPSCs are functionally similar to ESC-derived cardiomyocytes (Zhang et al., 2009). Furthermore, iPSC-derived cardiomyocytes have been engrafted successfully into the hearts of experimental animals (Zwi-Dantsis et al., 2013) and used to improve cardiac function after ischemic cardiomyopathy in a porcine model (Kawamura et al., 2012).

(b) Skeletal tissue regeneration with iPSCs

Skeletal tissue engineering includes bone and cartilage regeneration. Osteogenic differentiation of iPSCs for bone tissue regeneration has been reported using scaffolds such as macro-channeled polycaprolactone scaffolds (Jin et al., 2013), polyethersulfone nanofibrous scaffolds (Ardeshirylajimi et al., 2013) and fibrin or hydroxyapatite/β-tricalcium phosphate (Park and Im, 2013).

Osteogenic differentiation of hiPSCs could be conducted with EB formation (Ardeshirylajimi et al., 2013; Park and Im, 2013), or without the EB formation step, by using osteogenic factors, ascorbic acid, β-glycerophoshate and dexamethasone (Jin et al., 2013). Based on *in vitro* studies, iPSCs seem to have the similar characteristics to hESCs in osteogenic differentiation (Ardeshirylajimi et al., 2013). *In vivo* bone formation by iPSCs was also demonstrated in rats (Park and Im, 2013) and in nude mice (Duan et al., 2011). Studies have also shown that hiPSCs combined with gels containing an enamel matrix-derived protein complex from the amelogenin family provide a valuable tool for periodontal tissue engineering by promoting the formation of new alveolar bone and cementum formation, with normal periodontal ligament between them (Duan et al., 2011).

Cartilage tissue engineering using differentiated and purified iPSCs has also been reported (Diekman et al., 2012). Robust chondrogenic differentiation of iPSCs using BMP-4 treatment in micromass culture was observed. These iPSC-derived chondrocyte-like cells were effective at promoting the integration of nascent tissue with the surrounding adult cartilage in an *in vitro* cartilage injury model (Diekman et al., 2012). Besides direct differentiation from iPSCs, osteoblasts (Villa-Diaz et al., 2012) and chondrocytes (Koyama et al., 2013) could also be derived from iPSCs via a selection of cells that can adapt to MSC growth conditions. MSCs could be derived from iPSCs through EB formation, with typical expression of MSC surface markers and the potential to differentiate into adipocytes, chondrocytes, and osteoblasts (Tang et al., 2014).

(c) Tooth regeneration with iPSCs

iPSCs have the capacity to differentiate into oral tissue cells including dental epithelial and mesenchymal cells. miPSCs cultured with dental epithelial cell line cells display an epithelial cell–like morphology expressing the ameloblast markers ameloblastin and enamelin (Arakaki et al., 2012). miPSCs can differentiate into neural crest–like cells (NCLCs) (Lee et al., 2007), and if cocultured with dental epithelium, they express dental mesenchymal cell markers (Otsu et al., 2012). If culturing NCLCs in the conditioned medium of mouse dental epithelium cultures, their differentiation into odontoblasts is enhanced (Otsu et al., 2012). Such findings have led to a proposed protocol for whole-tooth regeneration using iPSCs (Figure 1.2) (Otsu et al., 2014). Using a tooth germ reconstitution and transplantation model, miPSCs were able to participate in the regeneration of alveolar bone and pulp of the engineered tooth unit *in vivo* (Wen et al., 2012). Human iPSC-derived epithelial cells combined with mouse dental mesenchyme can give rise to tooth-like structures *in vivo* (Cai et al., 2013; Liu et al., 2014). These results suggest that iPSCs may be a useful cell source for tooth regeneration and tooth development studies.

Neural regeneration with iPSCs

Many neurological disorders await therapeutic strategies including cell-based therapies. A good example would be Parkinson's disease, a common chronic progressive neurodegenerative disorder characterised primarily by major loss of nigrostriatal dopaminergic neurons. In a proof-of-principle experiment using a mouse model, iPSCs were

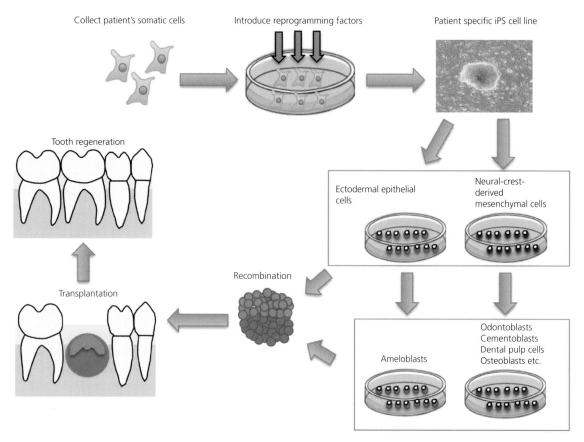

Figure 1.2 Schematic representation of a strategy for whole-tooth regeneration using iPSCs. The patient's somatic cells are harvested and reprogrammed into patient-specific iPSCs, which are then induced to form ectodermal epithelial cells and neural crest-derived mesenchymal cells. They may be further induced to form odontogenic cells *in vitro*. The two cell populations are combined by direct contact, mimicking the *in vivo* arrangement. Interaction of these cells leads to formation of an early-stage tooth germ. Once transplanted into the edentulous region, the recombinants develop into a functional tooth. (Adapted from Otsu et al., 2014. Used under CC-BY 3.0. http://creativecommons.org/licenses/by/3.0/.)

first guided to differentiate into neural precursor cells and transplanted into the fetal mouse brain. These iPSC-derived cells migrated into various brain regions and differentiated into glia and neurons, including glutamatergic, GABAergic, and catecholaminergic subtypes (Wernig et al., 2008a). These grafted neurons showed mature neuronal activity and were functionally integrated in the host brain. iPSC-derived dopamine neurons transplanted into a rat model of Parkinson's disease improved behavior (Wernig et al., 2008a; Wernig et al., 2008b). Furthermore, iPSCs reprogrammed from fibroblasts of Parkinson's disease patients can be guided to differentiate into dopaminergic neurons (Soldner et al., 2009). hiPSCs can be differentiated to form motor neurons with a similar efficiency as hESCs. The differentiation

of iPSCs appeared to follow a normal developmental progression associated with motor neuron formation and possessed prototypical electrophysiological properties (Hu et al., 2010; Karumbayaram et al., 2009). A recent report using a mouse model showed that transplantation of neural precursor cells derived from transgene-/vector-free hiPSCs into the mouse brain that had suffered ischemic stroke injury enhanced functional recovery (Mohamad et al., 2013a).

Protocols of neural regeneration using iPSCs

In vitro differentiation of iPSCs to neural cells has been achieved using various approaches. There are three major methods (summarised in Table 1.1): (a) EB

Table 1.1 Neural differentiation protocols of ESCs/iPSCs.

Protocol	Culturing Method	Differentiation Strategy	Reference
EB formation and rosette isolation	EB formation in suspension and following adherent culture of EBs	Induction and isolation of neural rosettes without morphogens	(Zhang et al., 2001)
Dual-SMAD inhibition	Adherent single cell culture of dissociated iPSCs	Inhibition of BMP/Nodal signals	(Chambers et al., 2009; Morizane et al., 2011)
SFEBq	EB-like formation by reaggregation of dissociated iPSCs	Inhibition of WNT/BMP/Nodal signals	(Mariani et al., 2012b; Watanabe et al., 2005; Watanabe et al., 2007)

Note: EB = embryoid body; SFEBq = serum-free culture of EB-like aggregates, quick method.
Source: Adapted from Kim et al., 2014. Reproduced with permission.

formation and rosette isolation method, (b) dual-SMAD inhibition method, and (c) SFEB method (serum-free culture of EB-like aggregates) (Kim et al., 2014).

(a) EB formation and rosette isolation method

One popular and powerful approach to mobilising iPSC/ESC differentiation through to a neural lineage is the EB formation and rosette isolation method (Dimos et al., 2008; Wang et al., 2011; Zhang et al., 2001), or even using a rotary cell culture protocol to increase EB homogeneity (Mohamad et al., 2013b). Four types of colonies can develop at the rosette stage of iPSCs, namely, colonies with rosette structure, colonies with differentiated neurons, colonies with myofibroblasts, and a small number of undifferentiated colonies. The unique cellular arrangement of epithelial cells is reminiscent of cross-sections of the developing neural tube and is considered a hallmark of successful neural induction. These rosette colonies are positive for neural crest markers AP-2, nestin, and p75, and may be used for nerve regeneration (Wang et al., 2011). Timely treatment with particular morphogens such as Shh and Wnts or their agonists/antagonists, redirects the regional identity of these progenitor cells to either ventral or caudal fate, leading to many methods for generating different neuronal subtypes. iPSCs have been shown to differentiate into dopaminergic neurons (Kwon et al., 2014; Wernig et al., 2008b) and motor neurons (Dimos et al., 2008; Hu et al., 2010; Karumbayaram et al., 2009). The schematic representation of EB-mediated neurogenesis is depicted in Figure 1.3 with Protocol 1.2 describing steps for EB-mediated neuronogenesis to generate neuronlike cells *in vitro* (Hu et al., 2010; Zou et al., 2012).

(b) Dual-SMAD inhibition method

A representation of the dual-SMAD inhibition method is illustrated in Figure 1.4. Chambers et al. (2009) first reported this method using hESCs/hiPSCs. Here, the hESCs/iPSCs are dissociated to single cells and grown as adherent cultures for neuroectodermal cell differentiation. PAX6+ cells emerge and form neural rosettes in 11 days. Subsequent differentiation into neural cells that express PAX6, FOXG1 (BF1), and OTX2 indicate dorsal telecephalic identity (Chambers et al., 2009). With slight modification of this protocol, iPSCs are able to convert to dopaminergic neurons (Morizane et al., 2011). Adding the BMP signaling inhibitor dorsomorphin and a TGF-β/activin/nodal signaling inhibitor SB431542 into single cell cultures of iPSCs/ESCs was shown to promote highly efficient neural differentiation. This method is referred to as the dual-SMAD inhibition approach because each signaling pathway recruits SMAD proteins as intracellular signal transducers. The small molecule compounds dorsomorphin and SB431542 are stable and cost effective, and this method may provide a promising strategy for controlled production of neurons in regenerative medicine (Morizane et al., 2011; Wattanapanitch et al., 2014).

(c) Serum-free EB-like (SFEB) method

Watanabe et al. (2005) first reported the SFEB method using mESCs. Here, the ESC colonies are dissociated into single cells and allowed to grow in suspension. Approximately 90% of cells spontaneously form aggregates of defined size in cultures, and the Wnt inhibitor Dkk1 and nodal signaling antagonist LeftyA are present to guide cells toward neural differentiation (Watanabe et al., 2005). Cells can be further guided into subpopulations of neuronal lineage with different growth factors.

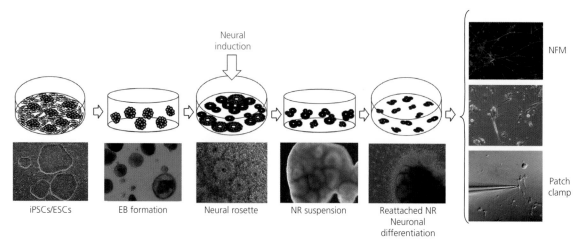

Figure 1.3 Embryoid body (EB)-mediated neurogenesis. iPSC/ESC colonies are lifted into suspension to form EBs, followed by growth in adherent culture in defined media containing N2 supplement and basic fibroblast growth factor (bFGF) and allowed to form neural rosettes (NR). Cells in the NRs express many neural stem cell markers such as Nestin, Musashi-1, and polysialylated-neuronal cell adhesion molecule. NRs are then detached and grown in suspension followed by reattachment onto a laminin-coated dish under neurogenic stimulation for further neural differentiation prior to functional assessment through patch clamp electrophysiology. (Patch clamp image courtesy of Dr. Kristen O'Connell, University of Tennessee Health Science Center. Reproduced with permission from K. O'Connell.)

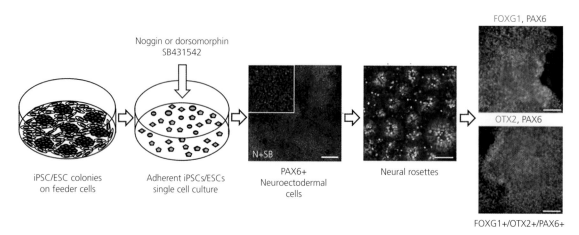

Figure 1.4 Dual-SMAD inhibition method for neural differentiation. Under serum-free conditions, adherent single cell-cultures of iPSCs/hESCs are treated with Noggin or dorsomorphin (BMP inhibitor) and SB431542 (Activin/Nodal inhibitor) to convert iPSCs/hESCs to largely PAX6-positive (green) neuroectodermal cells that subsequently form neural rosettes (Ki67, green phosphor-histone H3, red) following 11 days of differentiation. Neural cells generated express FOXG1 (red) and OTX2 (red), along with PAX6 (green). (Scheme based on Chambers et al., 2009. Reproduced with permission from Nature Publishing Group).

This group later tested this protocol on hESCs and had to use a ROCK inhibitor to increase survival of cells during culture (Watanabe et al., 2007). The modified protocol is depicted in Figure 1.5, showing that hESCs/hiPSCs are dissociated into single cells and allowed to form floating EB-like aggregates in the presence of

Dkk1, LeftyA, and BMPRIA-Fc, followed by reattachment onto coated dishes/wells. Under further differentiation stimulation, different populations of neurons emerge in response to certain signals. For example, Shh treatment for ventralisation leads to an increased population of NKx2.1+ cells (basal region of

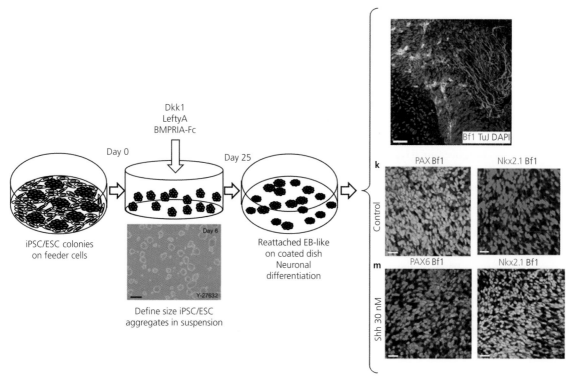

Figure 1.5 Serum-free EB-like (SFEB) method for neural differentiation. iPSC/ESC colonies are dissociated to single cells (2×10^5 cells/mL) and cultured in nonadherent dishes. Cell aggregates form spontaneously in the presence of a ROCK inhibitor. Dkk1 (Wnt inhibitor), LeftyA (Nodal signaling antagonist), and soluble BMPRIA-Fc (BMP-4 antagonist) are added to the culture from Day 0 to Day 24. The cell aggregates are then replated *en bloc* on dishes coated with poly-D-lysine, laminin, and fibronectin, and cultured until Day 35 in a neural differentiation medium (Neurobasal + B27 and glutamine). For ventralisation experiments, Shh is added. On Day 35, hESC-derived neural cells express Bf1 (32.9% ± 2.6%, far right image panel, top). The early embryonic telencephalon is subdivided into the pallial (Bf1+/PAX6+ cortical anlage) and basal (e.g., Nkx2.1+) regions. The majority of Bf1+ cells derived from Y-27632-treated hES cells coexpressed PAX6 (95.8 ± 0.7%), whereas Nkx2.1 was detected in only a few Bf1+ cells (1% or less) (far right middle image panel). Shh treatment (Days 15–35) decreased the PAX+ population (23.2% ± 5.3%) and increased the proportion of Nkx2.1+ cells among the Bf1+ cells (41.5% ± 14.5%) (far right bottom image panel). (Scheme based on Watanabe et al., 2007. Reproduced with permission from Nature Publishing Group.)

telencephalon) among BF1+ cells (Watanabe et al., 2007). Mariani et al. (2012a) adopted this protocol to use with hiPSCs, which were able to form multilayered structures expressing a gene profile typical of the embryonic telencephalon region.

iPSCs as disease study models

iPSCs can be generated from patients with specific diseases. If the generated iPSCs recapitulate the disease phenotype either *in vitro* or *in vivo*, these cells can be used to establish a patient iPSC library that can be used to study the disease mechanisms and novel drug development (Nishikawa et al., 2008; Park et al., 2008a). iPSCs generated from cells of patients with Hutchinson-Gilford progeria syndrome, caused by a single-point mutation in the lamin A (LMNA) gene, recapitulate the disease phenotype at the cellular and molecular level, providing an *in vitro* iPSC-based model to study the pathogenesis of this disease (Liu et al., 2011).

Genetic disease

Park et al. (2008a) established a disease iPSC library from patients with a variety of genetic diseases of Mendelian or complex inheritance. Examples include adenosine deaminase deficiency-related severe combined immunodeficiency, Shwachman-Bodian-Diamond syndrome, Duchenne and Becker muscular dystrophy, Parkinson's disease, Huntington disease, juvenile-onset, type 1 diabetes mellitus, and Down syndrome/trisomy 21 (Park et al., 2008a). iPSCs generated from patients with single-gene disorders can not only be used to study disease mechanisms, but can also be used to correct the genetic defect *ex vivo* such that the correct cells may be transplanted back to the patient. In the case of Huntington disease, iPSCs from such patients that carry the mutant Huntingtin gene (mHTT) can be differentiated into NSCs or neural progenitor cells (NPCs). mHTT expression in NSC and NPCs can be silenced by using RNAi or antisense oligonucleotides. The corrected cells can then be transplanted into the brain of the patient to replenish the lost cell population (Chen et al., 2014).

For genetic diseases involving haematopoietic systems, Hanna et al. (2007) first showed that in a humanised sickle cell anemia mouse model, iPSCs can be generated from the diseased mouse fibroblasts and the mutation corrected *in vitro* followed by differentiating the corrected iPSCs into haematopoietic progenitors for transplantation and curing the disease (Hanna et al., 2007). Similarly, in a human model, fibroblasts from Fanconi anaemia patients after genetic correction can be reprogrammed into pluripotency to generate patient-specific iPSCs. Corrected Fanconi-anaemia-specific iPS cells can give rise to haematopoietic progenitors of the myeloid and erythroid lineages that are phenotypically normal (Raya et al., 2009).

iPSCs have also been established from patients with various neurological disorders, including Rett syndrome, Fragile X syndrome, Angelman syndrome, Timothy syndrome, familial Alzheimer's disease, and Parkinson's disease (Israel et al., 2012; Wang and Doering, 2012; Yagi et al., 2011; Soldner et al., 2009;). iPSCs have additionally been used as a tool to study X-linked genes with mutations that are either dominant or recessive. The situation is not clear-cut. For example, the X-linked neurodevelopmental disorder, Rett syndrome (RTT), has been studied using iPSCs from cells of patients with Rett syndrome. The disease affects girls due primarily to heterozygous mutations in the X-linked gene encoding methyl-CpG binding protein 2 (MECP2) (Cheung et al., 2012). X-chromosome inactivation (XCI) status of RTT-hiPSCs has been inconsistent with some reports showing that RTT-hiPSCs retain the inactive X-chromosome of the founder somatic cells, retaining their allele specific expression patterns. Conversely, other reports show reactivation of the inactive X-chromosome in RTT-hiPSCs derived from the founder somatic cells. Subsequently, random XCI ensues with RTT-hiPSCs undergoing differentiation, resulting in cellular mosaicism with cells either expressing MECP2-WT or MECP2-Mut transcripts (Cheung et al., 2012).

Cancer-iPSCs

Reprogramming specific cancer cells into pluripotent state followed by differentiating into different lineages may help develop cancer vaccines, be applied in drug screening, or be used to understand the biological nature of cancer cells. For example, KBM7 cells derived from chronic myeloid leukemia have been reprogrammed into iPSCs. These cancer-iPSCs, in contrast to parental KBM7 cells, were completely resistant to the therapeutic drug Imatinib (Carette et al., 2010). Miyoshi and colleagues (2010b) reprogrammed cancer cells of endodermal origin including esophageal, stomach, colorectal, liver, pancreatic, and cholangio-cellular cancer cells. The reprogrammed cancer-iPSCs express morphological patterns of ectoderm, mesoderm, and endoderm, which were not expressed in the parental cells (Miyoshi et al., 2010b). These cancer-iPSCs showed slow proliferation, were sensitised to differentiation-inducing treatment, and had reduced tumorigenesis in NOD/SCID mice. Additionally, the tumor-suppressor gene P16 (INK4A) was repressed in induced pluripotent cancer (iPC) cells while its expression increased in differentiated iPC cells. The findings suggest that the reactivation of tumor suppressor genes by reprogramming may play a role in increased chemosensitivity to 5-FU and the regression of cell proliferation and invasiveness under differentiation-inducing conditions (Miyoshi et al., 2010b). Since cancer cells can potentially be reprogrammed into pluripotency and be capable of differentiation into multiple cell lineages of all three germ layers, it has been speculated that converting cancer cells into highly immunogenic tumor antigen–presenting dendritic cells for cancer immunotherapy may be a distinct possibility (Lin and Chui, 2012).

Protocol 1.1 Reprogramming oral MSCs into transgene-free iPSCs (Based on Sommer et al., 2010; Zou et al., 2012).

Materials

- Lentiviral vectors hSTEMCCA-LoxP (EMD Millipore Corporation. USA. http://www.emdmillipore.com/US/en/life-science-research/cell-culture-systems/stem-cell-research/cellular-reprogramming/stemcca/AV2b.qB.Zj4AAAE_c08RHeO2,nav
- TransIT-HelaMonster transfection kit (Mirus, Madison, WI, USA)
- Puromycin resistant Mouse Embryonic Fibroblasts (MEF) feeder cells (DR4 MEF, GlobalStem, Rockville, MD, USA)

1. Preparation of oral MSCs

- Seed approximately 10^5 cells (passage <5) into wells of 12-well plates (or wait till about 70%–80% confluent). Cells should show typical signs of oral MSCs with fast proliferation rate (population doubling time ~20 h).

2. Preparation and addition of virus mixture

- Thaw virus stored in −80°C on ice.
- Prepare 0.5 or 1 mL of fresh culture medium for each well in a separate tube.
- Add virus (viral titers of ~1×10^8 TU [transducing unit]/mL) into the tube with gentle pipetting to mix. (Lentiviral vectors hSTEMCCA-LoxP—a polycistronic single vector carrying all four human reprogramming factors c-Myc, Klf4, Oct4, Sox2)
- Add polybrene to a final concentration of 4-5 μg/mL.
- Remove the culture medium in the well, wash cells with PBS once.
- Add the viral mixture into the well. Incubate for 12–24 h, then change to fresh medium.

3. Preparation of feeder cells (MEFs)

- Coat the dish (10 cm) with 0.1% gelatin.
- Seed MEFs (mouse embryonic fibroblasts at passage <3 or 4 as feeder cells that have been treated with mitomycin C to inactivate their proliferation) into the dish about 1–2 days before.

4. Seed the transduced cells to MEFs

- Within 6 days of adding virus, pass the cells onto the feeder layer. Passage cells to new wells if they become confluent.
- Detach transduced cells and resuspend into the fresh cell culture medium and seed $1–5 \times 10^4$ transduced cells into the 10-cm dish with feeder cells (MEFs). Freeze down extra transduced cells for possible use if more reprogramming is needed.
- Next day, change the medium to human (h)ESC medium containing FGF (4 ng/mL).
- Change hESC medium every other day until the emergence of ESC-like colonies appear.
- ESC-like colonies should appear within 30 days. If no ESC-like colonies after 40 days, it is considered failed.

5. Subclone iPSC colonies

- Pick each ESC-like colony manually into a new well (12-well plate) containing MEFs.
- Expand the iPSCs and freeze some.

6. Preparation for excising transgenes with Cre

- Day 1: Pass iPSCs onto DR4-MEFs in wells of 6-well plates. Try to control the colonies number to reach about 60%–70% confluence before the next step.
- Days 2–4: Observe cells condition: confluence rate, colony size, and number. Do the excision procedure when the colony size is medium.
- Day 4: Take pictures of iPSC before Cre-mediated excision.

7. Cre-mediated excision of transgenes (for one well of 6-well plates)

- Warm TransIT-Hela and MONSTER (from transfection kit) to room temperature, vortex gently before use.
- Place 250 μL DMEM/F12 in a sterile 50-mL tube. Add 2.5 μg DNA (pHAGE2-Cre-IRES-PuroR plasmid), pipette gently. Add 7.5 μL Trans IT Hela, pipette gently. Add 5 μL MONSTER, pipette gently. Incubate at RT for 30 min.
- Add 2.5 mL/well of hESC medium. Add 2.5 mL mixture of above to each well. Record the time.
- After 24 h, wash the well with PBS once gently. Change to hESC medium and incubate for about 6 h.

8. Selection of iPSC colonies with Puromycin

- During the 6-h period, prepare hESC medium containing PUROMYCIN (PURO; 1.2µg/mL).
- After 6 h, change the medium to hESC medium with PURO to each well. Record the time.
- After 24 h, change to fresh hESC medium with PURO.
- Treat cells with PURO for 48 h total. After 48 h of PURO treatment, wash cells with PBS once gently. Change to hESC medium without PURO. (Several hours after the PURO treatment, the colonies begin dying.)
- Take pictures after PURO treatment. Mark the location of the remaining colonies underneath the well (To record that these colonies are not the reemerging ones). Observe and change medium daily.
- On about Days 2–4, small new colonies should reemerge from the edge of the previous colony that died out. Mark and take pictures of new colonies.
- Days 11–14, subclone the newly emerged colonies onto new MEF feeder layers and begin cell expansion.

9. Verification of transgene excision

- Extract genomic DNA from each subclone and perform PCR to detect presence or absence of transgenes.
- The primers for the PCR are as follows: c-MYC (forward primer): 5′ –GGA ACT CTT GTG CGT AAG TCG ATA G-3′; WPRE (reverse primer) 5′-GGA GGC GGC CCA AAG GGA GGA GAT CCG-3′;
- PCR steps: 95°C for 3 min; followed by 33 cycles of 94°C for 30 sec, 60°C for 30 sec, and 72°C for 5 min.
- The PCR products examined by electrophoresis on an agarose gel.

10. Verification of lack of integration of Cre plasmid

- Transgene-free iPSC clones are grown on DR4 MEFs in the presence of PUROMYCIN (1.2 µg/mL). Total cell death indicates the lack of plasmid integration into the genome.

Protocol 1.2 Pluripotent stem cell neurogenesis (based on Hu et al., 2010, and Zou et al., 2012)

Materials

hESC medium: DMEM/F12, 20% FBS/KOSR, 1% NEAA, 1 mM L-glutamine, 0.1 µM β-mercaptoethanol, 4 ng/mL bFGF
Neurogenic medium A: DMEM/F12, NEAA 1X, N2 1X, Noggin (500 ng/mL), SB4352 (10 nM)
Neurogenic medium B: DMEM/F12, NEAA 1X, N2 1X, Noggin (500 ng/mL)
Neurogenic medium C: DMEM/F12, NEAA 1X, N2 1X, Noggin (500 ng/mL), Retinoic acid (0.1 µM)
Neurogenic medium D: DMEM/F12, NEAA 1X, N2 1X, Retinoic acid (0.1 µM), SHH (100 ng/mL)

1. Culturing hESCs/iPSCs

- hESCs/iPSCs are cultured on a feeder layer of inactivated MEFs with a daily change of hESC medium.

2. Embryoid body (EB) formation

- Aspirate media off cell culture plate. Wash twice with PBS.
- Treat cells with collagenase IV (1 mg/mL). Incubate for 15–20 min at 37°C to detach the cell colonies.
- Pipette gently to dissociate the colonies. Collect cells into a conical tube.
- Remove the supernatant and wash the cells gently with 5 mL hESC medium [without bFGF, bFGF(-), hereafter denotes as hESC(-) medium]. Spin down at 500 rpm for 1 min.
- Resuspend cells in 3.5 mL/well (6-well plate) of hESC(-) medium. Break up cells by gently pipetting up and down.
- Plate cells into ultra-low attachment 6-well plates at a concentration of ~10^5 cells/cm^2 (estimated by digesting some iPSC/ESC colonies into single cells and count) to allow cell colonies to float in the medium. Change the hESC(-) medium every day.
After 2 days, cell colonies aggregate to form EBs, continue for 7 days.

3. Neurodifferentiation first step—neural rosette (NR) formation

- Collect EBs and spin down at 1000 rpm for 30 sec.
- Resuspend EBs in hESC(-) medium. Plate EBs into Matrigel coated wells to allow EB attachment on Matrigel.

- Culture attached EBs for 14 days with a neural induction medium (DMEM supplemented with B27 and 20 ng/mL bFGF). Change half of the media every 2 days and do a complete medium change every week.
- After 15 days of culture the clusters of NRs should appear.

4. Isolation and culture of neural rosettes (NR) in suspension

- Mark the NRs with marker pen under the microscope.
- With a sterile scissor, cut the bottom of few pipette tips. Smear petroleum jelly on uncut edge and place over individual NRs to form individual cloning wells.
- Triturate gently the NRs and aspirate them. Transfer the NRs into wells of 24-well ultra-low attachment plates (~5 NRs per well, the NRs will form large clusters).
- Cultivate NRs in suspension with a neurogenic medium (guide cells into neural progenitor cells) for the next 25 days with the following 4 steps:

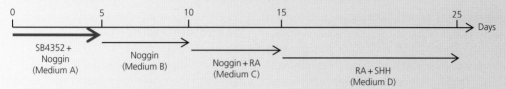

- During this period triturate gently the large clusters (>300 µm) with a cut pipette tip.

5. Differentiation toward a neuronogenic phenotype

- For a patch clamp assay, dissociate gently the cluster and seed a few cells onto a round glass cover slip coated with polylysine.
- Cultivate cells in Neurobasal medium supplemented with N2 supplement (1x), 1 µM cAMP (basic medium).
- For motoneuron differentiation add the following to the basic medium: BDNF (10 ng/mL)/GDNF (10 ng/mL)/IGF1 (10 ng/mL). Change the medium twice a week.
- Continue for up to 5 weeks. Observe morphological changes and search for neuron-like cells.
- Perform neuronal gene expression analysis and electrophysiology analysis.

Preclinical considerations

Transgene-/vector-free iPSCs

Various approaches have been developed to generate transgene-/vector-free iPSCs including transient expression using adenoviral or nonviral vectors (Gonzalez et al., 2009; Stadtfeld et al., 2008), nonintegrating episomal vectors (Yu et al., 2009a), (Okita et al., 2011; Okita et al., 2008; Yu et al., 2009b), minicircle DNA (Jia et al., 2010), Sendai virus (Ban et al., 2011), and removing the integrated vectors using piggyBac transposition or loxP/Cre-recombinase excisable viral vector system (Gonzalez et al., 2009; Kaji et al., 2009; Soldner et al., 2009; Woltjen et al., 2009). Nonvector approaches include synthetic modified mRNAs and recombinant protein-based four factors to generate iPSCs in the mouse and human system (Kim et al., 2009; Park et al., 2014; Zhou et al., 2009). Protein-based mouse iPSC reprogramming leads to greater genomic integrity compared to viral-induced strategies (Park et al., 2014). Protocol 1.1 details the methodology for

the application of the loxP/Cre-recombinase excisable viral vector system which has been used to generate dental iPSCs (Somers et al., 2010; Sommer et al., 2010; Zou et al., 2012). The method is consistent, efficient, and reliable.

Memory of hiPSCs as potential advantage

As discussed earlier, reprogramming cells into iPSCs was found to be incomplete, leaving behind a residual DNA methylation signature related to their cell of origin, termed "epigenetic memory". This epigenetic memory renders the iPSCs with a greater propensity to differentiate into the lineages of the original cell type rather than alternative lineages (Ghosh et al., 2010). Nonetheless, in the mouse system, such memory is mainly detected in iPSCs between passages 4 and 6, fading away by passage 10, and is entirely eliminated at passage 16 (Kim et al., 2010; Polo et al., 2010). hiPSCs, however, retain such memory up to passage 65 (Lister et al., 2011). The epigenetic memory may be utilised for specific clinical purposes if a particular cell type is needed that may be derived from iPSCs. For example, human limbal-derived iPSCs may be used to give rise to limbal-like epithelium more readily than fibroblast-derived iPSCs for medical applications (Sareen et al., 2014). Differentiation efficiency was also found to be higher in cardiac progenitor cell-derived iPSCs differentiating into cardiomyocytes than in fibroblast-derived-iPSCs, although it does not contribute to improved functional outcome *in vivo* (Sanchez-Freire et al., 2014). Likewise, dental cells may be obtained from dental stem cell–derived iPSCs for dental tissue regeneration.

Development of an iPSC library

Generation of individual iPSCs under good manufacturing practice (GMP) guidelines is costly, but a bank of allogenic clinical grade GMP cell lines is being considered to overcome this issue. It is proposed that a haplobank comprising the 100 iPSC lines with the most frequent HLA in each population would match 78% of European Americans, 63% of Asian Americans, 52% of Hispanic Americans, and 45% of African Americans (Gourraud et al., 2012; Turner et al., 2013). To achieve such a haplobank of iPSCs, lines would require a large-scale concerted worldwide collaboration.

Conclusion and prospects

iPSC technology allows us to further understand the plasticity of cells along the pathways of differentiation and de-differentiation. It also brings our attention to the remodeling of the epigenetic machinery during the stem cell immature state and its differentiation stages. Most importantly, it offers many possibilities for medical applications, one of which is cell-based therapy. Customised iPSC lines can be established from each individual for autologous as well as for allogenic use. Their pluripotent nature gives them the capacity to generate any cell types for therapies. iPSCs can be easily generated and can differentiate into a broad spectrum of cell lineages originating from all three embryonic germ layers and can replace the use of ESCs. While the understanding of the molecular status of iPSCs at genetic and epigenetic levels is still incomplete, investigation of their therapeutic capacities is needed to eventually apply these cells for clinic applications including their safety. Neural tissue regeneration has been a great challenge in the field of regenerative medicine as neural tissues have

low regenerative capacities and neural disorders are extremely difficult medical conditions to treat and manage. There has been significant progress in differentiating specific neural and neuronal cells from hESC/iPSCs, as some mentioned in this chapter. Further research is required to clarify the molecular events occurring during reprogramming that are essential to improving the safety and efficiency of culture protocols, and also to define the state-of-the-art differentiation steps for generating safe, effective, and functional cells of specific lineages for cell therapies.

Acknowledgements

This work was supported in part by a grant from the National Institutes of Health R01 DE019156-01 (G.T.-J.H.).

Author disclosure statement

There are no any commercial associations that might create a conflict of interest in connection with submitted manuscripts.

References

AASEN, T., RAYA, A., BARRERO, M. J., GARRETA, E., CONSIGLIO, A., GONZALEZ, F., et al. 2008. Efficient and rapid generation of induced pluripotent stem cells from human keratinocytes. *Nat Biotech*, 26, 1276–1284.

AGARWAL, S., LOH, Y. H., MCLOUGHLIN, E. M., HUANG, J., PARK, I. H., MILLER, J. D., et al. 2010. Telomere elongation in induced pluripotent stem cells from dyskeratosis congenita patients. *Nature*, 464, 292–296.

ARAKAKI, M., ISHIKAWA, M., NAKAMURA, T., IWAMOTO, T., YAMADA, A., FUKUMOTO, E., et al. 2012. Role of epithelial-stem cell interactions during dental cell differentiation. *J Biol Chem*, 287, 10590–10601.

ARDESHIRYLAJIMI, A., HOSSEINKHANI, S., PARIVAR, K., YAGHMAIE, P., & SOLEIMANI, M. 2013. Nanofiber-based polyethersulfone scaffold and efficient differentiation of human induced pluripotent stem cells into osteoblastic lineage. *Mol Biol Rep*, 40, 4287–4294.

BAN, H., NISHISHITA, N., FUSAKI, N., TABATA, T., SAEKI, K., SHIKAMURA, M., et al. 2011. Efficient generation of transgene-free human induced pluripotent stem cells (iPSCs) by temperature-sensitive Sendai virus vectors. *Proc Natl Acad Sci U S A*, 108, 14234–14239.

BOLAND, M. J., HAZEN, J. L., NAZOR, K. L., RODRIGUEZ, A. R., GIFFORD, W., MARTIN, G., et al. 2009. Adult mice generated from induced pluripotent stem cells. *Nature*, 461, 91–94.

CAI, J., YANG, M., POREMSKY, E., KIDD, S., SCHNEIDER, J. S., & IACOVITTI, L. 2010. Dopaminergic neurons derived from human induced pluripotent stem cells survive and integrate into 6-OHDA lesioned rats. *Stem Cells and Develop*, 9, 1017–1023.

CAI, J., ZHANG, Y., LIU, P., CHEN, S., WU, X., SUN, Y., et al. 2013. Generation of tooth-like structures from integration-free human urine induced pluripotent stem cells. *Cell Regen*, 2, 6.

CARETTE, J.E., PRUSZAK, J., VARADARAJAN, M., BLOMEN, V. A., GOKHALE, S., CAMARGO, F. D., et al. 2010. Generation of iPSCs from cultured human malignant cells. *Blood*, 115, 4039–4042.

CHAMBERS, S. M., FASANO, C. A., PAPAPETROU, E. P., TOMISHIMA, M., SADELAIN, M., & STUDER, L. 2009. Highly efficient neural conversion of human ES and iPS cells by dual inhibition of SMAD signaling. *Nat Biotechnol*, 27, 275–280.

CHEN, Y., CARTER, R. L., CHO, I. K., & CHAN, A. W. 2014. Cell-based therapies for Huntington's disease. *Drug Discov Today*, 19, 980–984.

CHEUNG, A. Y., HORVATH, L. M., CARREL, L. & ELLIS, J. 2012. X-chromosome inactivation in Rett syndrome human induced pluripotent stem cells. *Fronts Psychiatry*, 3, 24.

CHOI, K. D., YU, J., SMUGA-OTTO, K., SALVAGIOTTO, G., REHRAUER, W., VODYANIK, M., et al. 2009. Hematopoietic and endothelial differentiation of human induced pluripotent stem cells. *Stem Cells*, 27, 559–567.

COWAN, C. A., ATIENZA, J., MELTON, D. A. & EGGAN, K. 2005. Nuclear reprogramming of somatic cells after fusion with human embryonic stem cells. *Science*, 309, 1369–1373.

CYRANOSKI, D. 2013. Stem cells cruise to clinic. *Nature*, 494, 413.

DIEKMAN, B. O., CHRISTOFOROU, N., WILLARD, V. P., SUN, H., SANCHEZ-ADAMS, J., LEONG, K. W., et al. 2012. Cartilage tissue engineering using differentiated and purified induced pluripotent stem cells. *Proc Natl Acad Sci U S A*, 109, 19172–19177.

DIMOS, J. T., RODOLFA, K. T., NIAKAN, K. K., WEISENTHAL, L. M., MITSUMOTO, H., CHUNG, W., et al. 2008. Induced pluripotent stem cells generated from patients with ALS can be differentiated into motor neurons. *Science*, 321, 1218–1221.

DUAN, X., TU, Q., ZHANG, J., YE, J., SOMMER, C., MOSTOSLAVSKY, G., et al. 2011. Application of induced pluripotent stem (iPS) cells in periodontal tissue regeneration. *J Cell Physiol*, 226, 150–157.

DURRUTHY-DURRUTHY, J., BRIGGS, S. F., AWE, J., RAMATHAL, C. Y., KARUMBAYARAM, S., LEE, P. C., et al. 2014. Rapid and efficient conversion of integration-free human induced pluripotent stem cells to GMP-grade culture conditions. *PLoS One*, 9, e94231.

EFTHYMIOU, A. G., CHEN, G., RAO, M., CHEN, G., & BOEHM, M. 2014. Self-renewal and cell lineage differentiation strategies in human embryonic stem cells and induced pluripotent stem cells. *Expert Opin Biol Ther*, 14, 1333–1344.

FENG, Q., LU, S. J., KLIMANSKAYA, I., GOMES, I., KIM, D., CHUNG, Y., et al. 2010. Hemangioblastic derivatives from human induced pluripotent stem cells exhibit limited expansion and early senescence. *Stem Cells*, 28, 704–712.

GALLICANO, G. I., & MISHRA, L. 2010. Hepatocytes from induced pluripotent stem cells: A giant leap forward for hepatology. *Hepatology*, 51, 20–22.

GERMANGUZ, I., SEDAN, O., ZEEVI-LEVIN, N., SHTRICHMAN, R., BARAK, E., ZISKIND, A., et al. 2011. Molecular characterization and functional properties of cardiomyocytes derived from human inducible pluripotent stem cells. *J Cell Mol Med*, 15, 38–51.

GHOSH, Z., WILSON, K. D., WU, Y., HU, S., QUERTERMOUS, T., & WU, J. C. 2010. Persistent donor cell gene expression among human induced pluripotent stem cells contributes to differences with human embryonic stem cells. *PLoSOne*, 5, e8975.

GIORGETTI, A., MONTSERRAT, N., AASEN, T., GONZALEZ, F., RODRÍGUEZ-PIZÀ, I., VASSENA, R., et al. 2009. Generation of induced pluripotent stem cells from human cord blood using OCT4 and SOX2. *Cell Stem Cell*, 5, 353–357.

GIORGETTI, A., MONTSERRAT, N., RODRÍGUEZ-PIZÀ, I., AZQUETA, C., VEIGA, A., & BELMONTE, J. C. I. 2010. Generation of induced pluripotent stem cells from human cord blood cells with only two factors: OCT4 and SOX2. *Nat Protocols*, 5, 811–820.

GÓMEZ, M. C., POPE, C. E., & DRESSER, B. L. 2006. Nuclear transfer in cats and its application. *Theriogenology*, 66, 72–81.

GONZALEZ, F., BARRAGAN MONASTERIO, M., TISCORNIA, G., MONTSERRAT PULIDO, N., VASSENA, R., BATLLE MORERA, L., et al. 2009. Generation of mouse-induced pluripotent stem cells by transient expression of a single non-viral polycistronic vector. *Proc Natl Acad Sci U S A*, 106, 8918–8922.

GORE, A., LI, Z., FUNG, H. L., YOUNG, J. E., AGARWAL, S., ANTOSIEWICZ-BOURGET, J., et al. 2011. Somatic coding mutations in human induced pluripotent stem cells. *Nature*, 471, 63–67.

GOURRAUD, P. A., GILSON, L, GIRARD, M., & PESCHANSKI, M. 2012. The role of human leukocyte antigen matching in the development of multiethnic "haplobank" of induced pluripotent stem cell lines. *Stem Cells*, 30, 180–186.

HANNA, J., WERNIG, M, MARKOULAKI, S., SUN, C.-W., MEISSNER, A., CASSADY, J. P., et al. 2007. Treatment of sickle cell anemia mouse model with iPS cells generated from autologous skin. *Science*, 318, 1920–1923.

HIRSCHI, K. K, LI, S., & ROY, K. (2014). Induced pluripotent stem cells for regenerative medicine. *Ann Rev Biomed Eng*, 16, 277–294.

HU, B. Y., WEICK, J. P., YU, J., MA, L. X., ZHANG, X. Q., THOMSON, J. A., et al. 2010. Neural differentiation of human induced pluripotent stem cells follows developmental principles but with variable potency. *Proc Natl Acad Sci U S A*, 107, 4335–4340.

HUANG, G. T., GRONTHOS, S., & SHI, S. 2009. Mesenchymal stem cells derived from dental tissues vs. those from other sources: Their biology and role in regenerative medicine. *J Dent Res*, 88, 792–806.

ISRAEL, M. A., YUAN, S. H., BARDY, C., REYNA, S. M., MU, Y., HERRERA, C., et al. 2012. Probing sporadic and familial Alzheimer's disease using induced pluripotent stem cells. *Nature*, 482, 216–220.

JIA, F., WILSON, K. D., SUN, N., GUPTA, D. M., HUANG, M., LI, Z., et al. 2010. A nonviral minicircle vector for deriving human iPS cells. *Nature Methods*, 7, 197–199.

JIANG, G., DI BERNARDO, J., DELONG, C. J., MONTEIRO DA ROCHA, A., O'SHEA, K. S., & KUNISAKI, S. M. 2014. Induced pluripotent stem cells from human placental chorion for perinatal tissue engineering applications. *Tissue Engineering Part C, Methods*, 20, 731–734.

JIN, G. Z., KIM, T. H., KIM, J. H., WON, J. E., YOO, S. Y., CHOI, S. J., et al. 2013. Bone tissue engineering of induced pluripotent stem cells cultured with macrochanneled polymer scaffold. *J Biomed Mats Res Part A*, 101, 1283–1291.

KAJI, K., NORRBY, K., PACA, A., MILEIKOVSKY, M., MOHSENI, P., & WOLTJEN, K. 2009. Virus-free induction of pluripotency and subsequent excision of reprogramming factors. *Nature*, 458, 771–775.

KANG, L., WANG, J., ZHANG, Y., KOU, Z., & GAO, S. 2009. iPS cells can support full-term development of tetraploid blastocyst-complemented embryos. *Cell Stem Cell*, 5, 135–138.

KARUMBAYARAM, S., NOVITCH, B. G., PATTERSON, M., UMBACH, J. A., RICHTER, L., LINDGREN, A., et al. 2009. Directed differentiation of human-induced pluripotent stem cells generates active motor neurons. *Stem Cells*, 27, 806–811.

KAWAMURA, M., MIYAGAWA, S., MIKI, K., SAITO, A., FUKUSHIMA, S., HIGUCHI, T., et al. 2012. Feasibility, safety, and therapeutic efficacy of human induced pluripotent stem cell-derived cardiomyocyte sheets in a porcine ischemic cardiomyopathy model. *Circulation*, 126, S29–S37.

KIM, D., KIM, C.-H., MOON, J.-I., CHUNG, Y.-G., CHANG, M.-Y., HAN, B.-S., et al. 2009. Generation of human induced pluripotent stem cells by direct delivery of reprogramming proteins. *Cell Stem Cell*, 4, 472–476.

KIM, D. S., ROSS, P. J., ZASLAVSKY, K., & ELLIS, J. 2014. Optimizing neuronal differentiation from induced pluripotent stem cells to model ASD. *Front Cell Neurosci*, 8, 109.

KIM, J., LEE, Y., KIM, H., HWANG, K. J., KWON, H. C., KIM, S. K., et al. 2007. Human amniotic fluid-derived stem cells have characteristics of multipotent stem cells. *Cell Prolif*, 40, 75–90.

KIM, K., DOI, A., WEN, B., NG, K., ZHAO, R., CAHAN, P., et al. 2010. Epigenetic memory in induced pluripotent stem cells. *Nature*, 467, 285–290.

KOBAYASHI, Y., OKADA, Y., ITAKURA, G., IWAI, H., NISHIMURA, S., YASUDA, A., et al. 2012. Pre-evaluated safe human iPSC-derived neural stem cells promote functional recovery after spinal cord injury in common marmoset without tumorigenicity. *PLoS One* 7, e52787.

KOLF, C., CHO, E., & TUAN, R. (2007). Mesenchymal stromal cells. Biology of adult mesenchymal stem cells: Regulation of niche, self-renewal and differentiation. *Arthritis Res Ther*, 9, 204.

KOYAMA, N., MIURA, M., NAKAO, K., KONDO, E., FUJII, T., TAURA, D. et al. 2013. Human induced pluripotent stem cells differentiated into chondrogenic lineage via generation of mesenchymal progenitor cells. *Stem Cells and Devel*, 22, 102–113.

KWON, Y. W., CHUNG, Y. J., KIM, J., LEE, H. J., PARK, J., ROH, T. Y. et al. 2014. Comparative study of efficacy of dopaminergic neuron differentiation between embryonic stem cell and protein-based induced pluripotent stem cell. *PLoS One*, 9, e85736.

LEE, G., KIM, H., ELKABETZ, Y., AL SHAMY, G., PANAGIOTAKOS, G., BARBERI, T., et al. 2007. Isolation and directed differentiation of neural crest stem cells derived from human embryonic stem cells. *Nat Biotechnol*, 25, 1468–1475.

LENGNER, C. J. (2010). iPS cell technology in regenerative medicine. *Ann N Y Acad Sci*, 1192, 38–44.

LI, C., ZHOU, J., SHI, G., MA, Y., YANG, Y., GU, J., et al. 2009. Pluripotency can be rapidly and efficiently induced in human amniotic fluid-derived cells. *Hum Mol Genet*, 18, 4340–4349.

LIN, F. K., & CHUI, Y. L. 2012. Generation of induced pluripotent stem cells from mouse cancer cells. *Cancer Biother Radiopharm*, 27, 694–700.

LISTER, R., PELIZZOLA, M., KIDA, Y. S., HAWKINS, R. D., NERY, J. R., HON, G., et al. 2011. Hotspots of aberrant epigenomic reprogramming in human induced pluripotent stem cells. *Nature*, 471, 68–73.

LIU, G. H., BARKHO, B. Z., RUIZ, S., DIEP, D., QU, J., YANG, S. L., et al. 2011. Recapitulation of premature ageing with iPSCs from Hutchinson-Gilford progeria syndrome. *Nature*, 472, 221–225.

LIU, P., ZHANG, Y., CHEN, S., CAI, J., & PEI, D. 2014. Application of iPS cells in dental bioengineering and beyond. *Stem Cell Reviews*, 10, 663–670.

LOH, Y. H., AGARWAL, S., PARK, I. H., URBACH, A., HUO, H., HEFFNER, G. C., et al. 2009. Generation of induced pluripotent stem cells from human blood. *Blood*, 113, 5476–5479.

MARIANI, J., SIMONINI, M. V., PALEJEV, D., TOMASINI, L., COPPOLA, G., SZEKELY, A. M., et al. 2012a. Modeling human cortical development in vitro using induced pluripotent stem cells. *Proc Natl Acad Sci U S A*, 109, 12770–12775.

MARIANI, J., SIMONINI, M. V., PALEJEV, D., TOMASINI, L., COPPOLA, G., SZEKELY, A. M., et al. 2012b. Modeling human cortical development in vitro using induced pluripotent stem cells. *Proc Natl Acad Sci U S A*, 109, 12770–12775.

MASON, S., TARLE, S. A., OSIBIN, W., KINFU, Y., & KAIGLER, D. 2014. Standardization and safety of alveolar bone-derived stem cell isolation. *J Dent Res*, 93, 55–61.

MIYASHITA, N., SHIGA, K., YONAI, M., KANEYAMA, K., KOBAYASHI, S., KOJIMA, T., et al. 2002. Remarkable differences in telomere lengths among cloned cattle derived from different cell types. *Biol Reprod*, 66, 1649–1655.

MIYOSHI, K., TSUJI, D., KUDOH, K., SATOMURA, K., MUTO, T., ITOH, K., et al. 2010a. Generation of human induced pluripotent stem cells from oral mucosa. *J Biosci Bioeng*, 110, 345–350.

MIYOSHI, N., ISHII, H., NAGAI, K., HOSHINO, H., MIMORI, K., TANAKA, F., et al. 2010b. Defined factors induce reprogramming of gastrointestinal cancer cells. *Proc Natl Acad Sci U S A*, 107, 40–45.

MIZUNO, Y., CHANG, H., UMEDA, K., NIWA, A., IWASA, T., AWAYA, T., et al. 2010. Generation of skeletal muscle stem/progenitor cells from murine induced pluripotent stem cells. *FASEB J*, 24, 2245–2253.

MOHAMAD, O., DRURY-STEWART, D., SONG, M., FAULKNER, B., CHEN, D., YU, S. P., et al. 2013a. Vector-free and transgene-free human iPS cells differentiate into functional neurons and enhance functional recovery after ischemic stroke in mice. *PLoS One* 8, e64160.

MOHAMAD, O., YU, S. P., CHEN, D., OGLE, M., SONG, M., & WIE, L. 2013b. Efficient neuronal differentiation of mouse ES and iPS cells using a rotary cell culture protocol. *Differentiation*, 86, 149–158.

MORIZANE, A., DOI, D., KIKUCHI, T., NISHIMURA, K., & TAKAHASHI, J. 2011. Small-molecule inhibitors of bone morphogenic protein and activin/nodal signals promote highly efficient neural induction from human pluripotent stem cells. *J Neurosci Res*, 89, 117–126.

MORSCZECK, C., HUANG, G. T.-J., & SHI, S. 2013. Stem and progenitor cells of dental and gingival tissue origin. In *Stem Cells in Craniofacial Development and Regeneration*, Eds. G. T. J. Huang & I. Thesleff. Hoboken, NJ: Wiley-Blackwell, p. 285.

NAKAGAWA, M., KOYANAGI, M., TANABE, K., TAKAHASHI, K., ICHISAKA, T., AOI, T., et al. 2008. Generation of induced pluripotent stem cells without Myc from mouse and human fibroblasts. *Nat Biotech*, 26, 101–106.

NISHIKAWA, S.-I., GOLDSTEIN, R. A., & NIERRAS, C. R. 2008. The promise of human induced pluripotent stem cells for research and therapy. *Nat Rev Mol Cell Biol*, 9, 725–729.

NOGGLE, S., FUNG, H.-L., GORE, A., MARTINEZ, H., SATRIANI, K. C., PROSSER, R., et al. 2011. Human oocytes reprogram somatic cells to a pluripotent state. *Nature*, 478, 70–75.

OH, H. J., HONG, S. G., PARK, J. E., KANG, J. T., KIM, M. J., KIM, M. K., et al. (2009). Improved efficiency of canine nucleus transfer using roscovitine-treated canine fibroblasts. *Theriogenology*, 72, 461–470.

OKITA, K., MATSUMURA, Y., SATO, Y., OKADA, A., MORIZANE, A., OKAMOTO, S., et al. 2011. A more efficient method to generate integration-free human iPS cells. *Nat Methods*, 8, 409–412.

OKITA, K., NAKAGAWA, M., HYENJONG, H., ICHISAKA, T., & YAMANAKA, S. 2008. Generation of mouse induced pluripotent stem cells without viral vectors. *Science*, 322, 949–953.

OTSU, K., KISHIGAMI, R., OIKAWA-SASAKI, A., FUKUMOTO, S., YAMADA, A., FUJIWARA, N., et al. 2012. Differentiation of induced pluripotent stem cells into dental mesenchymal cells. *Stem Cells and Devel*, 21, 1156–1164.

OTSU, K., KUMAKAMI-SAKANO, M., FUJIWARA, N., KIKUCHI, K., KELLER, L., LESOT, H., et al. 2014. Stem cell sources for tooth regeneration: Current status and future prospects. *Front Physiol*, 5, 36.

PARK, H., KIM, D., KIM, C. H., MILLS, R. E., CHANG, M. Y., ISKOW, R. C., et al. 2014. Increased genomic integrity of an improved protein-based mouse induced pluripotent stem cell method compared with current viral-induced strategies. *Stem Cells Translat Med*, 3, 599–609.

PARK, I. H., ARORA, N., HUO, H., MAHERALI, N., AHFELDT, T., SHIMAMURA, A., et al. 2008a. Disease-specific induced pluripotent stem cells. *Cell*, 134, 877–886.

PARK, I. H., ZHAO, R., WEST, J. A., YABUUCHI, A., HUO, H., INCE, T. A., et al. 2008b. Reprogramming of human somatic cells to pluripotency with defined factors. *Nature*, 451, 141–146.

PARK, S., & IM, G. I. 2013. Embryonic stem cells and induced pluripotent stem cells for skeletal regeneration. *Tissue Eng Part B Rev*, 20, 381–391.

PETERSON, S. E., & LORING, J. F. 2014. Genomic instability in pluripotent stem cells: Implications for clinical applications. *J Biol Chem*, 289, 4578–4584.

POLO, J. M., LIU, S., FIGUEROA, M. E., KULALERT, W., EMINLI, S., TAN, K. Y. et al. 2010. Cell type of origin influences the molecular and functional properties of mouse induced pluripotent stem cells. *NatBiotechnol*, 28, 848–855.

RAO, M. S., & MALIK, N. 2012. Assessing iPSC reprogramming methods for their suitability in translational medicine. *J Cell Biochem*, 113, 3061–3068.

RAYA, A., RODRIGUEZ-PIZA, I., GUENECHEA, G., VASSENA, R., NAVARRO, S., BARRERO, M. J., et al. 2009. Disease-corrected haematopoietic progenitors from Fanconi anaemia induced pluripotent stem cells. *Nature*, 460, 53–59.

REVAZOVA, E. S., TUROVETS, N. A., KOCHETKOVA, O. D., KINDAROVA, L. B., KUZMICHEV, L. N., JANUS, J. D., et al. 2007. Patient-specific stem cell lines derived from human parthenogenetic blastocysts. *Cloning and Stem Cells*, 9, 432–449.

REVAZOVA, E. S., TUROVETS, N. A., KOCHETKOVA, O. D., AGAPOVA, L. S., SEBASTIAN, J. L., PRYZHKOVA, M. V., et al. 2008. HLA homozygous stem cell lines derived from human parthenogenetic blastocysts. *Cloning and Stem Cells*, 10, 11–24.

SANCHEZ-FREIRE, V., LEE, A. S., HU, S., ABILEZ, O. J, LIANG, P., LAN, F., et al. 2014. Effect of human donor cell source on differentiation and function of cardiac induced pluripotent stem cells. *J Am Coll Cardiol*, 64, 436–448.

SAREEN, D., SAGHIZADEH, M., ORNELAS, L., WINKLER, M. A., NARWANI, K., SAHABIAN, A., et al. 2014. Differentiation of human limbal-derived induced pluripotent stem cells into limbal-like epithelium. *Stem Cells Translat Med*, 3, 1002–1012.

SCHWARTZ, S. D., HUBSCHMAN, J. P., HEILWELL, G., FRANCO-CARDENAS, V., PAN, C. K., OSTRICK, R. M., et al. 2012. Embryonic stem cell trials for macular degeneration: A preliminary report. *Lancet*, 379, 713–720.

SCHWARTZ, S. D., REGILLO, C. D., LAM, B. L., ELIOTT, D., ROSENFELD, P. J., GREGORI, N. Z., et al. 2015. Human embryonic stem cell-derived retinal pigment epithelium in patients with age-related macular degeneration and Stargardt's macular dystrophy: Follow-up of two open-label phase 1/2 studies. *Lancet*, 385, 509–516.

SEKI, T., YUASA, S., KUSUMOTO, D., KUNITOMI, A., SAITO, Y., TOHYAMA, S., et al. 2014. Generation and characterization of functional cardiomyocytes derived from human T cell-derived induced pluripotent stem cells. *PLoS One* 9, e85645.

SI-TAYEB, K., NOTO, F. K., NAGAOKA, M., LI, J., BATTLE, M. A., DURIS, C., et al. 2010. Highly efficient generation of human hepatocyte-like cells from induced pluripotent stem cells. *Hepatology*, 51, 297–305.

SMITH, K. P., LUONG, M. X., & STEIN, G. S. 2009. Pluripotency: Toward a gold standard for human ES and iPS cells. *J Cell Physiol*, 220, 21–29.

SOLDNER, F., HOCKEMEYER, D., BEARD, C., GAO, Q., BELL, G. W., COOK, E. G., et al. 2009. Parkinson's disease patient-derived induced pluripotent stem cells free of viral reprogramming factors. *Cell*, 136, 964–977.

SOMERS, A., JEAN, J. C., SOMMER, C. A., OMARI, A., FORD, C. C., MILLS, J. A., et al. 2010. Generation of transgene-free lung disease-specific human induced pluripotent stem cells using a single excisable lentiviral stem cell cassette. *Stem Cells*, 28, 1728–40.

SOMMER, C. A., STADTFELD, M., MURPHY, G. J., HOCHEDLINGER, K., KOTTON, D. N., & MOSTOSLAVSKY, G. 2009. Induced pluripotent stem cell generation using a single lentiviral stem cell cassette. *Stem Cells*, 27, 543–549.

SONG, R. S., CARROLL, J. M., ACEVEDO, L., WU, D., LIU, Y., & SNYDER, E. Y. 2014. Generation, expansion, and differentiation of human induced pluripotent stem cells (hiPSCs) derived from the umbilical cords of newborns. *Curr Protoc Stem Cell Biol*, 6, 29:1C.16.1–1C.16.13.

STADTFELD, M., NAGAYA, M., UTIKAL, J., WEIR, G., & HOCHEDLINGER, K. 2008. Induced pluripotent stem cells generated without viral integration. *Science*, 322, 945–949.

STAERK, J., DAWLATY, M. M., GAO, Q., MAETZEL, D., HANNA, J., SOMMER, C. A., et al. 2010. Reprogramming of human peripheral blood cells to induced pluripotent stem cells. *Cell Stem Cell*, 7, 20–24.

SU, R. J., BAYLINK, D. J., NEISES, A., KIROYAN, J. B., MENG, X., PAYNE, K. J., et al. 2013. Efficient generation of integration-free ips cells from human adult peripheral blood using BCL-XL together with Yamanaka factors. *PLoS One*, 8, e64496.

SULLIVAN, G. J., HAY, D. C., PARK, I.-H., FLETCHER, J., HANNOUN, Z., PAYNE, C. M., et al. 2010. Generation of functional human hepatic endoderm from human induced pluripotent stem cells. *Hepatology*, 51, 329–335.

SUN, N., PANETTA, N. J., GUPTA, D. M., WILSON, K. D., LEE, A., JIA, F., et al. 2009. Feeder-free derivation of induced pluripotent stem cells from adult human adipose stem cells. *Proc Natl Acad Sci U S A*, 106, 15720–15725.

TAKAHASHI, K., TANABE, K., OHNUKI, M., NARITA, M., ICHISAKA, T., TOMODA, K., et al. 2007. Induction of pluripotent stem cells from adult human fibroblasts by defined factors. *Cell*, 131, 861–872.

TAKAHASHI, K., & YAMANAKA, S. 2006. Induction of pluripotent stem cells from mouse embryonic and adult fibroblast cultures by defined factors. *Cell*, 126, 663–676.

TAMAOKI, N., TAKAHASHI, K., TANAKA, T., ICHISAKA, T., AOKI, H., TAKEDA-KAWAGUCHI, T., et al. 2010. Dental pulp cells for induced pluripotent stem cell banking. *J Dent Res*, 89, 773–778.

TANG, M., CHEN, W., LIU, J., WEIR, M. D., CHENG, L., & XU, H. H. 2014. Human induced pluripotent stem cell-derived mesenchymal stem cell seeding on calcium phosphate scaffold for bone regeneration. *Tissue Eng Part A*, 20, 1295–1305.

THUAN, N. V., KISHIGAMI, S., & WAKAYAMA, T. 2010. How to improve the success rate of mouse cloning technology. *J Reprod Dev*, 56, 20–30.

TURNER, M., LESLIE, S., MARTIN, N. G., PESCHANSKI, M., RAO, M., TAYLOR, C. J., et al. 2013. Toward the development of a global induced pluripotent stem cell library. *Cell Stem Cell*, 13, 382–384.

VILLA-DIAZ, L. G., BROWN, S. E., LIU, Y., ROSS, A. M., LAHANN, J., PARENT, J. M., et al. 2012. Derivation of mesenchymal stem cells from human induced pluripotent stem cells cultured on synthetic substrates. *Stem Cells*, 30, 1174–1181.

WADA, N., WANG, B., LIN, N. H., LASLETT, A. L., GRONTHOS, S., & BARTOLD, P. M. 2011. Induced pluripotent stem cell lines derived from human gingival fibroblasts and periodontal ligament fibroblasts. *J Periodontal Res*, 46, 438–447.

WANG, A., TANG, Z., PARK, I. H., ZHU, Y., PATEL, S., DALEY, G. Q., et al. 2011. Induced pluripotent stem cells for neural tissue engineering. *Biomats*, 32, 5023–5032.

WANG, H., & DOERING, L. C. 2012. Induced pluripotent stem cells to model and treat neurogenetic disorders. *Neural Plast*, 2012, 346053.

WATANABE, K., KAMIYA, D., NISHIYAMA, A., KATAYAMA, T., NOZAKI, S., KAWASAKI, H., et al. 2005. Directed differentiation of telencephalic precursors from embryonic stem cells. *Nat Neurosci*, 8, 288–296.

WATANABE, K., UENO, M., KAMIYA, D., NISHIYAMA, A., MATSUMURA, M., WATAYA, T., et al. 2007. A ROCK inhibitor permits survival of dissociated human embryonic stem cells. *Nat Biotechnol*, 25, 681–686.

WATTANAPANITCH, M., KLINCUMHOM, N., POTIRAT, P., AMORNPISUTT, R., LORTHONGPANICH, C., Yaowalak, U.-P., et al. 2014. Dual small-molecule targeting of SMAD signaling stimulates human induced pluripotent stem cells toward neural lineages. *PLoS One*, 9, e106952.

WEN, Y., WANG, F., ZHANG, W., LI, Y., YU, M., NAN, X., et al. 2012. Application of induced pluripotent stem cells in generation of a tissue-engineered tooth-like structure. *Tissue Eng Part A*, 18, 1677–1685.

WERNIG, M., ZHAO, J.-P., PRUSZAK, J., HEDLUND, E., FU, D., SOLDNER, F., et al. 2008a. Neurons derived from reprogrammed fibroblasts functionally integrate into the fetal brain and improve symptoms of rats with Parkinson's disease. *Proc Natl Acad Sci U S A*, 105, 5856–5861.

WERNIG, M., ZHAO, J. P., PRUSZAK, J., HEDLUND, E., FU, D., SOLDNER, F., et al. 2008b. Neurons derived from reprogrammed fibroblasts functionally integrate into the fetal brain and improve symptoms of rats with Parkinson's disease. *Proc Natl Acad Sci U S A*, 105, 5856–5861.

WILMUT, I., SCHNIEKE, A. E., MCWHIR, J., KIND, A. J., & CAMPBELL, K. H. 1997. Viable offspring derived from fetal and adult mammalian cells. *Nature*, 385, 810–813.

WOLTJEN, K., MICHAEL, I. P., MOHSENI, P., DESAI, R., MILEIKOVSKY, M., & HAMALAINEN, R. et al. 2009. piggyBac transposition reprograms fibroblasts to induced pluripotent stem cells. *Nature*, 458, 766–770.

YAGI, T., ITO, D., OKADA, Y., AKAMATSU, W., NIHEI, Y., YOSHIZAKI, T., et al. 2011. Modeling familial Alzheimer's disease with induced pluripotent stem cells. *Hum Mol Genet*, 20, 4530–4539.

YAN, X., QIN, H., QU, C., TUAN, R. S., SHI, S., & HUANG, G. T.-J. 2010. iPS cells reprogrammed from human mesenchymal-like stem/progenitor cells of dental tissue origin. *Stem Cells and Devel*, 19, 469–480.

YU, J., HU, K., SMUGA-OTTO, K., TIAN, S., STEWART, R., SLUKVIN, I. I., et al. 2009a. Human induced pluripotent stem cells free of vector and transgene sequences. *Science*, 324, 797–801.

YU, J., HU, K., SMUGA-OTTO, K., TIAN, S., STEWART, R., SLUKVIN, I. I., et al. 2009b. Human induced pluripotent stem cells free of vector and transgene sequences. *Science*, 324, 797–801.

YU, J., VODYANIK, M. A., HE, P., SLUKVIN, I. I., & THOMSON, J. A. 2006. Human embryonic stem cells reprogram myeloid precursors following cell-cell fusion. *Stem Cells*, 24, 168–176.

YU, J., VODYANIK, M. A., SMUGA-OTTO, K., ANTOSIEWICZ-BOURGET, J., FRANE, J. L., TIAN, S., NIE, J., JONSDOTTIR, G. A., RUOTTI, V., STEWART, R., SLUKVIN, I. I., THOMSON, J. A. 2007. Induced pluripotent stem cell lines derived from human somatic cells. *Science*, 318, 1917–1920.

ZHANG, J., WILSON, G. F., SOERENS, A. G., KOONCE, C. H., YU, J., PALECEK, S. P., et al. 2009. Functional cardiomyocytes derived from human induced pluripotent stem cells. *Circ Res*, 104, e30–41.

ZHANG, S. C., WERNIG, M., DUNCAN, I. D., BRUSTLE, O., & THOMSON, J. A. 2001. In vitro differentiation of transplantable neural precursors from human embryonic stem cells. *Nat Biotechnol*, 19, 1129–1133.

ZHAO, X.-Y., LI, W., LV, Z., LIU, L., TONG, M., HAI, T., et al. 2009. iPS cells produce viable mice through tetraploid complementation. *Nature*, 461, 86–90.

ZHOU, H., WU, S., JOO, J. Y., ZHU, S., HAN, D. W., LIN, T., et al. 2009. Generation of induced pluripotent stem cells using recombinant proteins. *Cell Stem Cell*, 4, 381–384.

ZOU, X. Y., YANG, H. Y., YU, Z., TAN, X. B., YAN, X., HUANG, G. T. 2012. Establishment of transgene-free induced pluripotent stem cells reprogrammed from human stem cells of apical papilla for neural differentiation. *Stem Cell Res Ther*, 24, 43.

ZWI, L., CASPI, O., ARBEL, G., HUBER, I., GEPSTEIN, A., PARK, I. H., et al. 2009. Cardiomyocyte differentiation of human induced pluripotent stem cells. *Circulation*, 120, 1513–1523.

ZWI-DANTSIS, L., HUBER, I., HABIB, M., WINTERSTERN, A., GEPSTEIN, A., ARBEL, G. et al. 2013. Derivation and cardiomyocyte differentiation of induced pluripotent stem cells from heart failure patients. *Eur Heart J*, 34, 1575–1586.

CHAPTER 2

Immunomodulation by adult stem cells: Mechanisms of action and clinical applications

Lindsay C. Davies[1,2] and Katarina Le Blanc[1]

[1] *Centre for Hematology and Regenerative Medicine, Karolinska Institutet, Stockholm, Sweden*

[2] *School of Dentistry, Cardiff University, Heath Park, Cardiff, UK*

The craniofacial region is composed of a number of distinct tissue-specific mesenchymal stem or progenitor cell populations, of which some represent a more primitive neural crest phenotype, such as the oral mucosa lamina propria progenitor cells (OMLP-PCs) (Davies et al., 2010). Mesenchymal stem/stromal cell (MSC) populations have been isolated from numerous oral and dental tissues, including the dental pulp (of both permanent and deciduous teeth), the periodontal ligament, gingiva, apical papilla, and dental follicle (Gronthos et al., 2000, Morsczeck et al., 2005, Seo et al., 2004, Zhang et al., 2009).

The diversity in stem cell sources being called "mesenchymal stem cells", along with a lack in the definition of key properties a cell must possess in order to be termed an MSC, initially led to issues in accurately comparing results from a plethora of *in vitro* and *in vivo* experimental studies and clinical trials. Whilst a rare population of true self-renewing cells has been found within the bone marrow, it is unclear as to whether multipotent cells derived from other tissues, including those from the oral cavity, possess the same properties. This has led to adoption of the generic term *mesenchymal stromal cell* to standardise the classification of multipotent cells derived from mesenchymal tissues. In 2006, the International Society for Cellular Therapy (ISCT) published minimal criteria for the classification of a true MSC (Dominici et al., 2006). Based on these criteria, all cells defined as a tissue source of MSCs must be able to adhere to plastic, exhibit tri-lineage multipotency (differentiate upon appropriate stimuli into osteoblasts, chondrocytes, and adipocytes), and be phenotypically classified as $CD73^+CD90^+CD105^+$ and $CD11b^-CD14^-CD34^-CD45^-CD19^-CD79a^-$ and human leukocyte antigen (HLA) $-DR^-$.

MSCs as defined by the ISCT guidelines (Dominici et al., 2006) are HLA class I positive at low levels and HLA class II negative, with no expression of costimulatory molecules necessary for antigen presentation. These phenotypic characteristics contribute to the low inherent immunogenicity of MSCs and evasion of immune cells; properties crucial in the development of allogeneic cell-based therapies utilizing MSCs where the possibility of rejection and immune sensitisation are of serious concern.

Initial studies regarding the immunomodulatory properties of adult stem cells have been demonstrated using bone marrow–derived MSCs (BMMSCs). These foremost studies documented the primary evidence that MSCs, derived from multiple species, may be able to regulate immune cells, providing knowledge that activated MSCs could suppress lymphocyte proliferation *in vitro* in mixed lymphocytes cultures (Bartholomew et al., 2002, Maitra et al., 2004). This simplistic *in vitro* assay allows quantitative assessment of lymphocyte proliferation in response to alloantigen or mitogen and the potential of MSCs cocultured with the lymphocytes to modulate this proliferative response (Protocol 2.1).

Since these initial *in vitro* and *in vivo* experiments, much research has been undertaken to establish whether this property is unique to BMMSCs. Studies

---

Tissue Engineering and Regeneration in Dentistry: Current Strategies, First Edition. Edited by Rachel J. Waddington and Alastair J. Sloan.

Protocol 2.1 Evaluating immunomodulation by mixed lymphocyte cultures (Le Blanc et al., 2003).

1. Peripheral blood mononuclear cells (PBMCs) are isolated from heparinised blood by centrifugation on Ficoll-Isopaque (Lymphoprep™).
2. Isolated responder PBMCs (A) are combined with an equal number of irradiated PBMCs (pool of five donors acting as an alloantigen, Px) in RPMI-1640 medium supplemented with 10% heat-inactivated human AB serum in a 96-well culture plate.
3. Irradiated stem cells are added at a range of concentrations (10%–0.1%) to responder PBMCs.
4. A positive control for induction of lymphocyte proliferation (A combined with Px) and negative control for background lymphocyte proliferation (A + Ax) are run on each experimental plate.
5. Cultures are incubated at 37°C/5% CO_2 for 5 days.
6. 1uCi of ^{3}H-thymidine is added to each well and the plate incubated for a further 24 hours.
7. Cells are harvested onto glass fiber filters using a cell harvester, and solid scintillant is melted onto the filter before reading in a micro-β liquid scintillation counter.
8. Data are quantified by recording counts per minute (CPM) in experimental samples versus those of the positive (A + Px) and negative (A + Ax) controls.

have assessed the immunomodulatory properties of other adult stem cell sources, the exact mechanisms by which these cells exert this effect, and how these properties can be exploited for clinical use in the treatment of immunological disorders and allogeneic tissue regeneration. The mechanisms of MSC-mediated immunomodulation remain well debated, but it is generally accepted that cell-cell contact between BMMSCs and immune cells aids the MSCs in exerting their full immunosuppressive potential. This also holds true for some oral tissue–derived MSCs, such as gingival MSCs (GMSCs), with maximal immunosuppression of peripheral blood mononuclear cells (PBMCs) only demonstrated when GMSCs were in direct contact with the PBMC population (Zhang et al., 2009). Other oral stem cell sources, such as OMLP-PCs, do not require cell-cell contact, exerting their potent immunosuppressive effects through the secretion of soluble factors (Davies et al., 2012).

The potential for oral stem cell sources to modulate the immune system has received recent attention. Exposure to unique environmental cues from residing within the oral cavity certainly suggests the need for an immunomodulatory phenotype. An increasingly comprehensive list of reports and evidence is now accumulating with suggestions that the ability and mechanisms by which adult stem cells interact with immune cells is specific to the tissue of origin and microenvironment as well as the individual subsets of immune cells on which these cells act.

Certainly the environment from which the stem cells are derived plays a central role in determining their potential for immunomodulatory function. A recent study by Liu et al. demonstrated that periodontal ligament stem cells (PDLSC) isolated from inflamed tissue have a diminished capacity to inhibit T cell proliferation compared to PDLSCs derived from healthy periodontal ligament (Liu et al., 2012).

Inflammation arising from infection or tissue injury serves to protect the body. Initiation of this response pathway is associated with innate immune cells recognizing specific pathogenic or injury-associated molecules via Toll-like receptors (TLRs) expressed on their cell surface, leading to a cascade of immune responses and the release of inflammatory mediators. MSCs themselves can also sense this shift in the microenvironment, responding to the presence of proinflammatory cytokines such as interferon γ (IFNγ) with the upregulation of certain TLRs. Research supports the notion that MSCs are not constitutively immunomodulatory and that the anti-inflammatory MSC phenotype is induced by the exposure to the proinflammatory microenvironment (Bernardo and Fibbe, 2013). The nature of adult stem cell/immune cell interactions is complex and multifactorial. As understanding of these processes has evolved, it has been established that both cells of the innate and adaptive immunity are influenced by stem cells, with much information being gained with respect to the different types of cellular crosstalk and molecules implicated in these diverse pathways.

The effect of ageing on MSC function

Numerous reports have demonstrated the substantial loss of *in vivo* MSCs with ageing. Tuljapurkar et al. compared the bone marrow composition of a 22-year-old cadaver with that of an 86-year-old, illustrating the loss of red marrow and transformation into fatty degeneration with ageing (Tuljapurkar et al., 2011). This is not restricted to the bone marrow, with a similar age-related degeneration occurring within the dental pulp, where fatty deposition and loss of cellularity with increased fibrosis is evident with ageing within the pulp proper (Morse, 1991).

Studies evaluating MSCs have noted a loss in differentiation potency, growth factor secretion, and self-renewal capacity with ageing of the donor. Senescence, a state in which an aged cell is no longer capable of cellular division but remains metabolically active, is a phenomenon seen both *in vivo* with an accumulation of senescent cells within the bone marrow and *in vitro* where the osteogenic potential of dental pulp stem cells is lost with extended *in vitro* culture (Mehrazarin et al., 2011).

Furthermore, BMMSCs expanded extensively *in vitro* prior to infusion are more susceptible to triggering the instant blood-mediated inflammatory reaction (IBMIR), a cascade of proinflammatory events mediated by coagulation, complement components, and platelets, when exposed to whole blood *in vitro* (Moll et al., 2012). This destruction of the infused cells on contact with blood is less evident with low passage BMMSCs and is most likely due to a change in their cell surface receptor profile and expression of the prothrombotic tissue factor with *in vitro* ageing and passage. Triggering of IBMIR potentially results in a rapid clearance of the cells from the systemic circulation after infusion. It is estimated that 99% of infused cells are cleared within 5 minutes (Lee et al., 2009).

A recent *in vitro* study has identified that adipose-derived MSCs (ADMSCs) from "senior" donors have a reduced capacity to induce suppression of CD3+CD4+ T cell proliferation, with the results actually indicating a potential increase in immunogenicity. No difference in effect on CD8+ cells was reported, however, suggesting different mechanisms of actions between CD4 and CD8 T cell subsets. A decrease in immune suppressive soluble mediators (described below) indoleamine 2,3 dioxygenase (IDO), interleukin (IL) -10, and prostaglandin (PG) E2 secretion with MSCs from older donors confirms a shift in phenotype with ageing in adult stem cells (Wu et al., 2014).

This change in phenotype and proliferative capacity is of importance when considering the development of cell-based therapeutics where large numbers of cells are required for infusion. In the case of graft versus host disease (GvHD), a complication associated with hematopoietic stem cell transplantation, where donor T cells attack the recipient's organs, an average of 1–2 million cells/kg body weight of the patient are required per infusion (Le Blanc et al., 2008). The need for allogeneic therapies is therefore evident and key to the success of stem cell–based therapeutics for immune disorders.

Allogeneic versus autologous MSCs

The development of allogeneic cell-based therapies has made commercialisation of such technology more attractive. These cells can be generated in an "off the shelf" based approach, with large quantities of cells derived from various donors being cryopreserved ready for infusion to the patient. Many studies have demonstrated the efficacy of allogeneic stem cells for immune disorders without adverse side effects to the recipient. MSCs have no immunological restriction in their functionality, with similar suppressive effects observed with MSCs either autologous or allogeneic to the responder cells. The accepting nature of the body to these foreign stem cells may be attributed to their immune-privilege status and immunosuppressive properties or the fact that these infused cells are so rapidly cleared from the systemic circulation. In therapeutic situations where engraftment is not the primary aim, for example in the systemic infusion for the treatment of GvHD, allogeneic MSCs offer a practical therapeutic option.

In instances of tissue engineering, where both differentiation and engraftment of the cells is required for successful treatment, the potential for allogeneic MSCs is less well understood. The effects of differentiated MSC immunogenicity are not well characterised to date. *In vitro* assays suggest that differentiation of BMMSCs into adipocytes, chondrocytes, and osteoblasts does not affect their interaction with the immune system (Le Blanc et al., 2003). These data were supported by an *in vivo* rabbit study where allogeneic MSCs differentiated into osteoblasts remained immunosuppressive and functioned as osteoblasts *in vivo* (Liu et al., 2006). However, a recent report suggests that allogeneic MSCs can become immunogenic on differentiation, and this would limit their therapeutic benefit (Huang et al., 2010). It is clear that further research is required to establish whether allogeneic MSCs are suitable for all cell-based therapeutics or will remain limited to those treating inflammatory conditions and "reprogramming" of the patient's own immune system, where persistence of the cells is not a requirement.

Licensing of MSCs

Cellular licensing occurs when a cell develops a particular phenotype in response to being exposed to a defined chemical repertoire, normally of cytokines and/or chemokines. Studies have demonstrated the need for MSCs to be licensed in order to exert their full immunosuppressive potential (Le Blanc et al., 2003). MSCs can modulate the immune system both in a direct and indirect manner, heavily dependent on continuous interplay between innate and adaptive immune cells. Through these interactions with different cell types of the immune system, it has been demonstrated that MSCs can exhibit both proinflammatory and anti-inflammatory effects, leading to a subclassification system of MSC1 (proinflammatory) and MSC2 (anti-inflammatory) cell types (Figure 2.1) (Bernardo and Fibbe, 2013; Waterman et al., 2010). It is thought that through balancing this activating or suppressive phenotype, MSCs may be central to regulating immune control and tissue repair and regeneration.

MSC1

TLR4 activation is primarily associated with the generation of a proinflammatory MSC phenotype, known as an MSC1 (Figure 2.1). This is associated with the production of proinflammatory cytokines such as IL-6, IL-8, and transforming growth factor beta 1 (TGFβ1). Studies with murine MSCs have also indicated that activation of TLR2 signaling, associated with peptidoglycan derived from the cell wall of Gram-positive bacteria, may also induce an MSC1 phenotype, with increased IL-6 secretion via the NF-κB pathway (Tomchuck et al., 2008).

MSC1 cells are associated with early-stage infection and inflammation, migrating to the site of injury and promoting immune induction in a rapid response to microbial infection (Waterman et al., 2010). This process is associated with the secretion of chemokine (C-X-C motif) ligand (CXCL) 9, CXCL10, macrophage inflammatory protein (MIP)-1α, MIP-1β and Rantes, factors enhancing the recruitment of lymphocytes to the site of injury. The pro-inflammatory effects of MSC1

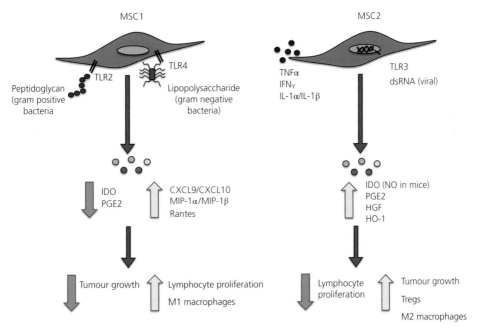

Figure 2.1 Licensing of MSCs. Environmental cues trigger the recruitment and licensing of MSCs to a proinflammatory (MSC1) or anti-inflammatory (MSC2) phenotype. MSC1 are essential to the early immune response, recruiting and activating innate and adaptive immune cells in response to microbial products such as lipopolysaccharide and peptidoglycan. Activated lymphocytes and M1 macrophages secreting proinflammatory cytokines such as TNFα and IFNγ (or exposure to viral double-stranded RNA) switches the MSC profile to an MSC2. Licensed MSC2 secrete anti-inflammatory cytokines central to reducing lymphocyte proliferation, controlling the inflammatory immune response and switching immune cells to a regulatory phenotype (M2 macrophage and Treg induction) to initiate a repair response.

cells have been demonstrated in *in vitro* assays, supporting induction of immune cell proliferation and in murine models of inflammatory lung injury, where evidence of aggravated inflammatory injury was observed (Waterman et al., 2010). Induction of the MSC1 phenotype can be beneficial in the regulation of tumor growth, however. Reports have indicated that a proinflammatory MSC1 can attenuate cancer cell growth, whilst induction of the MSC2 anti-inflammatory phenotype aids in the promotion of cancer growth and spreading (Waterman et al., 2012a).

MSC2

Licensing or pretreating MSCs with proinflammatory cytokines and/or TLR3 ligands such as double-stranded RNA (dsRNA) and viral infection induces an MSC2 phenotype, as evidenced by a clear enhancement of the production of immunosuppressive cytokines by MSCs (Figure 2.1). Both tumor necrosis factor alpha (TNFα) and IFNγ have central roles in licensing MSCs towards an MSC2, immunosuppressive phenotype. IFNγ, mainly produced by activated T cells, works in synergy with other proinflammatory mediators such as TNFα, IL-1α, and IL-1β in promoting MSC2 induction, triggering the synthesis and secretion of immunosuppressive soluble mediators including IDO and PGE2 by the licensed MSCs (Bernardo and Fibbe, 2013). Prelicensing of MSCs towards this immunosuppressive phenotype has been suggested to increase the efficacy of MSC action in murine models of GvHD, exerting a protective effect in preventing donor T cells from attacking host tissue (Bernardo and Fibbe, 2013). It could therefore be postulated that this may be an explanation for the increased efficacy of MSCs in the treatment of acute GvHD clinical studies, where IFNγ amongst other inflammatory mediators is increased. Based on this understanding, it would be reasonable to suggest that MSCs may be most efficacious in therapies if administered after induction of the inflammatory phase, rather than prophylactically. Certainly studies in murine models of GvHD demonstrated that infusion of MSCs on the same day as the hematopoietic stem cells (HSCs) has no preventive effect, whereas administration post-HSC significantly reduced GvHD-associated complications (Bernardo and Fibbe, 2013).

In support of this, the addition of MSC2 cells to *in vitro* assays suppressed lymphocyte proliferation as expected for MSCs. Furthermore, a murine model of inflammatory lung injury confirmed a decrease in inflammation and improvement of the injury with infusion of prelicensed MSC2 (Waterman et al., 2010). In this manner MSC2 cells could be seen to promote the reduction in inflammation and enhancement of tissue repair and regeneration. This is also evident in MSC2-based treatment of diabetic peripheral neuropathy, where licensed MSC2 cells infused in a murine model of diabetes attenuated the immune response to a greater extent than unprimed MSCs (Waterman et al., 2012b).

MSCs and TLRs

MSCs express TLRs, a family of receptors able to recognise molecules conserved amongst many pathogens, known as pathogen-associated molecular patterns (PAMPs). PAMP triggering of a particular TLR pathway results in specific cytokine production and antigen presentation. Human BMMSCs express TLRs 1–10, although TLR3 and 4 are the most prevalent, with TLR3 activated by dsRNA (normally associated with viruses) and TLR4 activated by lipopolysaccharide (LPS) from Gram-negative bacteria.

Expression levels of the different TLRs are regulated by the microenvironment. Under hypoxic conditions TLR 1/2/5 and 9 are upregulated, whilst under inflammatory conditions (exposure to IFNγ, TNFα, IL-1β, or IFNα) levels of TLR 2/3 and 4 are upregulated (Raicevic et al., 2010). It has been demonstrated within ADMSCs that TLR activation leads to downstream activation of MAPK, PI3K, and NF-κB pathways. Short-term activation of TLR signaling induces the directional migration of MSCs, supposedly mimicking MSCs homing to a site of injury. With long-term TLR stimulation the migration of MSCs is reduced, most likely as they are within the tissue and therefore will switch to a more reparative and regulatory role (Waterman et al., 2010).

Stimulation of the TLR4 pathway results in an increased resistance to oxidative stress within MSCs, much like the effect seen with complement binding, linked to the increased expression of antioxidants such as members of the superoxide dismutase family (Le Blanc and Mougiakakos, 2012; Lombardo et al., 2009; Yu et al., 2008). Triggering of the TLR3 pathway results in polarisation of MSCs to an MSC2 phenotype, with an anti-inflammatory cytokine profile and TLR4 triggering its opposite MSC1, proinflammatory phenotype (Bernardo and Fibbe, 2013). Several of the MSC2 immunomodulatory soluble factors are downstream of TLR signaling, including IDO and IL-6.

A direct comparative of the MSC1/MSC2 phenotype identified for BMMSCs has not been made for other stem cell sources at present. However, limited data do suggest the potential for TLR activation to also manipulate the immunomodulatory phenotype of some dental stem cell populations including dental pulp stem cells (DPSCs) and dental follicle MSCs (Tomic et al., 2011). Activation of the TLR3 pathway within these stem cell sources (known to induce an MSC2 phenotype in BMMSCs) increased the suppressive potential of both stem cell populations associated with an increased secretion of TGFβ1 and IL-6, thereby supporting induction of an MSC2-like phenotype. In contrast, activation of the TLR4 pathway (indicative of an MSC1 phenotype) also increased the immunosuppressive potential of the dental follicle MSCs but decreased the suppressive potential of the DPSCs, as indicated by a decrease in TGFβ1 and IDO (Tomic et al., 2011). These data indicate that there are fundamental differences between individual oral stem cell populations, especially when they are compared with BMMSCs.

It has been suggested that TLR signaling may provide a link between the cellular microenvironment and control of MSC homeostasis. Downregulation of MYD88 (an adaptor molecule involved in mediating TLR signaling, except in the case of TLR3) affects both the proliferation and differentiation potential of MSCs. TLR2 induction promotes the proliferation of BMMSCs, in contrast to activation of TLR9, which results in BMMSC cell cycle arrest at G1 (Pevsner-Fischer et al., 2007).

Adult stem cells and the innate immune system

The innate immune system is the first line of defense, responding to nonspecific pathogens such as bacterial and viral infection.

The innate immune response serves three major purposes *in vivo*:
- To respond to pathogens to prevent, control, and eliminate infections
- To recognise the components of damaged or dead cells and remove these whilst initiating a tissue repair response

- To stimulate the adaptive immune response for a T and B cell mediated response

This subset of the immune system is composed of a number of distinct immune cells, including dendritic cells (DCs), mast cells, and macrophages. Numerous studies have reported the direct influence on innate immune cell behavior by adult stem cells, including those of oral sources as discussed below.

Cells of the innate immune system

Neutrophils

Inflammation within the early stages of immune triggering is crucial, with initial responses driven by the migration of neutrophils into the inflammatory site. It has been demonstrated within mice that tissue resident stem cells are central to the recruitment of these neutrophils and supporting their activity by secreting chemotactic cytokines such as IL-6, IL-8, granulocyte-macrophage colony-stimulating factor (GM-CSF), and macrophage inhibitory factor (Brandau et al., 2010).

Neutrophils are the most prevalent innate immune cell type, responding to microbial challenge by accumulating at the wound site within minutes of the injury occurring. These phagocytic cells respond to microbial presence by releasing bactericidal molecules and producing neutrophil extracellular traps, webs of chromatin derived from the neutrophil nucleus that are laced with proteases.

BMMSCs act to promote survival of both resting and activated neutrophils through the secretion of IL-6, IFNβ, and GM-CSF as evidenced by an increased expression of the antiapoptotic factor MCL1 and downregulation of the proapoptotic molecule BAX within neutrophils on exposure to MSCs. Neutrophils are also maintained "healthy" by BMMSC enhancement of neutrophil burst activity, which in combination with increased survival enables maintenance of a neutrophil store for rapid release on detection of pathogen (Cassatella et al., 2011). Upon sense of microbial pathogens such as LPS, MSCs increase their secretion of IL-6, IL-8, and macrophage migration inhibitory factor, thereby attracting the neutrophils to the site of inflammation and promoting their proinflammatory response whilst ensuring their survival (Brandau et al., 2010). These findings are further evidenced by results from a murine sepsis model where infusion of MSCs was shown to aid bacterial clearance through enhancing the phagocytic activity of neutrophils (Hall et al., 2013).

Mast Cells

Mast cells are the key innate responder cells in allergic inflammation. They reside in tissues, close to the external environment–facing barrier. Although primarily known for their role in allergy, mast cells have been shown to play a key role in defense and in autoimmunity.

Mast cells mediate anaphylaxis in allergy through the release of histamine during degranulation. Histamine has been demonstrated to stimulate the secretion of a number of cytokines including IL-1α and IL-6 in different cell types. Nemeth et al. demonstrated that BMMSCs express the necessary histamine receptors 1, 2, and 4 to interact with histamine (Nemeth et al., 2012). This study illustrated the interaction between histamine and BMMSCs via cell surface expression of the H1 receptor, inducing IL-6 production within the MSCs in a dose- and time-dependent manner. This was regulated by induction of members of the MAPK pathway including p38, ERK, and JNK. In addition, PGD2, a mast cell lipid mediator, further stimulates IL-6 secretion by BMMSCs. These enhanced levels of IL-6 secretion aided in the prevention of pro-apoptotic activity on neutrophils whilst increasing superoxide production within these phagocytic cells (Nemeth et al., 2012).

MSCs can suppress allergic responses and chronic inflammation in experimental models of asthma (Nemeth et al., 2010) and allergic rhinitis (Cho et al., 2009). The activation of mast cells promotes the recruitment of neutrophils and DCs by enhancing T cell activation and regulating the cytokine microenvironment. It has been recently demonstrated that GMSCs, like BMMSCs, can reduce the number of mast cells in a murine model of contact hypersensitivity by reducing mast cell migration as well as the percentage of degranulated mast cells (Su et al., 2011). *In vitro*, this inhibitory effect on mast cells can be reversed by inhibiting the production of PGE2 by the GMSCs. This corresponds with the evidence for BMMSCs, where an effective suppression of mast cell functions both *in vitro* and *in vivo* has been demonstrated. When in direct contact with mast cells, BMMSCs are able to suppress degranulation, proinflammatory cytokine production, chemotaxis, and chemokinesis. These effects were also demonstrated to be dependent on the upregulation of cyclooxygenase (COX) 2 within BMMSCs and

the binding of secreted PGE2 to the EP4 receptor on mast cells (Brown et al., 2011).

Natural killer cells

Natural killer (NK) cells have a surveillance role in eliminating both virally infected and stressed cells. This subset of innate immune cells is of particular interest in understanding the mechanisms of rejection as they play a central role in the regulation of cytotoxicity in response to HLA molecules.

NK cells are activated by exposure to IL-2 or IL-15, resulting in the secretion of proinflammatory cytokines, IFNγ, and TNFα. NK cells target cells lacking expression of HLA class I, a characteristic of tumor and virally infected cells, as recognised by the NK inhibitor receptor NKG2, resulting in cytolysis of the target cell. Activation of NK cells in response to recognizing an infected cell is characterised by the release of IFNγ and TNFα by the NK cells, with cytolysis mediated by perforins, granzyme, and Fas ligand (Reviewed by Le Blanc and Mougiakakos, 2012).

BMMSCs directly interfere with the proliferation, cytokine production, and in some cases cytotoxicity of NK cells. These interactions between NK cells and stem cells are complex and largely dependent on the microenvironment and activation status of the NK cells when BMMSCs are present. BMMSCs suppress IL-2 and IL-15 induced proliferation and IFNγ production, but not the cytotoxicity of freshly isolated NK cells. In contrast, when confronted with previously activated NK cells, MSCs can interfere with NK-mediated cytotoxicity, cytokine production, and the expression of activating receptors on the cells surface of the NK cells (including NKp30, NKp44 and NKG2D), in addition to granzyme B release. This is primarily mediated by cell-cell contact and the secretion of IDO, PGE2, TGFβ1, and HLA-G5 by MSCs. HLA-G5 interacts with the inhibitory receptors (such as ILT2, KIR2DL4, and CD94-NKG2A) on the surface of NK cells, inhibiting cytolysis and IFNγ secretion (Reviewed by Le Blanc and Mougiakakos, 2012).

It is important to note that HLA mismatched MSCs are not immune to NK-mediated cytotoxicity. Human BMMSCs also express a number of ligands capable of activating NK cell receptors, such as ULBP-3 as well as the DNAM-1 ligand nectin-2 and/or PVR. These MSCs are susceptible to lysis by IL-2 and/or IL-15 activated or IL-12 and/or IL-18 activated NK cells, but not resting NK cells (Rasmusson et al., 2003; Sotiropoulou et al., 2006; Spaggiari et al., 2006; Gotherstrom et al., 2011).

Licensed MSCs (MSC2) pre-exposed to IFNγ are protected from NK-mediated cell killing, primarily thought to be due to their upregulated cell surface expression of HLA I (an inhibitory signal to the NK cells) and downregulation of ULBP-3 (an activating signal), which alongside an increased production of both IDO and PGE2 dampens the NK cell responsiveness to the MSCs (Francois et al., 2012). These findings demonstrate the importance of IFNγ in mediating MSC-NK crosstalk.

Dendritic cells

DCs provide a link between the innate and adaptive immune systems, presenting antigen to T cells and regulating their activation. The effect of adult stem cells on DC function has been demonstrated in both BMMSCs and GMSCs (Spaggiari et al., 2009, Su et al., 2011). Both stem cell sources can directly inhibit both the maturation of monocytes to DCs and the direct activation of DCs via the secretion of PGE2, IL-6, and Jagged-2 (a member of the Notch signaling family) mediated signaling (Zhang et al., 2009). Immature DCs through their exposure to MSCs are unable to effectively induce the activation of T cells, suggesting an indirect mechanism of MSC-mediated immunosuppression (Beyth et al., 2005).

MSCs modulate DC behavior in three main ways:

a *Promotion of a T helper cell 2 (Th2; anti-inflammatory T cell) response in preference to Th1 (proinflammatory T cell):* The cytokine profiles of DCs are dramatically altered, with lower production and secretion of proinflammatory cytokines such as TNFα, IFNγ, and IL-12 and an increased production of the anti-inflammatory cytokine IL-10 (Beyth et al., 2005). This is associated with activation of the Notch 2 pathway on the surface of T cells (see point C).

b *Promote the generation of regulatory T cells (Tregs)*

c *Reduce stimulation of CD8+ T cells by activation of the Notch pathway:* DCs produced in the presence of MSCs express high levels of the Notch transmembrane ligand, Jagged (Cheng et al., 2007). Binding of Jagged on the surface of DCs to the Notch 2 receptor on the surface of the T cells suppresses the proliferation and activation of cytotoxic CD8+ T cells (Eagar et al., 2004).

MSCs also act directly on mature DCs, reverting them to an immature phenotype associated with a downregulation of their cell surface expression of antigen-presenting and costimulatory molecules, IL-12 secretion, and an inability to stimulate lymphocyte proliferation *in vitro* (Maccario et al., 2005).

Macrophages

Macrophages, originating from monocytes, form part of both the innate and adaptive immune systems. These phagocytic cells are further characterised into two phenotypes, the M1 proinflammatory macrophage with antimicrobial activity and the M2 anti-inflammatory macrophage. These categories relate primarily to the differential secretion of cytokines and expression of cell surface markers by the macrophages. The interactions between macrophages and BMMSCs have been demonstrated within their environmental origin, the bone marrow, working in symbiosis for stem cell homeostatic maintenance and potential microbial challenge. BMMSCs promote movement of monocytes out of the bone marrow space after detecting microbial pathogens by secretion of chemokine (C-C motif) ligand 2 (CCL2). Within inflamed tissue, MSCs play a role in the recruitment of both monocytes and M1 macrophages by the secretion of factors such as CCL3, CXCL2, and CCL12 (Figure 2.2) (Reviewed by Le Blanc and Mougiakakos, 2012). Monocytes entering the inflammatory environment will respond to local chemical signals, differentiating into either M1 macrophages secreting IFNγ and TNFα to support and enhance inflammation, or M2 macrophages promoting transition to the reparative stage of wound healing by secreting anti-inflammatory factors such as IL-10 and TGFβ1, supporting tissue repair. In addition to this, the secretion of IL-10 by both monocytes and M2 polarised macrophages can prevent neutrophils migrating into the inflamed tissue, thereby reducing oxidative damage and indirectly aiding bacterial clearance due to a resulting higher number of neutrophils within the blood (Figure 2.2) (Hall et al., 2013). This illustrates the role of MSCs in orchestrating the inflammatory response, enhancing neutrophil migration into the inflamed environment during the early phases to promote an innate immune response and switching to a inhibitory, inflammation-dampening role later to prevent prolonged damage to the tissue through chronic inflammation.

MSCs directly protect monocytes, with gene expression studies demonstrating a downregulation of apoptosis-related genes, through the release of constitutive soluble factors such as macrophage colony-stimulating factor

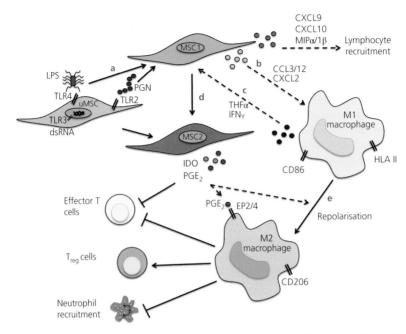

Figure 2.2 MSC crosstalk with macrophages regulates innate and adaptive immunity. (a) Unprimed MSC (uMSC) respond to bacterial stimuli such as lipopolysaccharide and peptidoglycan (PGN) through Toll-like receptors (TLRs) 2/4 by licensing to a proinflammatory MSC1 phenotype. (b) MSC1 secrete chemokine (C-C motif) ligand 3 and 12 and CXCL12 to recruit proinflamma-tory M1 macrophages to the site of inflammation. M1 macrophages in turn secrete (c) proinflammatory cytokines such as TNFα and IFNγ, triggering (d) the phenotypic switch of the MSCs to an anti-inflammatory MSC2. The secretion of immunomodulatory soluble factors such as indoleamine 2,3-dioxygenase (IDO) and prostaglandin E2 (PGE2) by MSC2 leads to (e) the repolarisation of M1 macrophages to regulatory M2 macrophages. MSC2 and M2 macrophages subsequently work both directly and indirectly to suppress effector T cell proliferation and neutrophil recruitment, whilst increasing the ratio of Tregs dampening the immune response and enhancing the wound healing process.

(Melief et al., 2013). Recent studies have reported the ability of adult stem cells, including GMSCs, to modulate the phenotype of macrophages by inducing a shift from the proinflammatory M1 to a functional anti-inflammatory M2 phenotype (Zhang et al., 2010, Bernardo and Fibbe, 2013). This shift to an M2 phenotype by exposure to GMSCs has been demonstrated to be instrumental in accelerating the wound healing process (Zhang et al., 2010). Co-cultures of human BMMSCs with macro-phages led to the expression of CD206 on the cell surface of macrophages, suggesting an M2 phenotype, accompa-nied by high-level secretion of IL-10 and IL-6, low levels of IL-12 and TNFα, and a functionally higher phagocytic activity (Kim and Hematti, 2009).

MSCs have also been reported to directly induce an M2 phenotype from immature monocytes. This directed maturation process is thought to be regulated partially via direct cell contact but also by BMMSC secretion of PGE2 and IDO; PGE2 binds to both EP2 and/or EP4

PGE2 receptor subsets expressed on the cell surface of the macrophage (Figure 2.2). Secretion of PGE2 by MSCs simultaneously stimulates the proliferation of epithelial cells, and therefore it has been hypothesised that the MSC role as an immunomodulator and healing promoting cell may be linked (Reviewed by Le Blanc and Mougiakakos, 2012). Changes in concentrations of these soluble signaling molecules may aid in the regula-tion and balancing of both the shift from M1 to M2 mac-rophages and the transition of MSC1 to MSC2.

A strong link between polarisation of macrophages by MSCs and modulation of T cell behavior has been demonstrated. Proinflammatory cytokine release by acti-vated T cells, including IFNγ and TNFα, increases the expression of COX2 and IDO in MSCs, further enhancing macrophage polarisation (Bernardo and Fibbe, 2013). M2 polarisation of macrophages has recently been associated with the induction of Tregs (Figure 2.2) and therefore a direct link to regulation of the adaptive immune response

(Melief et al., 2013). Secretion of TGFβ1, in addition to CCL18, by M2 macrophages works in parallel to induce this immunosuppressive T cell subset. This is an additive effect to that seen with IL-1β, where secretion of this proinflammatory cytokine by monocytes promotes the secretion of TGFβ1 by the MSCs to suppress lymphocyte proliferation (Uccelli et al., 2008).

The relevance of these findings linking MSCs to macrophage polarity has been supported by *in vivo* investigations. In a mouse model of sepsis, infusion of murine BMMSCs only decreased lethality in the presence of active macrophages, with depletion of macrophages or the presence of IL-10 neutralizing antibodies preventing this response (Nemeth et al., 2009).

MSCs and the complement system

The complement system is a central component of the innate immune system, bridging the divide between innate and adaptive pathways. This cascade has been implicated in the rejection of transplanted allografts (Hughes and Cohney, 2011) and more recently has been linked to the rapid clearance of systemically circulating MSCs after infusion (Li and Lin, 2012). Triggering of the complement cascade can occur via three separate pathways (classical, lectin, or alternative). Activation of the complement cascade via one or more of these pathways results in the recruitment and activation of leukocytes, enhanced phagocytosis, and the formation of membrane attack complexes, which directly injure the target cells.

The complement components C3 and C5, found abundantly within the serum, are cleaved by specific convertases to the anaphylatoxins C3a and C5a, both of which are found extensively within inflamed and injured tissues. BMMSCs express the receptors for these anaphylatoxins (C3aR and C5aR), suggesting that these breakdown products are chemotactic agents for the MSCs, promoting their migration towards the site of inflammation. Binding of C3a and C5a to their receptors on the cell surface of MSCs enhances MSC resistance to oxidative stress and prolongs the activation of intracellular signaling pathways involved in MSC proliferation and protection from apoptosis (Schraufstatter et al., 2009). Cell surface expression of the complement inhibitors CD46, CD55, and CD59 and the secretion of complement factor H helps to protect the MSCs from the lytic activity

of complement components (Ignatius et al., 2011; Tu et al., 2010); however, this mechanism of defense can be ineffective in a complement-activated environment. Despite the presence of these cell surface complement inhibitors, MSCs are injured by the formation of membrane attack complexes (Li and Lin, 2012). It is interesting to note that infused autologous MSCs instigate less complement activation and therefore less cellular injury, but remain susceptible to a degree most probably due to a change in their cell surface profile due to *in vitro* expansion (Li and Lin, 2012).

MSCs themselves are able to trigger the complement cascade via all three pathways by secreting both C3 and C5 when exposed to ABO-compatible blood and serum (Li and Lin, 2012, Moll et al., 2014, Moll et al., 2011). It is noted that the alternative pathway appears to play a major role in MSC-induced complement activation (Li and Lin, 2012). As discussed previously, the rapid clearance of MSCs after systemic infusion suggests triggering of IBMIR (Moll et al., 2011). This may, however, not be necessarily a bad thing, as complement activation by the MSCs appears to promote the activation and interaction of MSCs with immune cells within the blood, potentially initiating a cascade of intrinsic immunosuppressive functions within both the MSCs and immune cells, including Treg and M2 macrophage induction, to generate a complex and sophisticated immunosuppressive environment.

The adaptive immune response

Unlike the initial unspecific nature of the innate immune response, the adaptive immune system is antigen-specific and leads to the development of immunological memory. The adaptive immune system consists primarily of two lymphocyte families, the T cell and the B cell. Activation of the adaptive immune response occurs by direct presentation of antigen by professional antigen presenting cells and signaling cues from the innate immune response.

Adult stem cell populations have been demonstrated to both directly and indirectly modulate both of these lymphocyte populations dependent on the microenvironment and their MSC1/MSC2 status. In the following section we explore the complex interactions between stem cells and different adaptive immune cells in modulating the immune response.

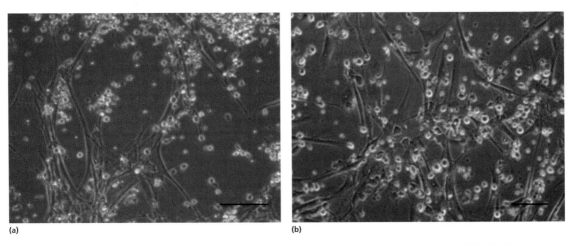

(a) (b)

Figure 2.3 BMMSC and OMLP-PC interaction with T cells. Photomicrographs of isolated (a) bone marrow MSCs (BMMSCs) and (b) oral mucosal lamina propria progenitor cells (OMLP-PCs) interacting in direct contact co-cultures with CD3+ T cells *in vitro*. Co-incubation of BMMSCs and OMLP-PCs with isolated T cells suppresses T cell proliferation (Protocol 2.2). Bar = 100 μm.

T cells

T cells, so named because their precursors migrate from the bone marrow into the thymus for maturation, consist of a number of subsets involved in both activating and suppressing adaptive immune responses. The two major subsets are the CD4+ T helper (Th) cell and the CD8+ cytotoxic lymphocyte (CTL). Most knowledge and mechanistic studies investigating the direct interaction of stem cells and T cells originate from *in vitro* experimentation. Both autologous and allogeneic MSCs have been demonstrated to inhibit T cell proliferation *in vitro* in response to a number of stimuli including mitogens such as phytohaemagluttinin (PHA); antibodies against CD2/CD3 and CD28 and allogeneic cells (PBMCs, lymphocytes, and DCs). Many studies utilise purified T cells, isolated from PBMCs by cell sorting (this is can be by flow cytometry cell sorting or magnetic cell selection), to demonstrate the suppression of T cell proliferation when in co-culture with stem cells (Figure 2.3). This is most frequently assessed by radioactive ^{3}H-thymidine uptake (as a measure of proliferation) or loss of the fluorescent dye carboxyfluorescein succinimidyl ester with division of the T cells (Protocol 2.2).

Th17 cells

Bordering the innate and adaptive immune systems are the Th17 cells. These originally classified adaptive immune cells have recently been demonstrated to be activated by innate immune cell receptors, evidencing

---

Protocol 2.2 Evaluating T cell suppression by flow cytometry.

1. CD3+ T cells are isolated from PBMCs (see Protocol 2.1 for isolation of PBMCs) using negative selection magnetic activated cell sorting. See manufacturer's details for specific details.

2. Isolated T cells are labeled with 0.25 μM Carboxyfluorescein succinimidyl ester (CFSE) for 7 minutes at 37°C/5% CO_2 before the reaction is halted by the addition of fetal calf serum (FCS).

3. Labeled T cells are washed 3 times in RPMI-1640 medium supplemented with 10% heat inactivated human AB serum.

4. CFSE-labeled T cells are combined with 10% irradiated stem cells and T cell activation beads (anti-CD2/anti-CD3/anti-CD28).

5. Co-cultures are incubated for 3 days before T cells are separated for flow cytometry (Figure 2.3).

6. Subsequent to co-culture, T cells can be stained for markers of activation (e.g., CD25) and for hallmarks of specific T cell subsets such as Tregs (CD4/CD25/FoxP3).

7. Samples are run on a flow cytometer and data analysed using the appropriate software.

Note: CFSE is used as a marker of cell division. Half of the fluorescence signal is lost with each division of the daughter cells, allowing accurate visualization and quantification of T cell division by flow cytometry.

their close link between the immune systems. IL-17 secreting T cells are typically protective in their mode of action, although they have been reported to persist in diseases of chronic inflammation such as multiple sclerosis (Kebir et al., 2009).

High levels of the proinflammatory cytokine IL-17 secretion coupled with high-level expression of the IL-17 receptor on the cell surface of BMMSCs promotes MSC proliferation and maintenance of an MSC2, anti-inflammatory phenotype (Huang et al., 2006). It is thought that this link between Th17 cells and BMMSCs may be a means of regulating the inflammatory response. In murine models of multiple sclerosis (experimental autoimmune encephalomyelitis), infusion of mouse BMMSCs suppressed both the migration and activation of Th17 cells (Rafei et al., 2009).

MSC licensing by exposure to IFNγ and TNFα results in an increased expression of intracellular adhesion molecule 1 (ICAM-1) on the cell surface of BMMSCs *in vitro*. This change in cell surface phenotype allows the MSCs to bind to Th17 cells in a chemokine receptor (CCR) 6-CCL20-dependent manner, prolonging their time in contact. This direct cell-cell contact suppresses the production of IL-17 and IL-22 by the Th17 cells and reprograms them into forkhead box (Fox) P3+ regulatory T cells, whilst blocking the production of *de novo* Th17 cells from naïve CD4+ T cells. Once again, MSC-derived PGE2, triggered by both cell contact and Th17 cell presence, is implicated in these processes, acting through the EP4 receptor expressed on the surface of the Th17 cells (Duffy et al., 2011, Ghannam et al., 2010). This inhibitory effect on Th17 cells has also been demonstrated with exposure to stem cells from human exfoliated teeth (SHED), both *in vitro* and in an *in vivo* model of systemic lupus erythematosus (SLE) (Yamaza et al., 2010). Within this study, SHED were shown to increase the ratio of Treg to Th17 cells, dampening autoimmune responses in addition to decreasing circulating Th17 cells within the peripheral blood.

The bidirectional state of MSCs in inducing T cells has also been demonstrated. When MSCs were cultured with apoptotic cells (mimicking the microenvironment of a rheumatoid arthritic bone marrow), the induction of Th17 cells was promoted in an IL-6 dependent manner (Tso et al., 2010). Furthermore, the persistence of Th17 cells in chronic inflammation further demonstrates the importance of the microenvironment in determining the response of MSCs. This is supported by

the knowledge that BMMSC-derived soluble factors alone promote the proliferation and induction of Th17 cells, confirming the need for MSCs to respond both to the environment and initiate direct cell-cell contact with these T cells to induce an inhibitory effect (Darlington et al., 2010). The effects of the microenvironment, especially the role of persistent inflammation on the phenotype of resident stem cell populations, is also of relevance here. A recent study isolating PDLSCs from both healthy and inflamed PDL demonstrated that those stem cells that had been exposed to chronic inflammatory signals had a reduced capacity to immunomodulate, losing their immunosuppressive phenotype even after removal from an inflammatory environment (Liu et al., 2012). This dampening in responsiveness of stem cells derived from inflammatory environments has also been shown in models of lupus and BMMSCs derived from SLE. Autologous MSCs derived from these studies were not effective after infusion in the treatment of lupus, with those derived from SLE patients reported to have a diminished response to recombinant IFNγ or CD8 stimulation, leading to insufficient IDO induction and therefore an inability to inhibit T cell proliferation (Gu et al., 2012).

Multiple adult stem cell populations, including BMMSCs, OMLP-PCs, GMSCs, and PDLSCs, are able to suppress the proliferation of activated T cells via both cell-contact-dependent and -independent mechanisms, the latter through the release of soluble factors such as IDO, TGFβ1, IL-10, hepatocyte growth factor (HGF), and PGE2 (Figure 2.3) (Davies et al., 2012, Zhang et al., 2009, Wada et al., 2009, Stagg and Galipeau, 2013), promoted by response to the proinflammatory cytokines IFNγ and TNFα secreted by activated T cells. This effect is dose dependent, except in the case of OMLP-PCs. Recent studies have indicated that oral stem cell sources, including SHED, DPSCs, and OMLP-PCs, may have differential mechanisms to BMMSCs in modulating T cell behavior, with some reports indicating that these novel stem cell sources demonstrate a higher efficacy for T cell immunosuppression in contact and contact-independent systems (Alipour et al., 2013, Sonoyama et al., 2008, Krampera et al., 2003, Davies et al., 2012). The mechanisms of action are wide-ranging with numerous factors indicated, including TGFβ1 for DPSC-mediated immunosuppression (Wada et al., 2009).

Within BMMSCs the central role of IFNγ in inducing the MSC2 phenotype, enabling the cells to exert their immunosuppressive effect, is exemplified by studies demonstrating that blocking of the IFNγ receptor in MSCs or inhibiting the secretion of IFNγ by T cells results in a decreased immunosuppressive MSC phenotype (Sheng et al., 2008, Krampera et al., 2006). The exposure of MSCs to these proinflammatory cytokines similarly promotes the secretion of chemokines CXCL9, CXCL10, and CXCL11, known to attract T cells and potentially promoting an early-stage interaction between the MSCs and T cells in an inflammatory environment, enabling MSCs to exert their immunosuppressive effects in close proximity to their target cells.

Cell contact mechanisms

Cell-cell contact between MSCs, including BMMSCs (Akiyama et al., 2012) and DPSCs (Zhao et al., 2012), and T cells has also been proposed as a mode of T cell–induced apoptosis via the FasL/Fas pathway, with FasL expressed on the surface of BMMSCs, GMSCs, and DPSCs (Xu et al., 2013). This mechanism of action is specific to Th cells but not Tregs, as neatly demonstrated by Zhao et al. in a murine model of ulcerative colitis where FasL knockdown in DPSCs reduced amelioration of colitis phenotypes, and that apoptosis was conserved to Th17 cells (Zhao et al., 2012). MSCs additionally express Fas, a death receptor, which controls the secretion of monocyte chemotactic protein-1 (MCP-1) to attract T cells and ensure their contact with MSCs (Wang et al., 2012). Interestingly, it was reported by Plumas et al. that MSCs induced T cell apoptosis only in activated T cells but not in resting T cells, suggesting that MSCs could support T cell survival in the G0 quiescent state (Plumas et al., 2005). This phenomenon was also demonstrated in a number of oral stem cell populations, including PDLSCs where the addition of PDLSCs to T cell cultures blocked T cell proliferation by inducing quiescence, not apoptosis (Kim et al., 2010). Davies et al. have also supported this theory, demonstrating that the addition of OMLP-PCs to suppress T cell–mediated proliferation actually decreases the level of T cell apoptosis in response to activation below that of the activated T cell controls (Davies et al., 2012).

When cultured in contact with one another, the Notch signaling pathway has been implicated in MSC-mediated immune cell suppression. Jagged 1 on the cell surface of MSCs can directly interact with its receptor, Notch on the surface of T cells, leading to NF-κB translocation and ultimately a decrease in IL-2 and IFNγ production in the T cells (Shi and Pamer, 2011; Eagar et al., 2004). Inactivation of TLRs 3 and 4 downregulates Jagged 1 on the MSC cell surface, impeding cell-cell contact with the T cells and therefore MSC contact-mediated inhibition of T cell proliferation (Liotta et al., 2008).

The role of cell-cell contact in mediating MSC effects may be situation and tissue specific. For example, resident MSCs can promote epithelial tissue repair after microbial damage within the gastrointestinal tract through the secretion of PGE2, but initiation of PGE2 secretion was dependent on TLR signaling (Brown et al., 2007).

Within human MSCs, suppression of both Th and CTL proliferation and the associated IFNγ production and cytotoxicity respectively is regulated primarily through IDO secretion. Whilst MSCs can act directly on T cells, it has been suggested that this effect is heightened in the presence of monocytes, with *in vitro* co-cultures of MSCs in the absence of monocytes demonstrating a reduced capacity to suppress the proliferation of T cells (Bernardo and Fibbe, 2013). Interestingly, differential expression levels of FasL on the surface of neural crest gingival stem cells (N-GMSCs) and their mesoderm-derived equivalents (M-GMSCs) have been used to establish the mechanism by which N-GMSCs are more immunosuppressive than M-GMSCs in T cell mediated suppression (Xu et al., 2013). OMLP-PCs, also of neural crest origin, have been reported to demonstrate potent immunosuppressive properties (Davies et al., 2012). Taken together, these findings suggest that more primitive neural crest stem cell populations may be a superior source of immunosuppressive cells for cell-based therapeutics targeting aberrant immune systems. Indeed this hypothesis is supported by the report that PDLSCs are less suppressive than BMMSCs and that this has been attributed to the partially committed phenotype of PDLSCs (Kim et al., 2010).

Tregs

Tregs are a subset of Th cells, able to suppress the immune response and dampen inflammation through the down-regulation of T cell proliferation. These cells are characterised by their expression of the transcription factor FoxP3 and can be subclassified into natural Tregs (thymus derived FoxP3$^+$ cells) and adaptive/inducible Tregs (derived from CD4$^+$CD25$^-$FoxP3$^-$ T cells circulating in the periphery). MSCs have been shown to increase the ratio of inducible Tregs aiding their function in regulating the inflammatory environment (Burr et al., 2013). This effect, through both direct cell contact and the secretion of TGFβ1, PGE2, and in some studies HLA-G5, is monocyte dependent with the removal of monocytes from co-cultures with MSCs preventing the induction of this Treg population (English et al., 2009, Maccario et al., 2005, Melief et al., 2013, Selmani et al., 2008). It has recently been demonstrated *in vitro* that induction of M2 macrophages from monocytes results in an increased secretion of CCL18, which induces Tregs in addition to the previously reported TGFβ1 Treg induction pathway (Melief et al., 2013). These findings have been supported by *in vivo* models of colitis and fibrillin-mutated systemic sclerosis, demonstrating the central role of macrophages in inducing Tregs (Akiyama et al., 2012). Here the mechanism of action was shown to be indirect, with infusion of murine BMMSCs inducing T cell apoptosis, triggering TGFβ1 production by macrophages and thereby the induction of FoxP3+ positive Tregs.

Hemeoxygenase (HO-1) is one of three isoenzymes involved in the oxidative degradation of haem to biliverdin, free iron, and carbon monoxide. Known primarily for its cytoprotective properties, HO-1 has been reported to play a pivotal role in immune regulation by promoting immunogenic tolerance. HO-1 is known to be expressed by DCs and has been demonstrated as necessary for Treg-mediated immunosuppression (George et al., 2008). HO-1 expression has recently been demonstrated in BMMSCs and involved in the generation of Treg cell subsets (Mougiakakos et al., 2011). Its mode of action has yet to be confirmed, but it is thought that HO-1 may deplete haem within the local environment required for certain enzyme activity. It may also have roles in inhibiting the production of proinflammatory cytokines as well as reactive oxygen species, whilst promoting the production of anti-inflammatory IL-10 (Chauveau et al., 2005, Remy et al., 2009). Despite the loss of HO-1 expression in licensed MSC2 cells, immunosuppression remains to be executed by PGE2. It is therefore hypothesised that BMMSC-mediated immunosuppression may be multistaged, with direct immune dampening at the site of inflammation and the generation of Tregs for long-term suppressive effects.

Cytotoxic lymphocytes (CTLs)

The immunosuppressive effects on T cells are not restricted to CD4+ cells. The effects of MSCs on modulating the function of CTLs are well characterised.

The primary role of a CTL is to kill cells producing foreign antigen or cells infected by viruses and other intracellular microorganisms.

As discussed above, MSCs can directly inhibit the maturation of DCs, thereby preventing the presentation of HLA I–associated alloantigen to the CTLs, a process required for their activation (Chiesa et al., 2011). This is one mechanism of indirect MSC-mediated immunosuppression. *In vitro* assays have demonstrated that inhibition of CTL proliferation induced by the T cell mitogen PHA does not affect their effector function, with those activated cells still able to induce a cytotoxic response (Ramasamy et al., 2008). This demonstrates the potential for MSCs in the treatment of conditions with a hyperactive immune system such as GvHD, where a dampening effect is required without affecting the functionality of the immune cells.

Recently, the role of IDO in modulating CTL function has been demonstrated in SLE, an autoimmune disease associated with abnormal T and B cell function (Wang et al., 2014). This previously undescribed CD8+-IDO axis demonstrated that high levels of IFNγ secretion by CD8+ T cells resulted in the induction of IDO and thereby immunosuppression by infused umbilical cord MSCs (UC-MSCs). These high levels of IFNγ, previously thought to originate from DC or NK cells, contribute to B cell activation and antibody production, linking to immunological memory.

MSCs have the capacity to alter the phenotype of CD8+ CTLs to a regulatory phenotype, as demonstrated for CD4+ Th cells (Prevosto et al., 2007). *In vivo* these regulatory cells are important in limiting the degree of self-reaction and controlling the immune response. These MSC-induced regulatory CD8+ cells can inhibit lymphocyte proliferation in mixed lymphocyte cultures, inhibit recall to alloantigen and mitogen or CD3 driven stimulation. They are characterised as CD25+ (the α chain of the IL-2 receptor and a marker of T cell activation) and CD28+ in the majority of cells (>85%). Regulatory CTLs have a lower level of FoxP3 mRNA expression than Tregs, however, suggesting different mechanisms in suppressing lymphocyte proliferation. This suggests that MSCs may operate two different immunosuppressive mechanisms dependent on the ratio of MSCs to immune cells. Soluble factors such as PGE2 operate at high stromal cell-lymphocyte frequencies (1:1–1:10), whereas the generation of CD8+ regulatory T cells allows immunosuppressive actions at lower frequencies of 1:2000 stromal cell-lymphocyte ratios, thus amplifying the effects of MSCs on blocking T cell proliferation (Poggi and Zocchi, 2008).

B cells

B cells form an essential part of the adaptive immune response by providing immunological memory. These immune cells produce antibodies and closely work alongside T cells, implicating their involvement in a number of autoimmune diseases such as MS. Naïve B cells are able to recognise antigen through the B cell receptor and present a processed version to Th2 cells via HLA class II. The Th2 cell, which has previously had this antigen presented to it by an antigen presenting cell, binds to the B cell and secretes cytokines triggering the process of B cell proliferation and differentiation into plasma cells. The plasma cells produce the antigen-specific antibodies for immunological memory. In addition to becoming plasma cells, B cells can remain as memory B cells.

The effect of MSCs on B cells remains controversial. Current findings indicate that MSCs inhibit the proliferation of B cells, their differentiation to immunoglobulin producing cells, and their production of cytokines, with most of these reports derived from *in vitro* systems and *in vivo* models of multiple sclerosis (De Miguel et al., 2012). These differing results may be attributed to the status of the MSCs tested and whether they were orientated towards a more MSC1 or MSC2 phenotype. Recent reports indicated that TLR4-primed MSC1 can enhance B cell proliferation by increasing expression of the B cell activating factor, BAFF. This factor is crucial in promoting the survival, proliferation, and differentiation of B lymphocytes (Yan et al., 2014).

MSC-originating soluble factors, released upon activation by B cells, have been reported to suppress the proliferation of B cells, with TGFβ1, HGF, PGE2, and IDO all implicated in mediating this role (Corcione et al., 2006). Antigen-presenting properties of the B cells appear not to be affected by the MSCs, with no change in the levels of HLA class II and cell surface expression of the co-stimulatory molecules CD40, CD86, and CD80. A downregulation of the chemotaxis receptors CXCR4 and CXCR5 suggests that MSCs may impede B cell migration in response to chemokine release (Corcione et al., 2006).

A recent report by Liu et al. has demonstrated the inhibitory effect of PDLSCs on B cell proliferation, apoptosis, chemotaxis, and differentiation into plasma cells (Liu et al., 2013). As reported by Corcione et al. in BMMSCs, expression of the co-stimulatory molecules HLA class II, CD40, CD80, and CD86 on the cell surface of the B cells was not affected by the presence of the PDLSCs, suggesting that the suppressed B cells retained their antigen-presenting function (Corcione et al., 2006). The chemokines CXCR4, CXCR5, and CCR7 were down-regulated in B cells postincubation with PDLSCs, and this was accompanied by decreased responsiveness of the B cells in attraction towards CXCL12, CXCL13, and CCL19 (Liu et al., 2013). The authors attribute this effect of PDLSCs on B cells to interactions between programmed cell death (PD)-1 and its ligand, PD-L1. This is different to the effect shown within BMMSCs, where PD-1 interacts with PD-L1 and PD-L2. High levels of PD-L1 on the surface of PDLSCs is linked to the elevated levels of IL-17, TNFα, and IFNγ within periodontitis tissue, as evidenced using a minipig model of periodontitis. These results indicate that PDLSC suppressive effects on B cells is multifactorial, acting through a contact-dependent mechanism (PD-1/PD-L1) to suppress the activity of B cells present within the inflammatory site, whereas soluble factors suppress the chemotaxis of additional B cells into the inflammatory area and inhibit B cell apoptosis (through the secretion of IL-6).

In vivo studies by Rafei et al. suggest this decrease in plasma cell immunoglobulin production is due to soluble factors released by MSCs affecting the CCL2 and CCL7 pathways (Rafei et al., 2008). It is suggested that matrix metalloproteinase (MMP) production by the MSCs cleaves CCL2 into a variant, which suppresses signal transducer and activator of transcription (STAT) 3 activation and plasma cell function. However, in some systems the reverse has been reported, with MSCs supporting the proliferation and differentiation of B cells (Rasmusson et al., 2007; Traggiai et al., 2008), indicating that we do not yet fully understand the mechanisms and complex interactions between B cells and adult stem cell populations.

Mediators of immunomodulation

Galectins

This group of molecules belongs to the lectin family and can be found at the cell surface and sequestered into the extracellular matrix. Galectins interact with glycans, such as N-linked glycans, post-translational modifications associated with cell membrane receptors and transporters.

MSC expression of galectins 1, 3, and 8 has been reported within the literature; galectin-1, a secretable form, has been implicated in MSC-mediated immunosuppression (Gieseke et al., 2010). Within this study, galectin-1 was demonstrated to have a direct role on the inhibition of T cell proliferation and production of IFNγ, with knockdown of galectin-1 within MSCs restoring the proliferation and effector function of T cells. These findings are substantiated by *in vivo* studies demonstrating that injection of BMMSCs and galectin-1 intraperitoneally into a mouse model of GvHD increased survival rate and decreased disease-associated symptoms. It has been suggested that galectins may exhibit an indirect effect on immunosuppression via induction of Tregs and/or the generation of tolergenic DCs (Baum et al., 2003; Ilarregui et al., 2009).

TNFα-stimulated gene/protein 6 (TSG-6)

Activated MSC2 cells express and secrete high levels of this immunomodulatory factor (Lee et al., 2009). As previously discussed, it is well acknowledged that on intravenous infusion, MSCs will rapidly be cleared from the circulation, move to the lungs, and be embolised. Despite this, MSCs continue to be reported to have therapeutic paracrine effects through the secretion of immunomodulatory factors. Lee et al. identified that MSCs trapped within the lungs after infusion within a murine model of myocardial infarction significantly upregulate mRNA levels of TSG-6, a factor not constitutively expressed by MSCs but induced upon receiving inflammatory signals (Lee et al., 2009). The study demonstrated the paracrine effects of TSG-6 in reducing inflammation within the heart and protecting the resident myocardiocytes, an effect lost on infusion of TSG-6 knockdown MSCs. These findings are supported by results from a rat model of corneal injury (Roddy et al., 2011). This study suggested that intravenous infusion of MSCs decreased neutrophil infiltration, the production of proinflammatory cytokines, and the development of opacity in the cornea. This was also seen if the MSCs were infused intraperitoneally. With <10 MSCs detected within the cornea at day 1 and 3 after either infusion technique, the data confirm the role of an MSC paracrine effect and that engraftment of the MSCs is not necessary for therapeutic benefit to be observed.

Infusion of TSG-6 knockdown MSCs within this model also confirmed a loss in the effectiveness of the MSCs (Roddy et al., 2011). Research suggests that TSG-6 may exert its immune dampening effects via action on innate immune cells, partially through inhibiting the migration of neutrophils (Getting et al., 2002). A more recent study on human MSCs utilised a murine model of zymogen (derived from the cell walls of yeast) induced peritonitis to demonstrate the mechanism of action of TSG-6. Zymogen binds to the TLR2 receptor on the macrophage cell surface, inducing the NF-κB pathway, resulting in downstream upregulation of proinflammatory cytokines such as TNFα. This study demonstrated that TSG-6 interacts directly with macrophages, binding to their CD44 cell surface receptor and inhibiting this zymogen-induced NF-κB activation (Shi et al., 2012). This negative feedback loop on the production of proinflammatory cytokines thereby prevents the recruitment of neutrophils.

Indoleamine 2,3-dioxygenase (IDO)

IDO is a rate-limiting enzyme implicated in tryptophan degradation. Expression of this immunomodulatory and antimicrobial enzyme is induced within macrophages, fibroblasts, and some stem cell populations by exposure to IFNγ and LPS (Ghannam et al., 2010; Hucke et al., 2004; O'Connor et al., 2009). IDO inhibits T cell proliferation by inducing a tryptophan-depleted environment not conducive to lymphocyte cell division.

Within human BMMSCs, IDO has been deemed the major immunomodulatory soluble factor, with experimental evidence supporting inhibition of T cell proliferation by IDO-secreting BMMSCs and restoration of T cell proliferation on replenishment of tryptophan or the addition of the IDO antagonist 1-methyl-L-tryptophan (1-MT) (Meisel et al., 2004; Ryan et al., 2007). IDO enzyme activity can be measured within the conditioned media of *in vitro* stem cell cultures by colorimetric assay. This simple plate assay allows quantification of the tryptophan metabolite, L-kynurenine within the stem cell secretome in response to exposure to IFNγ or co-culture with PBMCs/T cells (Protocol 2.3).

In addition to BMMSCs, the expression of IDO has been noted within several oral stem cell populations, with OMLP-PCs, GMSCs, and PDLSCs demonstrating immunosuppressive function through the induction of IDO in response to IFNγ secretion by activated PBMCs (Davies et al., 2012; Wada et al., 2009; Zhang et al., 2009).

Protocol 2.3 Quantification of IDO activity by colorimetric assay.

IDO activity is quantified by measuring the tryptophan metabolite L-kynurenine within conditioned media derived from stem cell co-culture with PBMCs or purified T cells (Davies et al., 2012).

1. One hundred microliters of conditioned media is combined with 50 μL of 30% (v/v) trichloroacetic acid.
2. Samples are centrifuged at 8000xg for 5 minutes at room temperature.
3. A standard curve of pure L-kynurenine (0–100 μM) is generated in unconditioned culture media.
4. Seventy-five μL of the supernatant/standard is plated into a 96-well microtitre plate and combined with an equal volume of Ehrlich's reagent.
5. Absorbance is read using a microplate reader at 492 nm.
6. Concentrations are calculated from the standard curve using a line of best fit.

In vivo IDO has been reported to be upregulated in chronic periodontitis within human gingival tissue, potentially due to increased levels of the proinflammatory cytokines IL-1 and TNFα (known to synergistically act with IFNγ in the induction of IDO) (Babcock and Carlin, 2000; Nisapakultorn et al., 2009). These results suggest that IDO induction by resident gingival cells may act in a protective manner to prevent excessive immune activation.

Hepatocyte growth factor (HGF)

HGF, also known as scatter factor, has been demonstrated to exhibit immunosuppressive actions against both innate and adaptive immune cells. HGF has an anti-inflammatory effect by preventing the migration of neutrophils and eosinophils into the wound/injury site and thereby limiting the release of proinflammatory cytokines and reactive oxygen species (Nakamura and Mizuno, 2010). The effects of HGF on T cells (Th cells) have also been documented, favoring the anti-inflammatory effects of Th2 cells by decreasing the release of proinflammatory factors from Th1 and increasing the release of the antagonizing anti-inflammatory factors from Th2 cells (Nakamura and Mizuno, 2010). Knowledge of this potential in HGF to skew the immune response towards a more regulatory phenotype has been exploited in mouse studies using HGF to treat acute GvHD (Rutella et al., 2006).

This growth factor is of particular interest within the oral context, as studies have indicated that HGF is strongly expressed within fibroblasts derived from the oral mucosa when compared to the skin (Enoch et al., 2010) and has been linked to the preferential wound healing response seen within the buccal mucosa, characterised by a reduced inflammatory phase, rapid re-epithelialisation, and modeling with minimal scar formation.

Prostaglandin E2 (PGE2)

PGE2 belongs to the prostanoid family, derived from arachidonic acid by COX-1, COX-2, and PGE2 synthase enzymes. PGE2 exhibits immunosuppressive activity against a number of immune cells, both innate and adaptive, and has been implicated in the immunomodulatory actions of BMMSCs and oral stem cell populations such as GMSCs (English et al., 2009; Su et al., 2011). PGE2 acts on the G-coupled E prostanoid receptors (EP1-4), of which EP2 and EP4 have been associated with the immunosuppressive actions on T cells (Sakata et al., 2010).

As described above for HGF, PGE2 preferentially supports the secretion of Th2 anti-inflammatory cytokines, whilst inhibiting Th1 action and promoting the production and activity of Tregs (Kalinski, 2012; Baratelli et al., 2005). These effects are both through direct interactions of PGE2 with the T cells and indirectly through an inhibition of DC maturation and thereby increasing Th2 presence (von Bergwelt-Baildon et al., 2006).

A symbiotic relationship between IDO and PGE2 appears to regulate the immunosuppressive action of MSCs. PGE2 has been reported to indirectly stimulate production of IDO, with IDO then leading to downstream activation of G protein coupled receptors (Penberthy, 2007; Spaggiari et al., 2008).

Human leukocyte antigen-G (HLA-G)

HLA-G is classified as a class I major histocompatibility complex, existing in seven isoforms, namely, the membrane bound HLA-G1, -G2, -G3, and -G4 and the soluble HLA-G5, -G6, and -G7. HLA-G5 is the most studied isoform with respect to stem cell–mediated immunomodulation. This isoform is found to be upregulated after treatment with IL-10 but not IFNγ in human BMMSCs (Selmani et al., 2008; Selmani et al., 2009). Interestingly, this increase in HLA-G5 expression and secretion by BMMSCs is also seen when in close contact with allo-stimulated PBMCs, hypothesised to be also through the secretion of IL-10 by the hematopoietic cells (Selmani et al., 2009). HLA-G's immunosuppressive effects are thought to be through the induction of Tregs when in close contact culture systems and also to inhibit NK cell-mediated cytolysis of third-party target cells and their secretion of IFNγ (Selmani et al., 2008).

Despite the major focus lying with HLA-G5, HLA-G1, a membrane-bound isoform, has been found to be expressed on the cell surface of BMMSCs and has been reported to be immunosuppressive through inhibition of DCs (Selmani et al., 2009). Positive expression of HLA-G on the cell surface of BMMSCs results in an inhibitory effect against both NK cells and CD8+ CTLs (Siegel et al., 2009). Such modes of actions have led to studies indicating that increased levels of HLA-G positively correlate with a decreased risk of graft rejection (Nasef et al., 2007).

Transforming growth factor Beta 1 (TGFβ1)
The immunosuppressive role of membrane-bound and soluble TGFβ1 is well established, with TGFβ1 on the surface of Tregs exerting an inhibitory effect on responder T cells. TGFβ1 secreted by MSCs has known immunomodulatory functions involving both immune cells of the adaptive and innate immune systems, primarily interacting with CD4+ Th cells and inducing a Treg phenotype and suppressing the production of cytokines from cytotoxic NK cells. TGFβ1 secretion by MSCs is induced by the presence of CD14+ monocytes and lymphocytes and/or proinflammatory cytokines such as IFNγ (Bernardo and Fibbe, 2013; Rubtsov et al., 2012). The mode of immune cell stimulation appears to play a role in how central TGFβ1 is in mediating MSC immunosuppression, with some studies reporting that TGFβ1 only suppresses T cell proliferation if T cell activation has been induced by mitogens such as PHA (Rasmusson et al., 2005).

Interleukin-6 (IL-6)
IL-6 expression is strongly correlated with PGE2. IL-6, through its inhibitory effect on the maturation of DCs as well as reverting mature DCs back to their immature state results in a decreased activation of T cells. This mode of action is further exerted by decreasing the action of reactive oxygen species, resulting in an anti-apoptotic effect on both neutrophils and lymphocytes (Ghannam et al., 2010).

The role of cell surface adhesion molecules in MSC-mediated immunosuppression

CD39/CD73
The inhibitory effects of CD39 and CD73 by Tregs in the regulation of T cell proliferation and the production of proinflammatory cytokines are well established. Cell surface CD39 promotes the conversion of adenosine triphosphate (ATP) and adenosine diphosphate (ADP) to the monophosphate form (AMP), which is subsequently hydrolysed to adenosine via CD73. Adenosine, released by damaged cells, is known to accumulate at injury sites and can directly induce immunosuppression via a number of receptors, including the A_{2A} adenosine receptor (Deaglio et al., 2007).

Recently GMSCs were demonstrated to express both CD73 and CD39 on their cell surface, promoting the production of adenosine, a mechanism by which the MSCs were able to inhibit mouse T cell proliferation (Chen et al., 2013). The authors demonstrated these inhibitory effects both *in vitro* and *in vivo* in a murine model of collagen-induced arthritis. It was noted that the GMSCs could both directly immunosuppress through the production of adenosine and indirectly through induction of immunosuppressive Tregs via CD39/CD73 signaling (Chen et al., 2013). This mechanism for immunosuppression has previously been demonstrated within BMMSCs, with cooperation between the T cells (expressing CD39) and MSCs (expressing CD73). These effects are beneficial not only in the induction of immunosuppression but also in wound healing as adenosine has been implicated in exerting both anti-inflammatory and antifibrotic effects.

ICAM-1/V-CAM-1
The cell surface receptors ICAM-1/CD54 and vascular cell adhesion molecule-1 (VCAM-1)/CD106 are known to play important roles in the activation and extravasation of T cells. MSCs upregulate both of these cell surface receptors in response to exposure to activated T cells and the level of expression on MSCs directly correlates with their immunosuppressive activity (Ren et al., 2010). Upregulation of these cell surface receptors is linked with exposure to proinflammatory cytokines such as IFNγ, TNFα and IL-1. These findings suggest an important mechanism in cell-cell contact-mediated immunosuppression, supported by the report that increased

expression of ICAM-1 and VCAM-1 on MSCs enhances adherence of the cells to Th17 cells, allowing effective suppression of Th17 cell function and differentiation (Ghannam et al., 2010).

Extracellular vesicles and immunomodulation

Exosomes (10–100 nm) and microvesicles (100–1000 nm) are secreted from the majority of living cells and have been reported to carry immunomodulatory factors, ranging from proteins to microRNAs encased within a phospholipid bilayer (Thery et al., 2009). The definition of these vesicles appears to be flexible within the literature due to the relative infancy of research into these entities. In light of this, the International Society for Extracellular Vesicles has suggested the use of the term *extracellular vesicles* (EVs) to encompass all types of vesicles present within the extracellular space, including both microvesicles and exosomes. The true difference between these vesicles, apart from their size, remains to be fully characterised.

These small entities are directly involved in cell-cell communication and in the transfer of cellular material from one cell to another. EVs have been proposed to signal via binding to cell surface receptors and by fusion or internalisation by the receiving cell (Temchura et al., 2008). EVs can be taken up by local target cells or travel to distant sites within the body via the blood system or other bodily fluids. EVs have become of particular interest again recently as a potential mechanism of how the paracrine effects of MSCs are exerted *in vivo*.

Within animal models, EVs have been demonstrated to have therapeutic potential in conditions such as acute kidney injury and myocardial ischemia (Katsuda et al., 2013). These properties appear to be mediated at least in part by mRNA cargo, as RNase treatment of the EVs to inactivate the contained mRNAs impeded their therapeutic benefit (Gatti et al., 2011). EVs derived from numerous cell sources have been demonstrated to modulate cells of both the innate and adaptive systems, including B cell–mediated tumor suppression, proapoptotic activity in CTLs, differentiation of monocytes in DCs, and induction of Tregs (Taylor et al., 2011).

Knowledge into the potential for EV-mediated therapies remains sparse and is a relatively new topic in regenerative medicine. It is thought that they may

represent a more defined therapy than using the cells themselves, and that they offer the advantage of being able to deliver target molecules intracellularly. In addition to this, EVs can avoid the lung barrier, a major obstacle for the systemic administration of MSCs (Katsuda et al., 2013). Preliminary data indicate that MSCs may transfer their immunosuppressive properties to their secreted EVs, with MSC EVs demonstrated to inhibit mitogen-induced PBMC proliferation *in vitro* (Yeo et al., 2013).

MSC EV–mediated immunomodulation has been reported to be through a direct interaction with monocytes through their TLR4 receptor (Zhang et al., 2014). In this study the MSC EVs contained the TLR4 ligand, FN1, which on binding to the monocytes induces intracellular TLR signaling via MYD88 within the monocyte. These monocytes differentiated into M2 macrophages associated with the secretion of IL-10 and were able to induce Treg polarisation. Further analysis using an *in vivo* model of allogeneic skin graft rejection demonstrated that these effects were only apparent in animals with an activated immune system, with no induction of Tregs in animals that did not receive skin grafts (Zhang et al., 2014).

Evidence that MSC EVs, like the MSCs themselves, will only suppress the activity of activated cells removes the risk of MSCs compromising the normal immune-surveillance functions of a healthy immunity and therefore may also be a suitable therapeutic for GvHD, where a hyperactive immune system is evident. In a recent study, MSC-derived EVs were derived for the treatment of GvHD (Kordelas et al., 2014). The EVs at the point of purification contained high levels of the antiinflammatory cytokines IL-10, TGFβ1, and HLA-G and demonstrated immunosuppressive activity against PBMCs and NK cells in *in vitro* mixed lymphocyte cultures. These EVs were systemically infused into a GvHD patient. After the third infusion, the patient's PBMCs demonstrated a repressed production of IL-1β, TNFα, and IFNγ, indicating that the infused MSC EVs may have dampened the inflammatory reactivity of the patient's PBMCs. This was accompanied by a reduction in GvHD-associated symptoms including diarrhea and mucosal and cutaneous GvHD.

For this to be translated into a mainstream clinical application, the isolation and purification of EVs must become cost and time effective (currently, isolation of sufficient quantities of EVs requires large-scale culturing of the cells from which the EVs are to be isolated and ultracentrifugation to purify them), with a higher degree of purity required. These issues are starting to be addressed, with current research investigating the potential immortalisation of human MSCs using the myc oncogene in providing a sustainable stem cell population for the production of immunomodulatory EVs (Chen et al., 2011).

The relevance of species in determining immunomodulatory mechanisms

Animal models are still of crucial value in evaluating and translating *in vitro* experimental findings to an *in vivo* system. It is important to note, however, that human and murine MSCs exhibit considerably different properties and mechanisms of action in terms of immunomodulation, and this should be taken into consideration when choosing appropriate model systems and evaluating *in vivo* results for extrapolation towards clinical testing.

Murine BMMSCs expand slower than human BMMSCs, with *in vitro* expansion resulting in transformation of the cells to a malignant state, associated with increased telomerase activity and proliferative rate, an altered cellular morphology, abnormal karyotype, and the ability to form tumors *in vivo*. It is therefore important to consider this altered phenotype in studies utilizing *in vitro* expanded murine MSCs and their distinct phenotypic and genotypic characteristics with their human counterparts. Human MSCs have not been demonstrated to undergo malignant transformation after long-term *in vitro* culture; however, their potential change in phenotype with ageing has been previously discussed within this review (Bernardo and Fibbe, 2013).

Distinct differences in the effector soluble factors implicated in suppression of T cell proliferation within these species have also been noted, with IDO important for human MSCs and nitric oxide primarily employed in murine MSCs (Bernardo and Fibbe, 2013). Within human MSCs, proinflammatory cytokines induce IDO expression, whereas in mice inducible nitric oxide synthase (iNOS) is upregulated. Interestingly it was reported that within the rhesus monkey, IDO is the immunomodulatory molecule of choice. Regardless of species, the effects downstream of these molecules are similar, with both IDO and iNOS resulting in the induction of T cell chemokines to induce immunosuppression.

Homing

Initial studies demonstrated that systemically and locally infused MSCs maintain the ability to home to sites of injury and cancer, most likely due to localised inflammatory mediators (Rojas et al., 2005; Ortiz et al., 2003; Kidd et al., 2009). MSCs express the necessary receptors for a number of growth factors including platelet-derived growth factor and insulin-like growth factor 1, in addition to chemokine receptors such as CCR2, CCR3, CCR4, and CCL5 to recognise specific mediators released in high concentrations after initiation of the inflammatory cascade (Ponte et al., 2007). This inherent capacity to home has also been demonstrated with *in situ* MSC mobilisation, as reported by an increase in circulating MSCs in response to bone fracture (Alm et al., 2010).

Among the chemokines central to MSC homing is stromal cell–derived factor 1 (SDF-1). Low levels of the SDF-1 receptor, CXCR4, are constitutively expressed on the cell surface of BMMSCs; however, upon stimulation, this expression level is upregulated. Data suggest that BMMSCs store high levels of CXCR4 intracellularly, ready to be translocated to the cell surface upon chemokine stimulation (Wynn et al., 2004). Furthermore, BMMSCs express numerous integrins on their cell surface, including α4 and β1 important in mediating cell-cell and cell–extracellular matrix interactions by binding to VCAM-1 and the V-region of fibronectin, respectively.

Despite their inherent capacity to home to the site of injury, both preclinical animal models and clinical trials have demonstrated very little if any engraftment of MSCs postinfusion, with less than 1% actually reaching their target tissue (Isakova et al., 2007). Despite this, the therapeutic effect is evident, with no correlation between engraftment and therapeutic efficacy, undoubtedly confirming the importance of MSC-originating trophic factors.

MSCs as modulators of the bacterial environment

Numerous immunosuppressive soluble factors described throughout this review also exhibit antibacterial actions, and therefore it is not surprising that the antibacterial properties of MSCs are starting to be reported. Evidence currently is limited, but both IDO and the cathelicidin,

LL-37, have been reported to play roles in MSC-mediated antibacterial responses (Meisel et al., 2011; Krasnodembskaya et al., 2010). LL-37 can directly bind LPS and inhibit LPS-induced cellular responses. This protein can be further processed into smaller peptides with enhanced antimicrobial activity. LL-37, synthesised by BMMSCs, has been demonstrated to act in an antimicrobial manner towards both Gram-positive and Gram-negative bacteria; working in a bacterial dose-dependent manner within both *in vitro* assays and in a murine model of *E. coli*–induced pneumonia (Krasnodembskaya et al., 2010). This study demonstrated that the infusion of MSCs reduced bacterial growth and enhanced clearance. This novel study has provided mechanistic insight into how MSCs can control bacterial infections as previously shown in different models of induced sepsis (Nemeth et al., 2009, Gonzalez-Rey et al., 2009).

IDO, through its ability to remove tryptophan from the environment, has been demonstrated to be antibacterial in response to tryptophan-sensitive bacteria such as B *streptococci, enterococci*, and *Staphylococcus aureus*. The antimicrobial effects of IDO are illustrated by studies demonstrating the protection against *Staphylococcus aureus* bacterial infection in human heart valves and vascular allografts by IDO induction (Saito et al., 2008).

As discussed previously, IDO is strongly induced within BMMSCs and some oral stem cell populations such as OMLP-PCs and DPSCs by IFNγ. This effect is enhanced by the presence of TNFα and IL-1, both of which are upregulated in chronic periodontitis (Graves and Cochran, 2003). It has been suggested that IDO induction by resident cells within gingival tissue in response to this cocktail of proinflammatory cytokines may prevent an excessive immune response mounting (Konermann et al., 2012).

Clinical applications of MSCs

To date, our primary information regarding the use of adult stem cells for the treatment of immune-related disorders is derived from clinical trials utilizing BMMSCs. According to the NIH website, http://clinicaltrials.gov, as of June 2014 there are 401 registered clinical trials utilizing "mesenchymal stem/stromal cells". The majority of these trials are focused on exploiting the immuno-modulatory or trophic properties of these cells, rather than their differentiation potential, earning MSCs the term *injury drugstore* (Caplan and Correa, 2011). Currently only four clinical trials are registered for the use of dental stem cells in the treatment of periodontal tissue regeneration, revitalisation of necrotic pulp in immature permanent teeth, and in alveolar bone tissue engineering. As we move towards the development of novel therapeutics utilizing newly characterised oral stem cell populations, valuable lessons can be learned from the MSC therapeutics currently being trialed.

MSCs have been evaluated for a number of diseases with immune involvement ranging from inflammatory to autoimmune disorders. In addition to their immuno-regulatory therapeutic effects, these cells have been demonstrated to positively affect tissue repair and regeneration both directly and through indirect effects on the tissue microenvironment. Much of the knowledge we have gained regarding the role of MSCs in tissue repair has been gleaned from preclinical models (Wei et al., 2013). Within the clinical arena, MSC therapy has shown beneficial effects in liver cirrhosis and liver failure patients (Peng et al., 2011; Kharaziha et al., 2009) as well as in periodontal tissue defect repair and diabetic limb ischaemia (Yamada et al., 2006; Lu et al., 2011). These multifaceted effects of MSCs are discussed below with, for the purposes of this review, focus placed on GvHD, multiple sclerosis as an autoimmune disease, and colitis as an inflammatory disease.

Graft versus host disease

As previously discussed, GvHD is a complication associated with hematopoietic stem cell transplantation, where donor T cells attack the recipient's organs. This is a disease primarily affecting the skin, oral mucosa, liver, and gut. Although generally considered a T cell–mediated disease, NK cell and macrophage involvement has been reported. Further indications towards an innate component in the pathophysiology of GvHD have also recently been reported through reaction with microbial peptides.

First-line treatment is steroids, but in the case of steroid-refractory GvHD, MSC systemic infusion has been successfully trialed. Le Blanc et al. (2004) first reported in 2004 that intravenous infusion of allogeneic MSCs may represent a novel therapeutic for the treatment of severe steroid-refractory acute GvHD. The exact mechanism of MSCs in the treatment of GvHD remains unknown; however, it is thought that the cells exert their therapeutic effects through skewing of the immune cell repertoire to a more tolerogenic phenotype (Zhao et al., 2015). Evidence of tissue repair due to MSC therapy is anecdotal, however. Ringdén et al. reported a pilot study where an MSC-treated patient with GvHD of the gut demonstrated reversal of perforated colon (Ringden et al., 2007).

Multiple sclerosis (MS)

MS is a debilitating immune-related disease of the central nervous system (CNS) characterised by the presence of immune cell infiltrated lesions leading to demyelination, inflammation, and axonal damage. The potential for MSCs in the treatment of MS has in the main come from murine studies using an experimental autoimmune encephalomyelitis (EAE) model for MS. Utilizing this model, Zappia et al. reported that systemic infusion of MSCs could decrease the severity of EAE, associated with a decrease in demyelination, T cell and macrophage infiltration, and enhanced functional recovery (Zappia et al., 2005). Supporting *in vitro* experiments demonstrated that MSCs secrete an antagonist form of CCL2 (known to have a central role in regulating immune cell infiltration within the CNS), reducing the secretion of IL-17 from Th cells. Furthermore, this study suggested that MSCs could also inhibit the recruitment of Th17 cells to the CNS (Park et al., 2005). Zappia also suggested that MSC infusions could induce T cell anergy, arresting Th cells in the G0/G1 phase of the cell cycle, a phenomenon that could only be partially restored by the addition of exogenous IL-2 (Zappia et al., 2005). These findings corroborate the hypothesis that MSCs improve MS effects via an immunomodulatory function. Hypotheses have also been put forward to indicate the potential for MSCs to exert a therapeutic effect via bystander effects on the fate and differentiation of endogenous stem cell populations at the site of the lesion to promote remyelination (Reviewed by Rivera and Aigner, 2012).

The utilisation of MSCs for the treatment of MS is now in clinical trials. Published studies are at this time limited but appear to confirm the potential for MSCs in the treatment of autoimmune disorders such as MS and the need to move towards placebo-controlled trials to assess the therapeutic potential of MSC infusion.

Colitis

Murine models of experimental colitis have demonstrated that symptoms could be reversed by the intraperitoneal injection of MSCs due to a decrease in proinflammatory Th1-derived cytokines (such as IL-2, TNFα and IFNγ), a switch to a Th2 phenotype associated with increased IL-10 secretion, and the induction of Tregs (Gonzalez et al., 2009). GMSCs have been reported to decrease the inflammatory response in experimental colitis via these mechanisms, resulting in both clinical and histopathological symptoms of the disease (Zhang et al., 2009). This effect has also been demonstrated with systemic infusion of MSCs. Injection of BMMSCs through the tail vein in a rat model of dextran sulphate sodium–induced colitis resulted in a reduction in weight loss, colon shortening, and microscopic injuries. At the mRNA level, MSCs significantly reduced the expression of TNFα, IL-1β, and COX2, confirming an anti-inflammatory effect as well as healing of the mucosal injuries (Tanaka et al., 2008). Direct injection of BMMSCs into the colonic submucosa was also found to accelerate healing of the intestinal tissue, associated with MSC-mediated secretion of vascular endothelial growth factor and TGFβ1 (Hayashi et al., 2008).

The role of the innate immune system and the protective effects of adipose-derived MSCs (ADMSCs) have also been demonstrated in reversing the effects of experimental colitis. ADMSCs induced an immunosuppressive macrophage phenotype associated with the production of IL-10 and an ability to suppress the activity of T cells as well as other macrophages. Reports suggest that induction of this regulatory macrophage phenotype is through the upregulation of COX2 and secretion of PGE2 by the ADMSCs (Anderson et al., 2013). Furthermore, systemic infusion of these macrophages exposed to ADMSCs or their conditioned media results in a reversal of colitis symptoms and protection from sepsis by reducing the infiltration of inflammatory cells and downregulating proinflammatory mediators *in vivo* (Anderson et al., 2013).

Summary

This chapter brings together the current knowledge regarding the immunomodulatory properties of adult stem cell populations. Stem cells derived from multiple adult tissues, including those from the oral cavity, have defined immunosuppressive characteristics that are regulated by the microenvironment and key paracrine signals. Here, the mechanisms of action in exerting key effects on different immune cell subsets have been discussed, with the potential to exploit this for the development of novel cell and soluble factor-based therapeutics in the treatment of immune-related disorders.

Acknowledgements

LD is supported by funding from Cardiff University and Karolinska Institutet. KLB is supported by grants from the Swedish Cancer Society, the Children's Cancer Foundation, the Swedish Medical Research Council, VINNOVA, Stockholm County Council (ALF), the Cancer Society in Stockholm, the Swedish Society of Medicine, the Tobias Foundation, and Karolinska Institutet.

References

AKIYAMA, K., CHEN, C., WANG, D., XU, X., QU, C., YAMAZA, T., CAI, T., CHEN, W., SUN, L., & SHI, S. 2012. Mesenchymal-stem-cell-induced immunoregulation involves FAS-ligand-/FAS-mediated T cell apoptosis. *Cell Stem Cell*, 10, 544–55.

ALIPOUR, R., ADIB, M., MASOUMI KARIMI, M., HASHEMI-BENI, B., & SERESHKI, N. 2013. Comparing the immunoregulatory effects of stem cells from human exfoliated deciduous teeth and bone marrow-derived mesenchymal stem cells. *Iran J Allergy Asthma Immunol*, 12, 331–44.

ALM, J. J., KOIVU, H. M., HEINO, T. J., HENTUNEN, T. A., LAITINEN, S., & ARO, H. T. 2010. Circulating plastic adherent mesenchymal stem cells in aged hip fracture patients. *J Orthop Res*, 28, 1634–42.

ANDERSON, P., SOUZA-MOREIRA, L., MORELL, M., CARO, M., O'VALLE, F., GONZALEZ-REY, E., & DELGADO, M. 2013. Adipose-derived mesenchymal stromal cells induce immunomodulatory macrophages which protect from experimental colitis and sepsis. *Gut*, 62, 1131–41.

BABCOCK, T. A., & CARLIN, J. M. 2000. Transcriptional activation of indoleamine dioxygenase by interleukin 1 and tumor necrosis factor alpha in interferon-treated epithelial cells. *Cytokine*, 12, 588–94.

BARATELLI, F., LIN, Y., ZHU, L., YANG, S. C., HEUZE-VOURC'H, N., ZENG, G., RECKAMP, K., DOHADWALA, M., SHARMA, S., & DUBINETT, S. M. 2005. Prostaglandin E2 induces FOXP3 gene expression and T regulatory cell function in human CD4+ T cells. *J Immunol*, 175, 1483–90.

BARTHOLOMEW, A., STURGEON, C., SIATSKAS, M., FERRER, K., MCINTOSH, K., PATIL, S., HARDY, W., DEVINE, S., UCKER, D., DEANS, R., MOSELEY, A., & HOFFMAN, R. 2002. Mesenchymal stem cells suppress lymphocyte proliferation in vitro and prolong skin graft survival in vivo. *Exp Hematol*, 30, 42–48.

BAUM, L. G., BLACKALL, D. P., ARIAS-MAGALLANO, S., NANIGIAN, D., UH, S. Y., BROWNE, J. M., HOFFMANN, D., EMMANOUILIDES, C. E., TERRITO, M. C., & BALDWIN, G. C. 2003. Amelioration of graft versus host disease by galectin-1. *Clin Immunol*, 109, 295–307.

BERNARDO, M. E., & FIBBE, W. E. 2013. Mesenchymal stromal cells: sensors and switchers of inflammation. *Cell Stem Cell*, 13, 392–402.

BEYTH, S., BOROVSKY, Z., MEVORACH, D., LIEBERGALL, M., GAZIT, Z., ASLAN, H., GALUN, E., & RACHMILEWITZ, J. 2005. Human mesenchymal stem cells alter antigen-presenting cell maturation and induce T-cell unresponsiveness. *Blood*, 105, 2214–19.

BRANDAU, S., JAKOB, M., HEMEDA, H., BRUDEREK, K., JANESCHIK, S., BOOTZ, F., & LANG, S. 2010. Tissue-resident mesenchymal stem cells attract peripheral blood neutrophils and enhance their inflammatory activity in response to microbial challenge. *J Leukoc Biol*, 88, 1005–15.

BROWN, J. M., NEMETH, K., KUSHNIR-SUKHOV, N. M., METCALFE, D. D., & MEZEY, E. 2011. Bone marrow stromal cells inhibit mast cell function via a COX2-dependent mechanism. *Clin Exp Allergy*, 41, 526–34.

BROWN, S. L., RIEHL, T. E., WALKER, M. R., GESKE, M. J., DOHERTY, J. M., STENSON, W. F., & STAPPENBECK, T. S. 2007. Myd88-dependent positioning of Ptgs2-expressing stromal cells maintains colonic epithelial proliferation during injury. *J Clin Invest*, 117, 258–69.

BURR, S. P., DAZZI, F., & GARDEN, O. A. 2013. Mesenchymal stromal cells and regulatory T cells: the Yin and Yang of peripheral tolerance? *Immunol Cell Biol*, 91, 12–18.

CAPLAN, A. I., & CORREA, D. 2011. The MSC: an injury drugstore. *Cell Stem Cell*, 9, 11–15.

CASSATELLA, M. A., MOSNA, F., MICHELETTI, A., LISI, V., TAMASSIA, N., CONT, C., CALZETTI, F., PELLETIER, M., PIZZOLO, G., & KRAMPERA, M. 2011. Toll-like receptor-3-activated human mesenchymal stromal cells significantly prolong the survival and function of neutrophils. *Stem Cells*, 29, 1001–11.

CHAUVEAU, C., REMY, S., ROYER, P. J., HILL, M., TANGUY-ROYER, S., HUBERT, F. X., TESSON, L., BRION, R., BERIOU, G., GREGOIRE, M., JOSIEN, R., CUTURI, M. C., & ANEGON, I. 2005. Heme oxygenase-1 expression inhibits dendritic cell maturation and proinflammatory function but conserves IL-10 expression. *Blood*, 106, 1694–702.

CHEN, M., SU, W., LIN, X., GUO, Z., WANG, J., ZHANG, Q., BRAND, D., RYFFEL, B., HUANG, J., LIU, Z., HE, X., LE, A. D., & ZHENG, S. G. 2013. Adoptive transfer of human gingiva-derived mesenchymal stem cells ameliorates collagen-induced arthritis via suppression of Th1 and Th17 cells and enhancement of regulatory T cell differentiation. *Arthritis Rheum*, 65, 1181–93.

CHEN, T. S., ARSLAN, F., YIN, Y., TAN, S. S., LAI, R. C., CHOO, A. B., PADMANABHAN, J., LEE, C. N., DE KLEIJN, D. P., & LIM, S. K. 2011. Enabling a robust scalable manufacturing process for therapeutic exosomes through oncogenic immortalization of human ESC-derived MSCs. *J Transl Med*, 9, 47.

CHENG, P., NEFEDOVA, Y., CORZO, C. A., & GABRILOVICH, D. I. 2007. Regulation of dendritic-cell differentiation by bone marrow stroma via different Notch ligands. *Blood*, 109, 507–15.

CHIESA, S., MORBELLI, S., MORANDO, S., MASSOLLO, M., MARINI, C., BERTONI, A., FRASSONI, F., BARTOLOME, S. T., SAMBUCETI, G., TRAGGIAI, E., & UCCELLI, A. 2011. Mesenchymal stem cells impair in vivo T-cell priming by dendritic cells. *Proc Natl Acad Sci U S A*, 108, 17384–9.

CHO, K. S., PARK, H. K., PARK, H. Y., JUNG, J. S., JEON, S. G., KIM, Y. K., & ROH, H. J. 2009. IFATS collection: Immunomodulatory effects of adipose tissue-derived stem cells in an allergic rhinitis mouse model. *Stem Cells*, 27, 259–65.

CORCIONE, A., BENVENUTO, F., FERRETTI, E., GIUNTI, D., CAPPIELLO, V., CAZZANTI, F., RISSO, M., GUALANDI, F., MANCARDI, G. L., PISTOIA, V., & UCCELLI, A. 2006. Human mesenchymal stem cells modulate B-cell functions. *Blood*, 107, 367–72.

DARLINGTON, P. J., BOIVIN, M. N., RENOUX, C., FRANCOIS, M., GALIPEAU, J., FREEDMAN, M. S., ATKINS, H. L., COHEN, J. A., SOLCHAGA, L., & BAR-OR, A. 2010. Reciprocal Th1 and Th17 regulation by mesenchymal stem cells: Implication for multiple sclerosis. *Ann Neurol*, 68, 540–5.

DAVIES, L. C., LOCKE, M., WEBB, R. D., ROBERTS, J. T., LANGLEY, M., THOMAS, D. W., ARCHER, C. W., & STEPHENS, P. 2010. A multipotent neural crest-derived progenitor cell population is resident within the oral mucosa lamina propria. *Stem Cells Dev*, 19, 819–30.

DAVIES, L. C., LONNIES, H., LOCKE, M., SUNDBERG, B., ROSENDAHL, K., GOTHERSTROM, C., LE BLANC, K., & STEPHENS, P. 2012. Oral mucosal progenitor cells are potently immunosuppressive in a dose-independent manner. *Stem Cells Dev*, 21, 1478–87.

DE MIGUEL, M. P., FUENTES-JULIAN, S., BLAZQUEZ-MARTINEZ, A., PASCUAL, C. Y., ALLER, M. A., ARIAS, J., & ARNALICH-MONTIEL, F. 2012. Immunosuppressive properties of mesenchymal stem cells: advances and applications. *Curr Mol Med*, 12, 574–91.

DEAGLIO, S., DWYER, K. M., GAO, W., FRIEDMAN, D., USHEVA, A., ERAT, A., CHEN, J. F., ENJYOJI, K., LINDEN, J., OUKKA, M., KUCHROO, V. K., STROM, T. B., & ROBSON, S. C. 2007. Adenosine generation catalyzed by CD39 and CD73 expressed on regulatory T cells mediates immune suppression. *J Exp Med*, 204, 1257–65.

DOMINICI, M., LE BLANC, K., MUELLER, I., SLAPER-CORTENBACH, I., MARINI, F., KRAUSE, D., DEANS, R., KEATING, A., PROCKOP, D., & HORWITZ, E. 2006. Minimal criteria for defining multipotent mesenchymal stromal cells. The International Society for Cellular Therapy position statement. *Cytotherapy*, 8, 315–7.

DUFFY, M. M., PINDJAKOVA, J., HANLEY, S. A., MCCARTHY, C., WEIDHOFER, G. A., SWEENEY, E. M., ENGLISH, K., SHAW, G., MURPHY, J. M., BARRY, F. P., MAHON, B. P., BELTON, O., CEREDIG, R., & GRIFFIN, M. D. 2011. Mesenchymal stem cell inhibition of T-helper 17 cell-differentiation is triggered by cell-cell contact and mediated by prostaglandin E2 via the EP4 receptor. *Eur J Immunol*, 41, 2840–51.

EAGAR, T. N., TANG, Q., WOLFE, M., HE, Y., PEAR, W. S., & BLUESTONE, J. A. 2004. Notch 1 signaling regulates peripheral T cell activation. *Immunity*, 20, 407–15.

ENGLISH, K., RYAN, J. M., TOBIN, L., MURPHY, M. J., BARRY, F. P., & MAHON, B. P. 2009. Cell contact, prostaglandin E(2) and transforming growth factor beta 1 play non-redundant roles in human mesenchymal stem cell induction of CD4+CD25(High) forkhead box P3+ regulatory T cells. *Clin Exp Immunol*, 156, 149–60.

ENOCH, S., PEAKE, M. A., WALL, I., DAVIES, L., FARRIER, J., GILES, P., KIPLING, D., PRICE, P., MOSELEY, R., THOMAS, D., & STEPHENS, P. 2010. 'Young' oral fibroblasts are geno/phenotypically distinct. *J Dent Res*, 89, 1407–13.

FRANCOIS, M., ROMIEU-MOUREZ, R., LI, M., & GALIPEAU, J. 2012. Human MSC suppression correlates with cytokine induction of indoleamine 2,3-dioxygenase and bystander M2 macrophage differentiation. *Mol Ther*, 20, 187–95.

GATTI, S., BRUNO, S., DEREGIBUS, M. C., SORDI, A., CANTALUPPI, V., TETTA, C., & CAMUSSI, G. 2011. Microvesicles derived from human adult mesenchymal stem cells protect against ischaemia-reperfusion-induced acute and chronic kidney injury. *Nephrol Dial Transplant*, 26, 1474–83.

GEORGE, J. F., BRAUN, A., BRUSKO, T. M., JOSEPH, R., BOLISETTY, S., WASSERFALL, C. H., ATKINSON, M. A., AGARWAL, A., & KAPTURCZAK, M. H. 2008. Suppression by CD4+CD25+ regulatory T cells is dependent on expression of heme oxygenase-1 in antigen-presenting cells. *Am J Pathol*, 173, 154–60.

GETTING, S. J., MAHONEY, D. J., CAO, T., RUGG, M. S., FRIES, E., MILNER, C. M., PERRETTI, M., & DAY, A. J. 2002. The link module from human TSG-6 inhibits neutrophil migration in a hyaluronan- and inter-alpha -inhibitor-independent manner. *J Biol Chem*, 277, 51068–76.

GHANNAM, S., PENE, J., MOQUET-TORCY, G., JORGENSEN, C., & YSSEL, H. 2010. Mesenchymal stem cells inhibit human Th17 cell differentiation and function and induce a T regulatory cell phenotype. *J Immunol*, 185, 302–12.

GIESEKE, F., BOHRINGER, J., BUSSOLARI, R., DOMINICI, M., HANDGRETINGER, R., & MULLER, I. 2010. Human multipotent mesenchymal stromal cells use galectin-1 to inhibit immune effector cells. *Blood*, 116, 3770–9.

GONZALEZ-REY, E., ANDERSON, P., GONZALEZ, M. A., RICO, L., BUSCHER, D., & DELGADO, M. 2009. Human adult stem cells derived from adipose tissue protect against experimental colitis and sepsis. *Gut*, 58, 929–39.

GONZALEZ, M. A., GONZALEZ-REY, E., RICO, L., BUSCHER, D., & DELGADO, M. 2009. Adipose-derived mesenchymal stem cells alleviate experimental colitis by inhibiting inflammatory and autoimmune responses. *Gastroenterology*, 136, 978–89.

GOTHERSTROM, C., LUNDQVIST, A., DUPREZ, I. R., CHILDS, R., BERG, L., & LE BLANC, K. 2011. Fetal and adult multipotent mesenchymal stromal cells are killed by different pathways. *Cytotherapy*, 13, 269–78.

GRAVES, D. T., & COCHRAN, D. 2003. The contribution of interleukin-1 and tumor necrosis factor to periodontal tissue destruction. *J Periodontol*, 74, 391–401.

GRONTHOS, S., MANKANI, M., BRAHIM, J., ROBEY, P. G., & SHI, S. 2000. Postnatal human dental pulp stem cells (DPSCs) in vitro and in vivo. *Proc Natl Acad Sci U S A*, 97, 13625–30.

GU, Z., CAO, X., JIANG, J., LI, L., DA, Z., LIU, H., & CHENG, C. 2012. Upregulation of p16INK4A promotes cellular senescence of bone marrow-derived mesenchymal stem cells from systemic lupus erythematosus patients. *Cell Signal*, 24, 2307–14.

HALL, S. R., TSOYI, K., ITH, B., PADERA, R. F., JR., LEDERER, J. A., WANG, Z., LIU, X., & PERRELLA, M. A. 2013. Mesenchymal stromal cells improve survival during sepsis in the absence of heme oxygenase-1: the importance of neutrophils. *Stem Cells*, 31, 397–407.

HAYASHI, Y., TSUJI, S., TSUJII, M., NISHIDA, T., ISHII, S., IIJIMA, H., NAKAMURA, T., EGUCHI, H., MIYOSHI, E., HAYASHI, N., & KAWANO, S. 2008. Topical implantation of mesenchymal stem cells has beneficial effects on healing of experimental colitis in rats. *J Pharmacol Exp Ther*, 326, 523–31.

HUANG, W., LA RUSSA, V., ALZOUBI, A., & SCHWARZENBERGER, P. 2006. Interleukin-17A: a T-cell-derived growth factor for murine and human mesenchymal stem cells. *Stem Cells*, 24, 1512–18.

HUANG, X. P., SUN, Z., MIYAGI, Y., MCDONALD KINKAID, H., ZHANG, L., WEISEL, R. D., & LI, R. K. 2010. Differentiation of allogeneic mesenchymal stem cells induces immunogenicity and limits their long-term benefits for myocardial repair. *Circulation*, 122, 2419–29.

HUCKE, C., MACKENZIE, C. R., ADJOGBLE, K. D., TAKIKAWA, O., & DAUBENER, W. 2004. Nitric oxide-mediated regulation of gamma interferon-induced bacteriostasis: inhibition and degradation of human indoleamine 2,3-dioxygenase. *Infect Immun*, 72, 2723–30.

HUGHES, P. D., & COHNEY, S. J. 2011. Modifiers of complement activation for prevention of antibody-mediated injury to allografts. *Curr Opin Organ Transplant*, 16, 425–33.

IGNATIUS, A., SCHOENGRAF, P., KREJA, L., LIEDERT, A., RECKNAGEL, S., KANDERT, S., BRENNER, R. E., SCHNEIDER, M., LAMBRIS, J. D., & HUBER-LANG, M. 2011. Complement C3a and C5a modulate osteoclast formation and inflammatory response of osteoblasts in synergism with IL-1beta. *J Cell Biochem*, 112, 2594–605.

ILARREGUI, J. M., CROCI, D. O., BIANCO, G. A., TOSCANO, M. A., SALATINO, M., VERMEULEN, M. E., GEFFNER, J. R., & RABINOVICH, G. A. 2009. Tolerogenic signals delivered by dendritic cells to T cells through a galectin-1-driven immunoregulatory circuit involving interleukin 27 and interleukin 10. *Nat Immunol*, 10, 981–91.

ISAKOVA, I. A., BAKER, K., DUTREIL, M., DUFOUR, J., GAUPP, D., & PHINNEY, D. G. 2007. Age- and dose-related effects on MSC engraftment levels and anatomical distribution in the central nervous systems of nonhuman primates: identification of novel MSC subpopulations that respond to guidance cues in brain. *Stem Cells*, 25, 3261–70.

KALINSKI, P. 2012. Regulation of immune responses by prostaglandin E2. *J Immunol*, 188, 21-8.

KATSUDA, T., KOSAKA, N., TAKESHITA, F., & OCHIYA, T. 2013. The therapeutic potential of mesenchymal stem cell-derived extracellular vesicles. *Proteomics*, 13, 1637–53.

KEBIR, H., IFERGAN, I., ALVAREZ, J. I., BERNARD, M., POIRIER, J., ARBOUR, N., DUQUETTE, P., & PRAT, A. 2009. Preferential recruitment of interferon-gamma-expressing TH17 cells in multiple sclerosis. *Ann Neurol*, 66, 390–402.

KHARAZIHA, P., HELLSTROM, P. M., NOORINAYER, B., FARZANEH, F., AGHAJANI, K., JAFARI, F., TELKABADI, M., ATASHI, A., HONARDOOST, M., ZALI, M. R., & SOLEIMANI, M. 2009. Improvement of liver function in liver cirrhosis patients after autologous mesenchymal stem cell injection: a phase I-II clinical trial. *Eur J Gastroenterol Hepatol*, 21, 1199–205.

KIDD, S., SPAETH, E., DEMBINSKI, J. L., DIETRICH, M., WATSON, K., KLOPP, A., BATTULA, V. L., WEIL, M., ANDREEFF, M., & MARINI, F. C. 2009. Direct evidence of mesenchymal stem cell tropism for tumor and wounding microenvironments using in vivo bioluminescent imaging. *Stem Cells*, 27, 2614–23.

KIM, H. S., KIM, K. H., KIM, S. H., KIM, Y. S., KOO, K. T., KIM, T. I., SEOL, Y. J., KU, Y., RHYU, I. C., CHUNG, C. P., & LEE, Y. M. 2010. Immunomodulatory effect of canine periodontal ligament stem cells on allogenic and xenogenic peripheral blood mononuclear cells. *J Periodontal Implant Sci*, 40, 265–70.

KIM, J., & HEMATTI, P. 2009. Mesenchymal stem cell-educated macrophages: a novel type of alternatively activated macrophages. *Exp Hematol*, 37, 1445–53.

KONERMANN, A., BEYER, M., DESCHNER, J., ALLAM, J. P., NOVAK, N., WINTER, J., JEPSEN, S., & JAGER, A. 2012. Human periodontal ligament cells facilitate leukocyte recruitment and are influenced in their immunomodulatory function by Th17 cytokine release. *Cell Immunol*, 272, 137–43.

KORDELAS, L., REBMANN, V., LUDWIG, A. K., RADTKE, S., RUESING, J., DOEPPNER, T. R., EPPLE, M., HORN, P. A., BEELEN, D. W., & GIEBEL, B. 2014. MSC-derived exosomes: a novel tool to treat therapy-refractory graft-versus-host disease. *Leukemia*, 28, 970–3.

KRAMPERA, M., COSMI, L., ANGELI, R., PASINI, A., LIOTTA, F., ANDREINI, A., SANTARLASCI, V., MAZZINGHI,

B., PIZZOLO, G., VINANTE, F., ROMAGNANI, P., MAGGI, E., ROMAGNANI, S., & ANNUNZIATO, F. 2006. Role for interferon-gamma in the immunomodulatory activity of human bone marrow mesenchymal stem cells. *Stem Cells*, 24, 386–98.

KRAMPERA, M., GLENNIE, S., DYSON, J., SCOTT, D., LAYLOR, R., SIMPSON, E., & DAZZI, F. 2003. Bone marrow mesenchymal stem cells inhibit the response of naive and memory antigen-specific T cells to their cognate peptide. *Blood*, 101, 3722–9.

KRASNODEMBSKAYA, A., SONG, Y., FANG, X., GUPTA, N., SERIKOV, V., LEE, J. W., & MATTHAY, M. A. 2010. Antibacterial effect of human mesenchymal stem cells is mediated in part from secretion of the antimicrobial peptide LL-37. *Stem Cells*, 28, 2229–38.

LE BLANC, K., FRASSONI, F., BALL, L., LOCATELLI, F., ROELOFS, H., LEWIS, I., LANINO, E., SUNDBERG, B., BERNARDO, M. E., REMBERGER, M., DINI, G., EGELER, R. M., BACIGALUPO, A., FIBBE, W., & RINGDEN, O. 2008. Mesenchymal stem cells for treatment of steroid-resistant, severe, acute graft-versus-host disease: a phase II study. *Lancet*, 371, 1579–86.

LE BLANC, K., & MOUGIAKAKOS, D. 2012. Multipotent mesenchymal stromal cells and the innate immune system. *Nat Rev Immunol*, 12, 383–96.

LE BLANC, K., RASMUSSON, I., SUNDBERG, B., GOTHERSTROM, C., HASSAN, M., UZUNEL, M., & RINGDEN, O. 2004. Treatment of severe acute graft-versus-host disease with third party haploidentical mesenchymal stem cells. *Lancet*, 363, 1439–41.

LE BLANC, K., TAMMIK, C., ROSENDAHL, K., ZETTERBERG, E., & RINGDEN, O. 2003. HLA expression and immunologic properties of differentiated and undifferentiated mesenchymal stem cells. *Exp Hematol*, 31, 890–6.

LEE, R. H., PULIN, A. A., SEO, M. J., KOTA, D. J., YLOSTALO, J., LARSON, B. L., SEMPRUN-PRIETO, L., DELAFONTAINE, P., & PROCKOP, D. J. 2009. Intravenous hMSCs improve myocardial infarction in mice because cells embolized in lung are activated to secrete the anti-inflammatory protein TSG-6. *Cell Stem Cell*, 5, 54–63.

LI, Y., & LIN, F. 2012. Mesenchymal stem cells are injured by complement after their contact with serum. *Blood*, 120, 3436–43.

LIOTTA, F., ANGELI, R., COSMI, L., FILI, L., MANUELLI, C., FROSALI, F., MAZZINGHI, B., MAGGI, L., PASINI, A., LISI, V., SANTARLASCI, V., CONSOLONI, L., ANGELOTTI, M. L., ROMAGNANI, P., PARRONCHI, P., KRAMPERA, M., MAGGI, E., ROMAGNANI, S., & ANNUNZIATO, F. 2008. Toll-like receptors 3 and 4 are expressed by human bone marrow-derived mesenchymal stem cells and can inhibit their T-cell modulatory activity by impairing Notch signaling. *Stem Cells*, 26, 279–89.

LIU, D., XU, J., LIU, O., FAN, Z., LIU, Y., WANG, F., DING, G., WEI, F., ZHANG, C., & WANG, S. 2012. Mesenchymal stem cells derived from inflamed periodontal ligaments exhibit impaired immunomodulation. *J Clin Periodontol*, 39, 1174–82.

LIU, H., KEMENY, D. M., HENG, B. C., OUYANG, H. W., MELENDEZ, A. J., & CAO, T. 2006. The immunogenicity and immunomodulatory function of osteogenic cells differentiated from mesenchymal stem cells. *J Immunol*, 176, 2864–71.

LIU, O., XU, J., DING, G., LIU, D., FAN, Z., ZHANG, C., CHEN, W., DING, Y., TANG, Z., & WANG, S. 2013. Periodontal ligament stem cells regulate B lymphocyte function via programmed cell death protein 1. *Stem Cells*, 31, 1371–82.

LOMBARDO, E., DELAROSA, O., MANCHENO-CORVO, P., MENTA, R., RAMIREZ, C., & BUSCHER, D. 2009. Toll-like receptor-mediated signaling in human adipose-derived stem cells: implications for immunogenicity and immunosuppressive potential. *Tissue Eng Part A*, 15, 1579–89.

LU, D., CHEN, B., LIANG, Z., DENG, W., JIANG, Y., LI, S., XU, J., WU, Q., ZHANG, Z., XIE, B., & CHEN, S. 2011. Comparison of bone marrow mesenchymal stem cells with bone marrow-derived mononuclear cells for treatment of diabetic critical limb ischemia and foot ulcer: a double-blind, randomized, controlled trial. *Diabetes Res Clin Pract*, 92, 26–36.

MACCARIO, R., PODESTA, M., MORETTA, A., COMETA, A., COMOLI, P., MONTAGNA, D., DAUDT, L., IBATICI, A., PIAGGIO, G., POZZI, S., FRASSONI, F., & LOCATELLI, F. 2005. Interaction of human mesenchymal stem cells with cells involved in alloantigen-specific immune response favors the differentiation of CD4+ T-cell subsets expressing a regulatory/suppressive phenotype. *Haematologica*, 90, 516–25.

MAITRA, B., SZEKELY, E., GJINI, K., LAUGHLIN, M. J., DENNIS, J., HAYNESWORTH, S. E., & KOC, O. N. 2004. Human mesenchymal stem cells support unrelated donor hematopoietic stem cells and suppress T-cell activation. *Bone Marrow Transpl*, 33, 597–604.

MEHRAZARIN, S., OH, J. E., CHUNG, C. L., CHEN, W., KIM, R. H., SHI, S., PARK, N. H., & KANG, M. K. 2011. Impaired odontogenic differentiation of senescent dental mesenchymal stem cells is associated with loss of Bmi-1 expression. *J Endod*, 37, 662–6.

MEISEL, R., BROCKERS, S., HESELER, K., DEGISTIRICI, O., BULLE, H., WOITE, C., STUHLSATZ, S., SCHWIPPERT, W., JAGER, M., SORG, R., HENSCHLER, R., SEISSLER, J., DILLOO, D., & DAUBENER, W. 2011. Human but not murine multipotent mesenchymal stromal cells exhibit broad-spectrum antimicrobial effector function mediated by indoleamine 2,3-dioxygenase. *Leukemia*, 25, 648–54.

MEISEL, R., ZIBERT, A., LARYEA, M., GOBEL, U., DAUBENER, W., & DILLOO, D. 2004. Human bone marrow stromal cells inhibit allogeneic T-cell responses by indoleamine 2,3-dioxygenase-mediated tryptophan degradation. *Blood*, 103, 4619–21.

MELIEF, S. M., SCHRAMA, E., BRUGMAN, M. H., TIEMESSEN, M. M., HOOGDUIJN, M. J., FIBBE, W. E., & ROELOFS, H. 2013. Multipotent stromal cells induce human regulatory T cells through a novel pathway involving skewing of monocytes toward anti-inflammatory macrophages. *Stem Cells*, 31, 1980–91.

MOLL, G., HULT, A., VON BAHR, L., ALM, J. J., HELDRING, N., HAMAD, O. A., STENBECK-FUNKE, L., LARSSON, S.,

TERAMURA, Y., ROELOFS, H., NILSSON, B., FIBBE, W. E., OLSSON, M. L., & LE BLANC, K. 2014. Do ABO blood group antigens hamper the therapeutic efficacy of mesenchymal stromal cells? *PLoS One*, 9, e85040.

MOLL, G., JITSCHIN, R., VON BAHR, L., RASMUSSON-DUPREZ, I., SUNDBERG, B., LONNIES, L., ELGUE, G., NILSSON-EKDAHL, K., MOUGIAKAKOS, D., LAMBRIS, J. D., RINGDEN, O., LE BLANC, K., & NILSSON, B. 2011. Mesenchymal stromal cells engage complement and complement receptor bearing innate effector cells to modulate immune responses. *PLoS One*, 6, e21703.

MOLL, G., RASMUSSON-DUPREZ, I., VON BAHR, L., CONNOLLY-ANDERSEN, A. M., ELGUE, G., FUNKE, L., HAMAD, O. A., LONNIES, H., MAGNUSSON, P. U., SANCHEZ, J., TERAMURA, Y., NILSSON-EKDAHL, K., RINGDEN, O., KORSGREN, O., NILSSON, B., & LE BLANC, K. 2012. Are therapeutic human mesenchymal stromal cells compatible with human blood? *Stem Cells*, 30, 1565–74.

MORSCZECK, C., GOTZ, W., SCHIERHOLZ, J., ZEILHOFER, F., KUHN, U., MOHL, C., SIPPEL, C., & HOFFMANN, K. H. 2005. Isolation of precursor cells (PCs) from human dental follicle of wisdom teeth. *Matrix Biol*, 24, 155–65.

MORSE, D. R. 1991. Age-related changes of the dental pulp complex and their relationship to systemic aging. *Oral Surg Oral Med Oral Pathol*, 72, 721–45.

MOUGIAKAKOS, D., JITSCHIN, R., JOHANSSON, C. C., OKITA, R., KIESSLING, R., & LE BLANC, K. 2011. The impact of inflammatory licensing on heme oxygenase-1-mediated induction of regulatory T cells by human mesenchymal stem cells. *Blood*, 117, 4826–35.

NAKAMURA, T., & MIZUNO, S. 2010. The discovery of hepatocyte growth factor (HGF) and its significance for cell biology, life sciences and clinical medicine. *Proc Jpn Acad Ser B Phys Biol Sci*, 86, 588–610.

NASEF, A., MATHIEU, N., CHAPEL, A., FRICK, J., FRANCOIS, S., MAZURIER, C., BOUTARFA, A., BOUCHET, S., GORIN, N. C., THIERRY, D., & FOUILLARD, L. 2007. Immunosuppressive effects of mesenchymal stem cells: involvement of HLA-G. *Transplantation*, 84, 231–7.

NEMETH, K., KEANE-MYERS, A., BROWN, J. M., METCALFE, D. D., GORHAM, J. D., BUNDOC, V. G., HODGES, M. G., JELINEK, I., MADALA, S., KARPATI, S., & MEZEY, E. 2010. Bone marrow stromal cells use TGF-beta to suppress allergic responses in a mouse model of ragweed-induced asthma. *Proc Natl Acad Sci U S A*, 107, 5652–7.

NEMETH, K., LEELAHAVANICHKUL, A., YUEN, P. S., MAYER, B., PARMELEE, A., DOI, K., ROBEY, P. G., LEELAHAVANICHKUL, K., KOLLER, B. H., BROWN, J. M., HU, X., JELINEK, I., STAR, R. A., & MEZEY, E. 2009. Bone marrow stromal cells attenuate sepsis via prostaglandin E(2)-dependent reprogramming of host macrophages to increase their interleukin-10 production. *Nat Med*, 15, 42–9.

NEMETH, K., WILSON, T., RADA, B., PARMELEE, A., MAYER, B., BUZAS, E., FALUS, A., KEY, S., MASSZI, T., KARPATI, S., & MEZEY, E. 2012. Characterization and function of

histamine receptors in human bone marrow stromal cells. *Stem Cells*, 30, 222–31.

NISAPAKULTORN, K., MAKRUDTHONG, J., SA-ARD-IAM, N., RERKYEN, P., MAHANONDA, R., & TAKIKAWA, O. 2009. Indoleamine 2,3-dioxygenase expression and regulation in chronic periodontitis. *J Periodontol*, 80, 114–21.

O'CONNOR, J. C., ANDRE, C., WANG, Y., LAWSON, M. A., SZEGEDI, S. S., LESTAGE, J., CASTANON, N., KELLEY, K. W., & DANTZER, R. 2009. Interferon-gamma and tumor necrosis factor-alpha mediate the upregulation of indoleamine 2,3-dioxygenase and the induction of depressive-like behavior in mice in response to bacillus Calmette-Guerin. *J Neurosci*, 29, 4200–9.

ORTIZ, L. A., GAMBELLI, F., MCBRIDE, C., GAUPP, D., BADDOO, M., KAMINSKI, N., & PHINNEY, D. G. 2003. Mesenchymal stem cell engraftment in lung is enhanced in response to bleomycin exposure and ameliorates its fibrotic effects. *Proc Natl Acad Sci U S A*, 100, 8407–11.

PARK, H., LI, Z., YANG, X. O., CHANG, S. H., NURIEVA, R., WANG, Y. H., WANG, Y., HOOD, L., ZHU, Z., TIAN, Q., & DONG, C. 2005. A distinct lineage of CD4 T cells regulates tissue inflammation by producing interleukin 17. *Nat Immunol*, 6, 1133–41.

PENBERTHY, W. T. 2007. Pharmacological targeting of IDO-mediated tolerance for treating autoimmune disease. *Curr Drug Metab*, 8, 245–66.

PENG, L., XIE, D. Y., LIN, B. L., LIU, J., ZHU, H. P., XIE, C., ZHENG, Y. B., & GAO, Z. L. 2011. Autologous bone marrow mesenchymal stem cell transplantation in liver failure patients caused by hepatitis B: short-term and long-term outcomes. *Hepatology*, 54, 820–8.

PEVSNER-FISCHER, M., MORAD, V., COHEN-SFADY, M., ROUSSO-NOORI, L., ZANIN-ZHOROV, A., COHEN, S., COHEN, I. R., & ZIPORI, D. 2007. Toll-like receptors and their ligands control mesenchymal stem cell functions. *Blood*, 109, 1422–32.

PLUMAS, J., CHAPEROT, L., RICHARD, M. J., MOLENS, J. P., BENSA, J. C., & FAVROT, M. C. 2005. Mesenchymal stem cells induce apoptosis of activated T cells. *Leukemia*, 19, 1597–604.

POGGI, A., & ZOCCHI, M. R. 2008. Role of bone marrow stromal cells in the generation of human CD8+ regulatory T cells. *Hum Immunol*, 69, 755–9.

PONTE, A. L., MARAIS, E., GALLAY, N., LANGONNE, A., DELORME, B., HERAULT, O., CHARBORD, P., & DOMENECH, J. 2007. The in vitro migration capacity of human bone marrow mesenchymal stem cells: comparison of chemokine and growth factor chemotactic activities. *Stem Cells*, 25, 1737–45.

PREVOSTO, C., ZANCOLLI, M., CANEVALI, P., ZOCCHI, M. R., & POGGI, A. 2007. Generation of CD4+ or CD8+ regulatory T cells upon mesenchymal stem cell-lymphocyte interaction. *Haematologica*, 92, 881–8.

RAFEI, M., CAMPEAU, P. M., AGUILAR-MAHECHA, A., BUCHANAN, M., WILLIAMS, P., BIRMAN, E., YUAN, S.,

YOUNG, Y. K., BOIVIN, M. N., FORNER, K., BASIK, M., & GALIPEAU, J. 2009. Mesenchymal stromal cells ameliorate experimental autoimmune encephalomyelitis by inhibiting CD4 Th17 T cells in a CC chemokine ligand 2-dependent manner. *J Immunol*, 182, 5994–6002.

RAFEI, M., HSIEH, J., FORTIER, S., LI, M., YUAN, S., BIRMAN, E., FORNER, K., BOIVIN, M. N., DOODY, K., TREMBLAY, M., ANNABI, B., & GALIPEAU, J. 2008. Mesenchymal stromal cell-derived CCL2 suppresses plasma cell immunoglobulin production via STAT3 inactivation and PAX5 induction. *Blood*, 112, 4991–8.

RAICEVIC, G., ROUAS, R., NAJAR, M., STORDEUR, P., BOUFKER, H. I., BRON, D., MARTIAT, P., GOLDMAN, M., NEVESSIGNSKY, M. T., & LAGNEAUX, L. 2010. Inflammation modifies the pattern and the function of Toll-like receptors expressed by human mesenchymal stromal cells. *Hum Immunol*, 71, 235–44.

RAMASAMY, R., TONG, C. K., SEOW, H. F., VIDYADARAN, S., & DAZZI, F. 2008. The immunosuppressive effects of human bone marrow-derived mesenchymal stem cells target T cell proliferation but not its effector function. *Cell Immunol*, 251, 131–6.

RASMUSSON, I., LE BLANC, K., SUNDBERG, B., & RINGDEN, O. 2007. Mesenchymal stem cells stimulate antibody secretion in human B cells. *Scand J Immunol*, 65, 336–43.

RASMUSSON, I., RINGDEN, O., SUNDBERG, B., & LE BLANC, K. 2003. Mesenchymal stem cells inhibit the formation of cytotoxic T lymphocytes, but not activated cytotoxic T lymphocytes or natural killer cells. *Transplantation*, 76, 1208–13.

RASMUSSON, I., RINGDEN, O., SUNDBERG, B., & LE BLANC, K. 2005. Mesenchymal stem cells inhibit lymphocyte proliferation by mitogens and alloantigens by different mechanisms. *Exp Cell Res*, 305, 33–41.

REMY, S., BLANCOU, P., TESSON, L., TARDIF, V., BRION, R., ROYER, P. J., MOTTERLINI, R., FORESTI, R., PAINCHAUT, M., POGU, S., GREGOIRE, M., BACH, J. M., ANEGON, I., & CHAUVEAU, C. 2009. Carbon monoxide inhibits TLR-induced dendritic cell immunogenicity. *J Immunol*, 182, 1877–84.

REN, G., ZHAO, X., ZHANG, L., ZHANG, J., L'HUILLIER, A., LING, W., ROBERTS, A. I., LE, A. D., SHI, S., SHAO, C., & SHI, Y. 2010. Inflammatory cytokine-induced intercellular adhesion molecule-1 and vascular cell adhesion molecule-1 in mesenchymal stem cells are critical for immunosuppression. *J Immunol*, 184, 2321–8.

RINGDEN, O., UZUNEL, M., SUNDBERG, B., LONNIES, L., NAVA, S., GUSTAFSSON, J., HENNINGSOHN, L., & LE BLANC, K. 2007. Tissue repair using allogeneic mesenchymal stem cells for hemorrhagic cystitis, pneumomediastinum and perforated colon. *Leukemia*, 21, 2271–6.

RIVERA, F. J., & AIGNER, L. 2012. Adult mesenchymal stem cell therapy for myelin repair in multiple sclerosis. *Biol Res*, 45, 257–68.

RODDY, G. W., OH, J. Y., LEE, R. H., BARTOSH, T. J., YLOSTALO, J., COBLE, K., ROSA, R. H., JR., & PROCKOP, D. J. 2011. Action at a distance: systemically administered adult stem/

progenitor cells (MSCs) reduce inflammatory damage to the cornea without engraftment and primarily by secretion of TNF-alpha stimulated gene/protein 6. *Stem Cells*, 29, 1572–9.

ROJAS, M., XU, J., WOODS, C. R., MORA, A. L., SPEARS, W., ROMAN, J., & BRIGHAM, K. L. 2005. Bone marrow-derived mesenchymal stem cells in repair of the injured lung. *Am J Respir Cell Mol Biol*, 33, 145–52.

RUBTSOV, Y. P., SUZDALTSEVA, Y. G., GORYUNOV, K. V., KALININA, N. I., SYSOEVA, V. Y., & TKACHUK, V. A. 2012. Regulation of Immunity via Multipotent Mesenchymal Stromal Cells. *Acta Naturae*, 4, 23–31.

RUTELLA, S., DANESE, S., & LEONE, G. 2006. Tolerogenic dendritic cells: cytokine modulation comes of age. *Blood*, 108, 1435–40.

RYAN, J. M., BARRY, F., MURPHY, J. M., & MAHON, B. P. 2007. Interferon-gamma does not break, but promotes the immunosuppressive capacity of adult human mesenchymal stem cells. *Clin Exp Immunol*, 149, 353–63.

SAITO, A., MOTOMURA, N., KAKIMI, K., NARUI, K., NOGUCHI, N., SASATSU, M., KUBO, K., KOEZUKA, Y., TAKAI, D., UEHA, S., & TAKAMOTO, S. 2008. Vascular allografts are resistant to methicillin-resistant *Staphylococcus aureus* through indoleamine 2,3-dioxygenase in a murine model. *J Thorac Cardiovasc Surg*, 136, 159–67.

SAKATA, D., YAO, C., & NARUMIYA, S. 2010. Emerging roles of prostanoids in T cell-mediated immunity. *IUBMB Life*, 62, 591–6.

SCHRAUFSTATTER, I. U., DISCIPIO, R. G., ZHAO, M., & KHALDOYANIDI, S. K. 2009. C3a and C5a are chemotactic factors for human mesenchymal stem cells, which cause prolonged ERK1/2 phosphorylation. *J Immunol*, 182, 3827–36.

SELMANI, Z., NAJI, A., GAIFFE, E., OBERT, L., TIBERGHIEN, P., ROUAS-FREISS, N., CAROSELLA, E. D., & DESCHASEAUX, F. 2009. HLA-G is a crucial immunosuppressive molecule secreted by adult human mesenchymal stem cells. *Transplantation*, 87, S62–6.

SELMANI, Z., NAJI, A., ZIDI, I., FAVIER, B., GAIFFE, E., OBERT, L., BORG, C., SAAS, P., TIBERGHIEN, P., ROUAS-FREISS, N., CAROSELLA, E. D., & DESCHASEAUX, F. 2008. Human leukocyte antigen-G5 secretion by human mesenchymal stem cells is required to suppress T lymphocyte and natural killer function and to induce CD4+CD25highFOXP3+ regulatory T cells. *Stem Cells*, 26, 212–22.

SEO, B. M., MIURA, M., GRONTHOS, S., BARTOLD, P. M., BATOULI, S., BRAHIM, J., YOUNG, M., ROBEY, P. G., WANG, C. Y., & SHI, S. 2004. Investigation of multipotent postnatal stem cells from human periodontal ligament. *Lancet*, 364, 149–55.

SHENG, H., WANG, Y., JIN, Y., ZHANG, Q., ZHANG, Y., WANG, L., SHEN, B., YIN, S., LIU, W., CUI, L., & LI, N. 2008. A critical role of IFNgamma in priming MSC-mediated suppression of T cell proliferation through up-regulation of B7-H1. *Cell Res*, 18, 846–57.

SHI, C., & PAMER, E. G. 2011. Monocyte recruitment during infection and inflammation. *Nat Rev Immunol*, 11, 762–74.

SHI, Y., SU, J., ROBERTS, A. I., SHOU, P., RABSON, A. B., & REN, G. 2012. How mesenchymal stem cells interact with tissue immune responses. *Trends Immunol*, 33, 136–43.

SIEGEL, G., SCHAFER, R., & DAZZI, F. 2009. The immunosuppressive properties of mesenchymal stem cells. *Transplantation*, 87, S45–9.

SONOYAMA, W., LIU, Y., YAMAZA, T., TUAN, R. S., WANG, S., SHI, S., & HUANG, G. T. 2008. Characterization of the apical papilla and its residing stem cells from human immature permanent teeth: a pilot study. *J Endod*, 34, 166–71.

SOTIROPOULOU, P. A., PEREZ, S. A., GRITZAPIS, A. D., BAXEVANIS, C. N., & PAPAMICHAIL, M. 2006. Interactions between human mesenchymal stem cells and natural killer cells. *Stem Cells*, 24, 74–85.

SPAGGIARI, G. M., ABDELRAZIK, H., BECCHETTI, F., & MORETTA, L. 2009. MSCs inhibit monocyte-derived DC maturation and function by selectively interfering with the generation of immature DCs: central role of MSC-derived prostaglandin E2. *Blood*, 113, 6576–83.

SPAGGIARI, G. M., CAPOBIANCO, A., ABDELRAZIK, H., BECCHETTI, F., MINGARI, M. C., & MORETTA, L. 2008. Mesenchymal stem cells inhibit natural killer-cell proliferation, cytotoxicity, and cytokine production: role of indoleamine 2,3-dioxygenase and prostaglandin E2. *Blood*, 111, 1327–33.

SPAGGIARI, G. M., CAPOBIANCO, A., BECCHETTI, S., MINGARI, M. C., & MORETTA, L. 2006. Mesenchymal stem cell-natural killer cell interactions: evidence that activated NK cells are capable of killing MSCs, whereas MSCs can inhibit IL-2-induced NK-cell proliferation. *Blood*, 107, 1484–90.

STAGG, J., & GALIPEAU, J. 2013. Mechanisms of immune modulation by mesenchymal stromal cells and clinical translation. *Curr Mol Med*, 13, 856–67.

SU, W. R., ZHANG, Q. Z., SHI, S. H., NGUYEN, A. L., & LE, A. D. 2011. Human gingiva-derived mesenchymal stromal cells attenuate contact hypersensitivity via prostaglandin E2-dependent mechanisms. *Stem Cells*, 29, 1849–60.

TANAKA, F., TOMINAGA, K., OCHI, M., TANIGAWA, T., WATANABE, T., FUJIWARA, Y., OHTA, K., OSHITANI, N., HIGUCHI, K., & ARAKAWA, T. 2008. Exogenous administration of mesenchymal stem cells ameliorates dextran sulfate sodium-induced colitis via anti-inflammatory action in damaged tissue in rats. *Life Sci*, 83, 771–9.

TAYLOR, D. D., ZACHARIAS, W., & GERCEL-TAYLOR, C. 2011. Exosome isolation for proteomic analyses and RNA profiling. *Methods Mol Biol*, 728, 235–46.

TEMCHURA, V. V., TENBUSCH, M., NCHINDA, G., NABI, G., TIPPLER, B., ZELENYUK, M., WILDNER, O., UBERLA, K., & KUATE, S. 2008. Enhancement of immunostimulatory properties of exosomal vaccines by incorporation of fusion-competent G protein of vesicular stomatitis virus. *Vaccine*, 26, 3662–72.

THERY, C., OSTROWSKI, M., & SEGURA, E. 2009. Membrane vesicles as conveyors of immune responses. *Nat Rev Immunol*, 9, 581–93.

TOMCHUCK, S. L., ZWEZDARYK, K. J., COFFELT, S. B., WATERMAN, R. S., DANKA, E. S., & SCANDURRO, A. B. 2008. Toll-like receptors on human mesenchymal stem cells drive their migration and immunomodulating responses. *Stem Cells*, 26, 99–107.

TOMIC, S., DJOKIC, J., VASILIJIC, S., VUCEVIC, D., TODOROVIC, V., SUPIC, G., & COLIC, M. 2011. Immunomodulatory properties of mesenchymal stem cells derived from dental pulp and dental follicle are susceptible to activation by Toll-like receptor agonists. *Stem Cells Dev*, 20, 695–708.

TRAGGIAI, E., VOLPI, S., SCHENA, F., GATTORNO, M., FERLITO, F., MORETTA, L., & MARTINI, A. 2008. Bone marrow-derived mesenchymal stem cells induce both polyclonal expansion and differentiation of B cells isolated from healthy donors and systemic lupus erythematosus patients. *Stem Cells*, 26, 562–9.

TSO, G. H., LAW, H. K., TU, W., CHAN, G. C., & LAU, Y. L. 2010. Phagocytosis of apoptotic cells modulates mesenchymal stem cells osteogenic differentiation to enhance IL-17 and RANKL expression on CD4+ T cells. *Stem Cells*, 28, 939–54.

TU, Z., LI, Q., BU, H., & LIN, F. 2010. Mesenchymal stem cells inhibit complement activation by secreting factor H. *Stem Cells Dev*, 19, 1803–9.

TULJAPURKAR, S. R., MCGUIRE, T. R., BRUSNAHAN, S. K., JACKSON, J. D., GARVIN, K. L., KESSINGER, M. A., LANE, J. T., BJ, O. K., & SHARP, J. G. 2011. Changes in human bone marrow fat content associated with changes in hematopoietic stem cell numbers and cytokine levels with aging. *J Anat*, 219, 574–81.

UCCELLI, A., MORETTA, L., & PISTOIA, V. 2008. Mesenchymal stem cells in health and disease. *Nat Rev Immunol*, 8, 726–36.

VON BERGWELT-BAILDON, M. S., POPOV, A., SARIC, T., CHEMNITZ, J., CLASSEN, S., STOFFEL, M. S., FIORE, F., ROTH, U., BEYER, M., DEBEY, S., WICKENHAUSER, C., HANISCH, F. G., & SCHULTZE, J. L. 2006. CD25 and indoleamine 2,3-dioxygenase are up-regulated by prostaglandin E2 and expressed by tumor-associated dendritic cells in vivo: additional mechanisms of T-cell inhibition. *Blood*, 108, 228–37.

WADA, N., MENICANIN, D., SHI, S., BARTOLD, P. M., & GRONTHOS, S. 2009. Immunomodulatory properties of human periodontal ligament stem cells. *J Cell Physiol*, 219, 667–76.

WANG, D., FENG, X., LU, L., KONKEL, J. E., ZHANG, H., CHEN, Z., LI, X., GAO, X., LU, L., SHI, S., CHEN, W., & SUN, L. 2014. A CD8 T cell-IDO axis is required for mesenchymal stem cell suppression of human SLE. *Arthritis Rheumatol*.

WANG, L., ZHAO, Y., & SHI, S. 2012. Interplay between mesenchymal stem cells and lymphocytes: implications for immunotherapy and tissue regeneration. *J Dent Res*, 91, 1003–10.

WATERMAN, R. S., HENKLE, S. L., & BETANCOURT, A. M. 2012a. Mesenchymal stem cell 1 (MSC1)-based therapy attenuates tumor growth whereas MSC2-treatment promotes tumor growth and metastasis. *PLoS One*, 7, e45590.

WATERMAN, R. S., MORGENWECK, J., NOSSAMAN, B. D., SCANDURRO, A. E., SCANDURRO, S. A., & BETANCOURT, A. M. 2012b. Anti-inflammatory mesenchymal stem cells (MSC2) attenuate symptoms of painful diabetic peripheral neuropathy. *Stem Cells Transl Med*, 1, 557–65.

WATERMAN, R. S., TOMCHUCK, S. L., HENKLE, S. L., & BETANCOURT, A. M. 2010. A new mesenchymal stem cell (MSC) paradigm: polarization into a pro-inflammatory MSC1 or an immunosuppressive MSC2 phenotype. *PLoS One*, 5, e10088.

WEI, X., YANG, X., HAN, Z. P., QU, F. F., SHAO, L., & SHI, Y. F. 2013. Mesenchymal stem cells: a new trend for cell therapy. *Acta Pharmacol Sin*, 34, 747–54.

WU, L. W., WANG, Y. L., CHRISTENSEN, J. M., KHALIFIAN, S., SCHNEEBERGER, S., RAIMONDI, G., COONEY, D. S., LEE, W. P., & BRANDACHER, G. 2014. Donor age negatively affects the immunoregulatory properties of both adipose and bone marrow derived mesenchymal stem cells. *Transpl Immunol*, 30, 122–7.

WYNN, R. F., HART, C. A., CORRADI-PERINI, C., O'NEILL, L., EVANS, C. A., WRAITH, J. E., FAIRBAIRN, L. J., & BELLANTUONO, I. 2004. A small proportion of mesenchymal stem cells strongly expresses functionally active CXCR4 receptor capable of promoting migration to bone marrow. *Blood*, 104, 2643–5.

XU, X., CHEN, C., AKIYAMA, K., CHAI, Y., LE, A. D., WANG, Z., & SHI, S. 2013. Gingivae contain neural-crest- and mesoderm-derived mesenchymal stem cells. *J Dent Res*, 92, 825–32.

YAMADA, Y., UEDA, M., HIBI, H., & BABA, S. 2006. A novel approach to periodontal tissue regeneration with mesenchymal stem cells and platelet-rich plasma using tissue engineering technology: a clinical case report. *Int J Periodontics Restorative Dent*, 26, 363–9.

YAMAZA, T., KENTARO, A., CHEN, C., LIU, Y., SHI, Y., GRONTHOS, S., WANG, S., & SHI, S. 2010. Immunomodulatory properties of stem cells from human exfoliated deciduous teeth. *Stem Cell Res Ther*, 1, 5.

YAN, H., WU, M., YUAN, Y., WANG, Z. Z., JIANG, H., & CHEN, T. 2014. Priming of Toll-like receptor 4 pathway in mesenchymal stem cells increases expression of B cell activating factor. *Biochem Biophys Res Commun*, 448, 212–7.

YEO, R. W., LAI, R. C., ZHANG, B., TAN, S. S., YIN, Y., TEH, B. J., & LIM, S. K. 2013. Mesenchymal stem cell: an efficient mass producer of exosomes for drug delivery. *Adv Drug Deliv Rev*, 65, 336–41.

YU, S., CHO, H. H., JOO, H. J., BAE, Y. C., & JUNG, J. S. 2008. Role of MyD88 in TLR agonist-induced functional alterations of human adipose tissue-derived mesenchymal stem cells. *Mol Cell Biochem*, 317, 143–50.

ZAPPIA, E., CASAZZA, S., PEDEMONTE, E., BENVENUTO, F., BONANNI, I., GERDONI, E., GIUNTI, D., CERAVOLO, A., CAZZANTI, F., FRASSONI, F., MANCARDI, G., & UCCELLI, A. 2005. Mesenchymal stem cells ameliorate experimental autoimmune encephalomyelitis inducing T-cell anergy. *Blood*, 106, 1755–61.

ZHANG, B., YIN, Y., LAI, R. C., TAN, S. S., CHOO, A. B., & LIM, S. K. 2014. Mesenchymal stem cells secrete immunologically active exosomes. *Stem Cells Dev*, 23, 1233–44.

ZHANG, Q., SHI, S., LIU, Y., UYANNE, J., SHI, Y., SHI, S., & LE, A. D. 2009. Mesenchymal stem cells derived from human gingiva are capable of immunomodulatory functions and ameliorate inflammation-related tissue destruction in experimental colitis. *J Immunol*, 183, 7787–98.

ZHANG, Q. Z., SU, W. R., SHI, S. H., WILDER-SMITH, P., XIANG, A. P., WONG, A., NGUYEN, A. L., KWON, C. W., & LE, A. D. 2010. Human gingiva-derived mesenchymal stem cells elicit polarization of m2 macrophages and enhance cutaneous wound healing. *Stem Cells*, 28, 1856–68.

ZHAO, K., LOU, R., HUANG, F., PENG, Y., JIANG, Z., HUANG, K., WU, X., ZHANG, Y., FAN, Z., ZHOU, H., LIU, C., XIAO, Y., SUN, J., LI, Y., XIANG, P., & LIU, Q. 2015. Immunomodulation effects of mesenchymal stromal cells on acute graft-versus-host disease after hematopoietic stem cell transplantation. *Biol Blood Marrow Transplant*, 21, 97–104.

ZHAO, Y., WANG, L., JIN, Y., & SHI, S. 2012. Fas ligand regulates the immunomodulatory properties of dental pulp stem cells. *J Dent Res*, 91, 948–54.

CHAPTER 3

Research advances in tissue regeneration by dental pulp stem cells

Rachel J. Waddington and Alastair J. Sloan

School of Dentistry, Cardiff Institute of Tissue Engineering and Repair, Cardiff University, Cardiff, UK

Mesenchymal stem cells (MSCs) are now fully recognised as the principle cell population ultimately responsible for the synthesis of the collagenous connective tissue, including dentine and bone. Within the dental pulp these MSCs have been reported to represent between 1% and 9% of the total cell population, depending on the marker used for their identification and population doubling in culture (Gronthos et al., 2002; Lizier et al., 2012). This is noticeably higher than estimates of MSCs in bone marrow, which represent 0.01% of the total bone marrow mononuclear cells (Jones et al., 2002). Dental pulp MSCs are heterogeneous in nature, partly due to the prediction that they fall into a hierarchical order of cell types that is seen in so many other connective tissues. The "true" or "mother" adult stem cells infrequently divide, but when signalled to do so, they will divide asymmetrically to give rise to a renewed mother stem cell and a daughter transit amplifying progenitor cell. Transit amplifying (TA) progenitor cell is a befitting description since these cells subsequently become cells that undergo rapid continued cell division to amplify the progenitor population to produce more mature progeny cells in transition from the stem cell to the differentiated cell (Figure 3.1). The long-lived mother cell is proposed to maintain its slow diving nature, where it is suggested to be beneficial in adult tissue for minimising possible DNA replication mutations in the genome (Reya et al., 2001; Riquelme et al., 2008). Cells expanded in culture are therefore highly likely to contain a predominance of TA cells. TA cells derived from MSCs have been shown to be multipotent in that they are able to differentiate into cells capable of synthesising a range of collagenous-based connective tissue structures. However, most excitement in relation to the clinical use of MSCs from dental pulp has focused on their ability to regenerate dentine, pulp, and bone-like tissues. Some researchers have also demonstrated some success in effecting their differentiation down myoblastic and neuronal lineages in synthesising muscle-like and nervous tissue, respectively, for use in craniofacial reconstruction.

Embryological origins of the stem cell pool in adult dental pulp

A fundamental difference between the cell populations of the dental pulp and bone marrows is that dental pulp is a non-haematopoietic tissue and, unlike bone marrow, it does not contain haematopoietic stem cells that function in mediating long-term repopulation of all blood-cell lineages. In addition, the embryological development of the dental pulp can also be considered to lead to a different profile of mesenchymal stem cells surviving into the adult tissue. The classical viewpoint is that the mesoderm, one of the three primary (embryonic) germ layers formed during gastrulation, ultimately provides the stem cell populations for the formation of the mesenchymal connective tissues. However, it is now well established that cells of the dental pulp also contain neural crest stem cells (NCCs) that derive from the external ectoderm. Early during embryogenesis NCCs from the neural tube migrate along relatively extensive distances to the ventral side of

Tissue Engineering and Regeneration in Dentistry: Current Strategies, First Edition. Edited by Rachel J. Waddington and Alastair J. Sloan.
© 2017 John Wiley & Sons, Ltd. Published 2017 by John Wiley & Sons, Ltd.

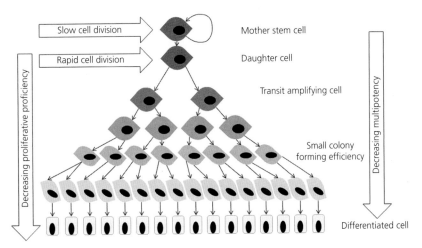

Figure 3.1 Hierarchy model of stem cell differentiation. The mother stem cell is able to divide for self-renewal to replace itself or give rise to transit amplifying cells, which eventually give rise to the committed progenitors. The model hypothesis is that early transit amplifying cells rapidly divide to produce large colonies. As cell division continues, proliferative rates decrease and only small progenitor cell colonies are able to form. This is associated with a reduction in multipotentiality as the cells become committed to a specific unipotential lineage and finally differentiate to produce a large number of terminally differentiated, nonmitotic cells. (Adapted from Chan et al., 2004.)

the head, producing the discrete swellings of the branchial arches. The first branchial arch contributes to the development of the proximal portion of the maxilla, the entire mandible, and the tooth structure within. During these early stages of embryogenesis, these NCCs are proposed to undergo an epithelial to mesenchymal transition to form ectomesenchymal cells which, through complex mesenchymal-epithelial cross-talk with the oral epithelium, give rise to the condensed dental mesenchyme capable of forming the dental pulp, dentine, and the periodontal supporting tissues of periodontal ligament, cementum, and bone.

The migration of the NCCs along specific migratory routes has been extensively investigated in the mouse (Miletich and Sharpe, 2004). As the NCCs migrate through the body, these cells appear to develop a biological diversity such that NCCs entering the first branchial arch either prepossess or acquire positional identity so that molecular signals and interaction with the oral epithelium induce only the formation of the craniofacial structures. Advancements in molecular biology have enabled the use of the Cre recombinase/lac Z reporter system to indelibly label the transient expression of Wnt1 in NCCs prior to migration from the central nervous system, which can then be lineage-tracked to examine the destiny of the neural crest cells in forming

the dental and periodontal tissues (Chai et al., 2000; Janebodin et al., 2011). These studies have demonstrated that NCCs contribute only to the formation of mesenchymal tissues, including the dentine and dental papilla. They do not appear to contribute to the cell populations of other ectodermally derived cells of the enamel organ responsible for the formation of enamel. These studies have also shown that as tooth development progresses, the percentage of NCCs decreases, although it is not clear if this is as a consequence of apoptosis or higher proliferation of neighbouring non-NCCs. Additionally, as the mature dental pulp forms, the NCC population becomes progressively restricted in terms of its multipotency (Tucker and Sharpe 1999). Nonetheless, an NCC population is retained within the postnatal dental pulp, which makes an attractive source of cells for tissue engineering of connective tissues and nervous system.

MSCs in primary dentinogenesis and dentine repair

During tooth development ectomesenchymal cells at the periphery of the developing dental papillae interface with the inner enamel epithelia cells, separated by a continuous basement membrane. Through complex reciprocal mesenchymal-epithelial signalling pathways, together with compositional and structural modification of the basement membrane, these preodontoblast cells sequentially withdraw from the cell cycle and overtly differentiate into odontoblasts (Ruch 1998) capable of synthesising first predentine, the matrix of which is remodelled to allow for deposition of mineralised dentine. Significantly, the mature odontoblast polarises and develops a cell body, rich in organelles, adopting a basal position of the cells lining the basement membrane. With the formation of primary dentine, the cell body retreats pulpally, away from the inner enamel epithelium producing a long cellular process, extending the entire width of the predentine and the dentine and is responsible for producing the "tubular" structure of the primary tissue. These odontoblasts remain viable within the adult tooth and protect the pulp by localised upregulation of dentine synthesis, called reactionary dentine, in response to mild caries or pathological trauma (Lesot et al., 1993). However, significant injury to the pulp may lead to odontoblast death. In this scenario, a population of dental pulp stem cells (DPSCs) resident within the pulpal tissue are recruited to the site of tissue injury, where they proliferate and subsequently differentiate into odontoblast-like cells that secrete a reparative dentine matrix representing either an atubular amorphous mineralised matrix or sometimes a semi-tubular mineralised matrix with globular and interglobular structures.

Tissue engineering of dentine aims to recapitulate the embryonic events of tooth development to produce a tubular dentine structure, and this has partially been achieved in *in vivo* transplantation studies (see below). *In vitro* studies have been more successful in the synthesis of mineralised matrix more akin to reparative dentine, confirmed through the expression of dentine siaolphosphoprotein gene. Within the dentine pulp complex, reparative dentinogenesis is regulated by various growth factors known to play a role in recruitment and functional control of dental pulp stem cells. Those growth factors believed to be responsible for pulpal stem cell control during repair are members of the transforming growth factor beta (TGF-β1) superfamily including BMPs, in addition to platelet-derived growth factor (PDGF), and insulin-like growth factor (IGF) (Tziafas et al., 2001; Iohara et al., 2004; Kim et al., 2010). Several studies have suggested that BMP-7 TGF-β1 and -β3 may

mediate dentine matrix secretion in a 3D organotypic culture system (Sloan and Smith, 1999; Sloan et al., 2000). Also crucial from a clinical translational aspect, but currently poorly understood, is the response of the DPSCs to the cells and proinflammatory cytokines as part of the inflammatory response following pulpal injury. Cytokines generated as part of the inflammatory response are proposed to contribute to the initiation of the reparative phase of wound healing, as established for tissue wound healing in general (Boleman et al., 2012). If prolonged or inappropriate, the inflammatory response may adversely affect the function of such growth factors (e.g., BMP-7), which become insufficient to induce dentine formation within the inflamed pulp compared with healthy tissue (Rutherford and Gu, 2000).

SHEDs, SCAPs, and DPSC

MSCs were first isolated from the dental pulp of adult teeth by Gronthos and Shi and coworkers (Gronthos et al., 2000, 2002; Shi and Gronthos, 2003). Isolated by digestion with collagenase, the DPSCs were capable of forming colonies with different density, growth rates, size, and morphology suggesting that clonal variation may exist. Some clones, but not all are capable of high proliferation even after extended culture (Gronthos et al., 2002). Clonal variation has been further confirmed by recent studies indicating that expression of MSC cell surface markers varies greatly between clones and expression levels change both up and down during extended culture (Harrington et al., 2014). DPSCs and selected clonal cell lines have successfully been differentiated to form adipogenic, chondrogenic, myogenic, neurogenic, and osteogenic lineages as determined by the detection of tissue-specific transcription or matrix markers at either the mRNA gene level or the protein level (Table 3.1) (Gronthos et al., 2002; Laino et al., 2005; Zhang et al., 2006; d'Aquino et al., 2007).

In vivo studies have suggested that DPSCs are more lineage restricted compared to bone marrow–derived MSCs (BMMSCs). When transplanted into the dorsal surface of immunocompromised mice, BMMSCs produced bone-like tissue, with osteocytes evident, whilst DPSC produced dentine-like tissue with cytoplasmic processes extending into the matrix interfacing with a vascularised pulplike material (Gronthos et al., 2000).

Table 3.1 Multipotentiality towards the formation of mesenchymal connective tissues is a principle characterisation for defining an MSC. Dental pulp stem cells (DPSCs), stem cells from human exfoliated teeth (SHEDs), and stem cells from apical papilla (SCAPs) have all demonstrated variable multipotential characteristics as determined by the appearance of cell surface markers, transcription factors, deposition of extracellular matrix proteins, minerals and fatty acids, and cell morphology, characterising a specified differentiation pathway. Ideally, characterisation of lineage commitment and the differentiated cell should utilise a triplicate of markers tracing the differentiation process. (Modified information from Huang et al., 2009.)

Differentiated Cell	Differentiation Marker	MSC Derivation
Osteoblast	Transcription factors RUNX2, Osterix, matrix proteins, osteonectin, bone sialoprotein, osteocalcin; alkaline phosphatase (not bone specific); histological staining of calcium mineral deposition with alizarin red or von Kossa	DPSCs SHEDs SCAPs
Adipocyte	Peroxisome proliferator-activated receptor gamma (PPAR-γ) lipoprotein lipase, fatty acid binding protein 4 (FABP4), adipocyte CCAAT/enhancer binding protein alpha (C/EBPα), adiponectin; histological staining of intracellular lipid globules with oil red O or LipidTOX™	DPSCs SHEDs SCAPs
Chondrocytes	Type II collagen, aggrecan, Sox9; histological staining of high glycosaminoglycan content with toluidine blue or safranin-O	DPSCs SHEDs
Myoblast	Expression of transcription factors MyoD1, myogenin, PAX7; formation of fused multinucleated, myocin heavy chain positive, myotubes	DPSCs SHEDs
Neuronal	Synapsin, synatophysin, neurofilament 1, MAP-2; histological observation of neurosphere-like bodies	DPSCs SHEDs SCAPs
Odontoblast	Osteoblast marker plus DSPP of dentine sialoprotein; formation of a dentinal tubule *in vivo*.	DPSCs SHEDs SCAPs

The additional presence of hydroxyapatite/tricalcium phosphate or dentine matrix, leads to similar results (Batouli et al., 2003). Compared to BMMSCs, DPSCs appear to be more restricted in their ability for multipotency, with the heterogeneous MSC populations preferring to differentiate to cells capable of forming dentine and pulp. This may relate to functional adaptation of the cells in the mature tissue, where cells in dental tissues are only required to synthesise reparative dentine and remodel pulp in response to trauma, whilst bony tissues require an MSC population for continual remodelling. Strategies to increase multipotency involve refinement of the culture media to stimulate the less restricted cell populations or reprogramming of the DSPCs to induce pluripotent stem cells by forced expression of embryonic genes such as Oct4 (Pou5f1), Sox2, cMyc, and Klf4 (see Chapter 1).

An alternative approach to increase multipotency has been to isolate MSCs from less aged teeth (Figure 3.2). Studies examining stem cells from human exfoliated teeth (SHEDs), suggested that these teeth do indeed contain a more immature MSC population compared with DPSCs. SHEDs are highly proliferative and clonogenic, readily forming into colonies. They also demonstrated greater potentiality in differentiating more readily into a variety

of cell types compared with DPSCs (Miura et al., 2003). Increased expression of nestin may suggest an increased presence of neural crest cells (Miura et al., 2003). *In vivo*, SHEDs still show greater commitment to the formation of a mineralised tissue resembling dentine (Luisi et al., 2007; Wei et al., 2007) following transplantation into mice. By virtue of their greater potentiality of the non-selected MSC populations, SHEDs have been promoted by some researchers as ideal for tissue banking with potential use in a wide range of cell-based therapies.

Researchers have also isolated "stem cells from apical papilla" of developing teeth (SCAPs) (Sonoyama et al., 2008) and the immature papilla root–forming stage of rat incisors (Lei et al., 2011). Isolated from an embryonic-like tissue of the developing root, the MSC pool is responsible for the formation of root dentine, dental papilla, cementum, and alveolar bone. SCAPs have a higher proliferation rate compared to DSPCs (Sonoyama et al., 2008) and readily differentiate down osteogenic, adipogenic, chondrogenic, and neurogenic lineages. However, as for SHEDs and DPSCs, they retain a preference to differentiate into odontoblasts when transplanted into immunocompromised mice (Sonoyama et al., 2008), and preliminary evidence suggests that

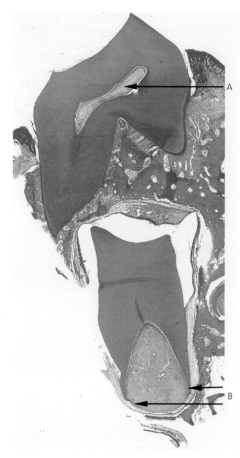

Figure 3.2 Resorbing deciduous tooth providing MSC source for SHEDs (A). The developing roots of the tooth below provide a potential source for SCAPs (B), which may be harvested during tooth eruption prior to closure of the root apices.

these cells are more effective in making primary dentine with increased odontoblast polarisation and tubular structure. Conversely, MSCs from DPSCs are more capable of differentiating into odontoblast-like cells capable of making tertiary reparative dentine, which has a less tubular and more amorphous structure compared with primary dentine.

Classical markers of a mesenchymal stem cell?

A clear issue within stem cell research is their characterisation. For the literature relating to just DPSCs alone, different methodologies are used for isolation, culture

expansion, and characterisation of mesenchymal stem cells. The presence of different cell populations means that caution should be made when directly comparing the various studies. An attempt was suggested in the year 2006 by the Mesenchymal and Tissue Stem Cell Committee of the International Society for Cellular Therapy, who proposed "minimal criteria" to define mesenchymal stem cells (Dominici et al., 2006). They proposed three criteria to define human mesenchymal stem cells used in laboratory-based investigations, although they recognised that standards may need revision as new data arise, and the criteria may not apply in non-human systems. The first criterion is that MSCs must be plastic adherent when being maintained with standard culture conditions in tissue culture flasks, which is a property well described in the literature (Colter et al., 2000). The second criterion states that greater than 95% MSCs should express specific surface antigens: CD73 (an ecto 5' nucleotidase), CD90 (Thy-1), and CD105 (endoglin). In addition, cells should be less than 2% positive for haematopoietic antigens CD45 (pan-leukocyte marker), CD34 (endothelial cells and primitive haematopoietic progenitors), CD14 or CD11b (both for monocytes and macrophages), CD79α or CD19 (B-cell markers), and HLA class II (although human leukocyte antigen can be expressed by mesenchymal stem cells when stimulated with interferon gamma). However, weaknesses in using this triplicate marker collection are now emerging with studies demonstrating the expression of CD73, CD90, and CD105 on mature fibroblastic cells (Brohem et al., 2013). CD105 is also known as endoglin or TGF-β receptor III. TGF-β signalling plays an important role from the very early stages of bone and dentine repair and throughout tissue healing period (Dimitriou, 2005). CD105 and CD73 are proposed to be involved in several MSC functions, but both are also present in endothelial lineage cells. CD90 has also been described to be involved in the adhesion of monocytes and leukocytes. Moreover, CD90 demonstrates a consistent expression in humans, but it is described as absent in sheep and goat, and two isoforms (Thy1.1 and Thy1.2, varying by one amino acid) have been observed in mice. As a word of warning here, the absence or low detection of the marker may relate to nature of the antibody used.

For the third and final criterion, MSCs must, as a minimum demonstrate tripotentiality, capable of differentiating into osteoblasts, chondroblasts, and adipocytes, using *in vitro* differentiating conditions (Protocol 3.4) or commercially available kits. The demonstration of differentiation is fairly basic in its requirement. Osteoblast differentiation is demonstrated using alizarin red or von Kossa staining to detect mineralisation; chondroblast differentiation is shown by alcian blue staining for glyco-proteins or immunohistochemical detection of collagen type II; oil red O staining for lipids demonstrates adipo-cyte differentiation. Many studies provide much further characterisation with the identification of specific tran-scription factors or matrix proteins defining the respec-tive cell differentiation pathways (Table 3.1). Ideally, this should be performed to demonstrate expression at gene level of the mRNA and followed through to confirm translation and synthesis of the protein.

Alternative markers for mesenchymal stem cells

Other cell surface antigens are available and their use in evaluating the presence of a mesenchymal stem cell present in dental pulp and other tissue sources, such as bone marrow and adipose tissue, have been well reported in the literature (Table 3.2). Initial studies heavily relied on the presence of Stro-1, a trypsin-resis-tant cell surface receptor, to characterise MSCs in dental pulp. However, Stro-1 positive cells are absent from adipose tissue, despite studies indicating that MSCs are found in relative abundance in this tissue (Kern et al., 2006). Studies in bone marrow have subsequently sug-gested that Sto-1 positive cells represent only a subpop-ulation of cells capable of osteogenic differentiation. Conscious that the adult MSC population derive from the ectomesenchymal tissue enriched by neural crest cells, the detection of cells positive for low affinity nerve growth factor receptor (LNGFR), also known as P75 or CD271, have been successful in detecting a subpopula-tion in dental pulp (Waddington et al., 2009). In BMMSCs, LNGFR is observed to be lost during culture expansion (Jones et al., 2002), which may indicate that either the inductive signals for its continued expression are lost or that other LNGFR MSC stem cell populations proliferate at a greater rate to become the predominant MSC population. Similar restraints may be applied when using other embryonic stem cell markers such as Oct4, Nanog, Twist, Snai1, and Sox2 to characterise the MSC population.

The search for a marker for MSCs has thus proved troublesome, but it has also been successful in establishing the heterogeneous nature of MSCs in dental pulp. That cells fall into a hierarchical structure (Figure 3.1) is now proposed for a number of stem cells derived from various tissue sources and may account for the observed heterogeneity. The model describes that those transit amplifying cells that closely derive from the mother stem cell demonstrate the greatest potential to form large colonies with high proliferation rates and the highest multipotentiality, capable of dif-ferentiating into multiple cell lineages. As the transit amplifying cells continue to expand and divide, cells are proposed to decrease in their proliferative potential, forming smaller colonies. At the same time the transit amplifying cells are proposed to become more lineage restricted, demonstrating quadri-potentiality through to tri-, bi-, and ultimately unipotentiality. The model allows for the proliferation of transit amplifying cells, giving rise to large numbers of terminally differentiated cells with no proliferative capacity. As the transit ampli-fying cells proliferate and alter their potentiality, the profile of cell surface markers would be expected to change to meet the new biological function of the cell. The model also helps explain the potential to lose cell surface markers, especially embryonic markers, during culture expansion.

Recognising that stem cells are heterogeneous in nature, the use of cell markers is better employed for understanding the biological activity of the cell and predicting its subsequent activity, allowing selection of cells to meet a therapeutic need. Consequently, a long list of cell surface markers is now available that characterises the function of the cell (Table 3.2, reviewed by Docheva et al., 2008). Growth factors such as FGF (fibroblast growth factor), PDGF, IGF, TGF-β, and EGF (epidermal growth factor) have all been identified as necessary for regulating colony formation, self-renewal, and early stages of cell com-mitment (Kuznetsov, 1997). The presence of the corresponding receptor on the surface of the MSC would be prerequisite for functional activity. Important cell-matrix receptors are the integrins, which collec-tively affect cellular processes including cell spreading, migration, proliferation differentiation, and apoptosis. The expression of α5β1 has been shown to be prefer-entially expressed on primitive cells where they are proposed to play a role in the constrained localisation

Table 3.2 Protein markers used to characterise mesenchymal stem cells. MSCs are now regarded as heterogeneous in nature; therefore, there is no one unifying mesenchymal stem cell marker as markers appear or disappear depending upon their proliferation rate and differentiation potentiality.

MSC Source	Marker	Purported Function
Classical mesenchymal markers	STRO-1, CD73 membrane bound ecto-5′-nucleotisidase, CD90 Thy1, CD105 endoglin, CD271 Low affinity nerve growth factor, CD146 MCAM	
Signal transduction molecules	SH2, SH3, SH4, Stat-3	Activated by protein tyrosine kinases
Cytoskeletal molecules	Smooth muscle α Actin, vimentin	
Telomere regulator	hTERT, hTR	Maintains telomere length of rapidly dividing cells
Growth factor receptors	EGFR, BFGFR, IGFR, PDGFR, TGF-βRI, and RII	Important for self-renewal and lineage commitment
Chemokine receptors	CCR1, CCR2, CCR4, CCR6, CCR7, CCR9, CCR10, CXR1, CXCR2, CXCR4, CXCR5, CXCR6, CX3CR1, CXCL12, HGFR (c-met)	Pivotal role in homing, migration, and engraftment of MSCs
Cytokine receptors	IL-1R, IL-3R, IL-4R, IL-6R, IL-7R, IFNγR and TNFI, and IIR	Migration via increased expression of chemokines
Cell matrix receptors	Integrin subunit α1, α2, α3, α5, α6, αV, β1 (CD29), β3, β5, CD44	Important for cell attachment and cell survival
Cell-cell receptors	Notch receptors and their ligands Jagged-1, Jagged-2, DLL-1, DLL-3, DLL-4	Cell-cell communication and control of multiple cell differentiation processes
Cell adhesion	CD34, CD106 (VCAM), CD166 (ALCAM)	
Immuno-modulatory	HLA-A, HLA-B, HLA-C, HLA-DR, HLA-I, HLA-DP, HLA-DQ; TLRs 1, 2, 3, 4, 5, 6, 9; soluble factors indoleamine 2,3-dioxygenase (IDO); IL-6, IL-10	T cell inhibition, antigen presentation, cytokine production
Transcription factors	E2F2, PTTG1, TWIST-1, LDB2, Oct4, Oct4A, Nanog, Sox2, Slug, Snai1	Cell growth and survival; positive regulator of cell maturation

of the MSC within its niche through its binding to fibronectin (Jones and Watt 1993). Chemokine receptors play a pivotal role in MSC homing, migration, and engraftment to wound repair sites. Cytokine receptors allow MSCs to respond to proinflammatory cytokines, for example, IL-1β and TNFα, stimulating MSCs to produce further cytokines and chemokines for autocrine and paracrine signalling to provide trophic support in the early stages of tissue regeneration. The presence of cell surface receptors of the immunoglobulin superfamily, such as ICAM-1 and -2, VCAM-1, and ALCAM, have been identified on MSCs where they facilitate an array of cell-cell interactions with immune and endothelial cells and potentially play a role in binding T cells and playing an immune-modulatory role. Following priming with IFN gamma, MSCs increase their expression of major histocompatibility complex (MHC) class 2 molecules, although low levels of MHC class 1 are constitutively expressed at low levels by MSCs (see Chapter 2).

Using MSC markers to identify potential stem cell niches

The mother stem cell sits within a stem cell niche where several physical and chemical factors within the micro-environment provide trophic support to maintain the stem cell characteristics. Unfortunately, the location of the stem cell niches has proved difficult to definitively identify. The original identification of STRO-1 positive MSCs, with high colony forming efficiency, from dental pulp also found the presence of vascular cell markers, CD146 and α smooth muscle actin, and pericyte antigen 3G5 in the same cell population (Shi and Gronthos, 2003; Miura et al., 2003). This lead to the proposal that stem cells resided in a perivascular niche for stem/progenitor cells within pulp. Activation of the stem cell niche following wounding has also indicated the presence of stem cell niches in other areas of the dental pulp. This has been achieved by the *in vivo* monitoring of members of the

Notch signalling family that are proposed to regulate stem cell fate specification and are activated in response to injury. Following a series of pulp capping experiments in mice and *in situ* hybridization, the upregulation of Notch expression has respectively identified potential niches in the subodontoblast layer near the wound site and in pulp stroma surrounded by coronal odontoblasts (Lovschall et al., 2005, 2007). The upregulation of Rgs5, a marker for pericytes, and coexpressing with Notch 3, additionally confirmed the importance of stem cell niches in perivascular structures (Lovschall et al., 2007). A characteristic of the mother cell is its slow cell division, and by the administration of a pulse of the thymidine homologue, BrdU, to prenatal animals, studies have indicated the presence of a slow-cycling putative stem or progenitor population that resides centrally in the postnatal dental pulp (Ishikawa et al., 2010). Of note, these studies have shown the presence of a dense label-retaining cell population, presumed to be DPSCs, which were identified throughout the dental pulp 2 weeks postnatally. The number of labelled cells subsequently decreased to reach a plateau low by 4 weeks, and these cells were mainly located in the central pulp, associated with the blood vessel. Interestingly, this population of cells did not always colocalise with STRO-1 or the vascular cell marker CD146, indicating differential expression of markers even within a stem cell niche. A more granular BrdU-staining cell population is also described as the presumed transit amplifying (TA) cells, which increase in number throughout the pulpal tissue as it develops postnatally. Injury and transplantation studies have led to the proposal that these TA cells are the first to differentiate into new odontoblast-like cells following cavity-induced injury. The DPSC population numbers remain static within the tissue and are assumed to actively proliferate to play a crucial role in the pulpal reorganisation of the healing tissue, following endogenous stimuli in cooperation with the TA cells as part of the wound healing process. Although requiring further definitive evidence, this hypothesis is strengthened by previous studies monitoring *ex vivo* BrdU uptake by proliferative cells responding to injury, that have suggested that the progenitor/stem cell niches reside in the perivascular regions of the pulpal cavity, from where they migrated to the site of injury (Tecles et al., 2005), possibly as replacement of the TA cells.

In vivo analysis of MSCs in dental pulp

In moving towards a translational goal, a number of studies have transplanted MSCs from dental pulp into immunocompromised mice and tissue defects. On the whole, these studies are looking towards the utilisation of DPSCs in cell-based therapies or in the organ generation of the tooth. As highlighted above, DPSCs or SHEDs have been transplanted either subcutaneously in immunocompromised mice (Gronthos et al., 2000, 2002, Seo et al., 2004, Huang et al., 2009) or seeded into rat renal capsules, which offer an immunocompromised capacity (Yu et al., 2007). In general, cells are seeded into either collagen sponges or using a hydroxyapatite/tricalcium phosphate to provide a scaffold and to help provide an osteoconductive-like environment. For both models the regeneration of a dentine-like tissue was observed, with evidence of odontoblast processes producing a tubular structure and the formation of a dentine-pulp complex. The host environment receiving the transplanted cells will be a major consideration in the success of these experiments. As discussed above, tooth development critically relies on the interaction of the ectomesenchymal cells with the oral epithelial cells in instructing their differentiation into polarised odontoblast cells, forming cells with a long cytoplasmic process traversing the entire width of dentine matrix and a cell body containing the nucleus and rich endoplasmic reticulum at the dentine-pulp interface. Post-development of the tooth bud, the ectomesenchymal cells are regarded to command the instructive signalling influence in directing tooth shape and development, whilst the signals of the epithelium provide a permissive signalling role. When cells are transplanted into mice, the availability of mesenchymal-epithelial interaction with cells within the dorsal surface or renal capsule has likely facilitated odontoblast formation, mirroring embryonic tooth developmental events. The observation that BMMSCs transplanted into the same sites develop into a bone-like tissue suggests that the DPSCs have retained some of this instructive power acquired in initiating the process of tooth development. When DPSCs or SHEDs are seeded into bone defects, the cells differentiate into bone-like tissue (Zheng et al., 2009; d'Aquino et al., 2009; Alkaisi et al., 2013).

Cell transplantation experiments into dorsal and renal surfaces provide not only for epithelial-mesenchymal interactions when required, but also a wound healing environment to promote tissue regeneration. The early events of the inflammatory phase result in the initiation of the clotting cascade, with the release of various soluble factors such as chemokines and cytokines, which facilitate migration of cells to the healing site. Angiogenesis will be initiated together with an influx of neutrophils and macrophages, all contributing to the ever-changing signalling environment. However, for cell transplantation into areas such as the renal capsule, immunocompromised animals are required, and an absence of T and B lymphocytes and NK cells will alter the immune response. Alternatively, cells can be transplanted into critical size defects made in bone tissue in animal models. Whilst these experiments do not require immunocompromised animals and thus repair mechanisms involve signalling from lymphocytes, these models invariably lead to the formation of a bone-like reparative tissue due to the absence of epithelial-mesenchymal interactions. It is also worth bearing in mind here the limitations or restrictions for data retrieval using any cell transplantation models. Whilst in *in vivo* experimental models all cells are *in situ*, the added complexity and the difficult task of extracting molecular mechanistic data justifies our equal reliance on *in vitro* studies for providing biological data to fully understand regulatory processes.

In vitro analysis of MSCs in dental pulp

A plethora of studies have examined dental pulp stem cells *in vitro*. Unfortunately, there is no one standardised protocol for the isolation of these cells, which has made for a literature reporting varied cell responses. Cells may be obtained from culture of pulp tissue explants or by the dissociation of the cells by digestion of the extracellular matrix components with trypsin or collagenase dispase. The former method has been developed on the principle that MSCs are adherent to plastic. Methodological studies have compared DPSC cultures established following enzymatic digestion from the extracellular matrix and by direct outgrowth from pulpal tissue explants (Bakopoulou et al., 2011) and determined that enzymatic digestion generated a cell population which was richer in STRO-1 and CD34, possibly as a consequence of the release of stem cells from the perivascular niche (Gronthos et al., 2000). The enzymatically released cells displayed an enhanced

mineralisation capacity, laying down an osteodentin-like matrix determined through the expression of dentine sialoprotein, indicating a more valuable MSC population for investigating dentinal repair processes. Whist regarded as a necessary step, enzymatic treatment of cells presents issues with removal of cell surface receptors, or the increased presence of matrix degradation components potentially influencing cell signalling networks and hence the short- or long-term cellular behaviour of the MSC. Release of cells from dental pulp tissue therefore utilised mild enzymatic conditions involving collagenase and dispase for periods up to 1 hour (Protocol 3.1).

Whilst cells released by enzymatic procedures do demonstrate the "classical" stem cell markers, they are likely to be heterogeneous in nature, representing all the different cells present within the hierarchical structure (Figure 3.1), with differences in proliferation rates and differentiation potentiality. Differentiated pulpal fibroblasts of MSC origin and therefore plastic adherent would also be expected to be present. A variety of methods have been adopted in an attempt to select for specific cell surface markers to produce an "enriched" cell population (Figure 3.3).

The high expression of ß1 integrins in primitive cells has been exploited through the preferential adherence to fibronectin-coated wells, selecting those cells which adhere within the first 20 minutes from seeding (Waddington et al., 2009; Jones and Watt, 1993) (Protocol 3.2). An MSC side population, selected through their failure to incorporate the DNA binding dye Hoechst 33342 due to low cell cycling has also been characterised from dental pulp (Iohara et al., 2006).

Using cell sorting, such as fluorescent activated or magnetic activated cell sorting, MSCs enriched for particular cell surface receptors have been have been isolated and characterised (Gronthos et al., 2011). Early studies by Shi and Gronthos (2003) derived STRO-1 positive DPSCs, which also possessed vascular antigens known to be expressed on endothelial cells such as CD146 and the pericyte antigen 3G5, localising these cells to a perivascular niche. While a high percentage of DPSCs expressed these markers, comparative studies indicated that only a minor population of STRO-1 positive cells from BMMSC were found to be positive for 3G5, suggested different cellular phenotypes representing different perivascular cell populations, although both populations were capable of differentiation into

Protocol 3.1 Enzymatic release of dental pulp progenitor cells.

1. Prepare antibiotic serum-free medium: αMEM (with ribonucleosides, deoxyribonucleosides), 100 units/mL penicillin, 1 µg/mL streptomycin sulphate and 0.25 µg/mL amphotericin.
2. Obtain caries-free teeth; growing incisors of 4 week-old rats or mice; 3rd molars or 1st/2nd premolars human teeth with appropriate ethics.
3. Sterilise by soaking in 70% ethanol; remove soft tissue from outer surface using a sterilised scalpel.
4. For rodent teeth, split longitudinally using a scalpel.
5. For human teeth cut a groove in the centre of three areas (mesial, distal, and occlusal) with a rotary diamond edged bone saw; fracture along grooves using a chisel and hammer on a dissection board.
6. Remove pulp and maintain hydration by placing into αMEM (pre-supplemented with DNA and RNA) plus antibiotics.
7. Mince pulp tissue on a glass slide in small amount of media and transfer into 5 mL bijoux tubes containing 1 mL of 4 µg/µL collagenase/dispase.
8. Incubate pulpal tissue for 1 h, with regular agitation every 20 min, to increase cell dissociation. Ensure that pulpal tissues from individual teeth are prepared separately.
9. Pass digested pulpal tissue through a 70 µm mesh cell strainer and collect single cell suspension in a 50 mL Falcon tube.
10. Pass a further 10 mL medium through the cell strainer to ensure all cells are collected.
11. Centrifuge cells at 1,800 rpm for 5 min and resuspend in 1 mL medium.
12. Take 10 µL aliquot of cell suspension and add 0.4% trypan blue stain; count vital and nonvital cells using a haemocytometer by light microscopy.

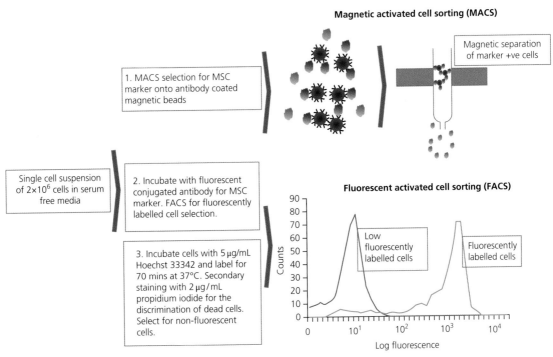

Figure 3.3 Application of FACS and MACS in the selection of side populations such as STRO-1, CD146, or CD34-positive cells. Cells can be dual labelled for the selection of cells, although neither method will provide the sole isolation of cells carrying both markers. Alternatively, the procedure can be repeated for the further selection of an MSC-positive cell within the isolated side population. FACS can also be used to characterise the presence of MSC markers. For detailed protocols, reader is best referred to manufacturer's instructions.

Protocol 3.2 Fibronectin adhesion selection of ß1 integrins expressing immature MSCs.

1. Prepare 10 µg/mL fibronectin (human plasma) in 0.1 M phosphate-buffered saline (PBS), pH 7.4 containing 1 mM Ca^{2+} and 1 mM Mg^{2+}.
2. Prepare culture media: αMEM (with ribonucleosides and deoxyribonucleosides), 20% heat-inactivated foetal calf serum, 4 mM L-glutamine, 100 µM L-ascorbate 2-phosphate and antibiotics/antimycotics. Also prepare approximately 50 mL of the same culture media containing no serum.
3. Precoat wells of 6 well plates with fibronectin (1 mL/well) and leave overnight.
4. Remove excess fibronectin solution and seed each well with 4,000 cells/cm² isolated in protocol 1 in 1 mL serum-free culture media. Leave cells to adhere at 37°C, 5% CO_2 for 20 min.
5. Remove nonadherent cells (save as nonadherent cells may be of interest) and add 2 mL fresh serum culture medium. Incubate at 37°C, 5% CO_2, changing the media every 2 days.
6. During culture, monitor cell appearance using an inverted light microscope at x10 magnification. Record daily the number of cells and colonies with >32 cells. Record the colony efficiency as the number of colonies on day x / 24 hr total cell count.
7. By day 12, isolated colonies should be identifiable. Cultures may be continued to allow cells to continue to expand as merged heterogeneous MSC population, or colonies may be isolated following Protocol 3.3.
8. At each passage count total cell numbers for each culture vessel. Calculate population doublings (PD) across each passage:

$$PD = \left(log_{10} \left[cell\ count\ at\ time\ of\ passage \right] - log_{10} \left[cell\ count\ originally\ seeded\ into\ culture\ vessel \right] \right) / log_{10}(2)$$

9. Plot cumulative PD against cumulative days in culture.

---

osteoblast-like cells producing a mineralised matrix. The positive selection for STRO-1 identified a population able to differentiate into an odontoblast-like phenotype, whilst negative cells showed a more fibroblast-like phenotype (Yang et al., 2007). In contract, selection of DPSCs for CD105+/CD31-/CD146- cells identified a cellular subfraction with enhanced potential for regeneration of the pulp tissue with enhanced vascular and neuronal potential (Nakashima and Iohara, 2011). Although c-kit and CD34 are regarded as markers for haematopoietic cells, DPSCs have been sorted for c-kit+/CD34+/CD45- cell population, which was highly clonigenic and in appropriate culture conditions differentiated into osteoblasts (Laino et al., 2005, 2006). The jury is still out for deliberations as to whether selection of side populations is advantageous for use in tissue engineering therapies. Recent studies have suggested that selection for STRO-1 was able to differentiate into an osteoblast phenotype similar to the non-selected cells (Yang et al., 2007).

Selection based on one marker may still yield a heterogeneous MSC population with variable clonal populations demonstrating variable proliferation rates and multipotentiality. The approach can, however, provide important data in elucidating the nature of the various MSC populations present in dental pulp and the importance of the various side populations in dentine repair process.

The study of clonal cell lines versus heterogeneous populations

Clonal isolation of MSC populations has been important in elucidating the heterogeneity of the MSC population present in dental pulp. Within these studies clonal cell lines have been established from a single cell isolated from the tissue matrix (Protocol 3.3). Early studies by Gronthos et al. (2000) demonstrated that only approximately 20% of single cell–derived DPSC colonies/clones were able to proliferate beyond 20 population doublings. Further, the odontogenic potential of 12 individual single-colony-derived DPSC strains demonstrated that two-thirds of clones generated abundant ectopic dentin *in vivo*, while only a limited amount of dentin was detected in the remaining one-third (Gronthos et al., 2002), thus suggesting that DPSCs have subset populations that differ in their ability for odontogenesis due to different proliferative capacities and developmental potential. More recent analysis has demonstrated that the colony-forming efficiency for DPSCs was 12 times greater than the colony-forming efficiency for BMMSCs (Harrington et al., 2014). This perhaps concurs with the higher stem cell population present in dental pulp; however, DPSCs formed smaller colonies with $<1.5 \times 10^3$ cells at day 12 compared with BMMSC colonies that averaged 3.3×10^3 cells. Moreover, only 10% of DPSC

Protocol 3.3 Isolation of clonal colonies following low density seeding onto fibronectin-coated plates.

1. Identify the colony under an inverted light microscope and with a marker pen draw an identification position on the underside of the plate. Smear petroleum jelly around one edge of a sterile cloning ring. Cutting a 1 mL pipette tip to obtain the collar as a cylindrical tube works equally well. Place over the colony jelly edge to plate to form a watertight seal.
2. Dissociate cells in the cloning ring with 100 μL accutase or trypsin, 5 min (37°C, 5% CO_2). Transfer each colony into one well of a 98-well plate and maintain cells in 5% CO_2, 37°C.
3. When cells are 80% confluent, passage cells. Wash cells with 0.1 M PBS, pH 7.4 before treating with 2 mL accutase, 37°C, 5 min or until cells become detached. Inactivate accutase by addition of equal volume of serum containing culture medium. Recover cells by centrifuging at 1800 rpm, 5 min. Keep cells recovered from individual wells separate.
4. Resuspend cells in culture medium and plate cells from 1 well of a 98-well plate into 1 well of a 48-well plate. Continue to culture expand by passaging into increasing well/flask size to T75.

clones were successfully propagated to over 40 population doublings, with high and low proliferative clones identifiable. By comparison, approximately 50% BMMSC clones were successfully expanded to beyond 40 population doublings and demonstrated a more consistently higher growth rate. Bone marrow clones demonstrated consistent tri-potentiality, whilst dental pulp clones were more bi- or uni-potential in forming a diffuse mineralised matrix. Of note for those clones that were successfully expanded in culture, the expression of the more immature MSC markers Snai1 and Nanog were maintained, although markers such as VCAM1 (CD106), MCAM (CD 145), and Msx2 did fluctuate greatly during the culture period. This perhaps indicates the sensitivity of MSCs to their niche environment; cell density and nutrient/growth factor concentration in the serum supplemented culture medium can greatly vary during a culture passage period, and this can greatly influence the levels of expression of cell surface receptors and transcription factors. If wishing to quantify such markers by methods such as qPCR, then rigorous standardised culture and sampling protocols need to be reported to allow repetition of results.

However, microarray analysis of clonal populations has led to initial identification of common gene expression signatures associated with high growth and high multipotential MSC populations, highlighting high expression of transcription factors with critical roles in cell growth and survival such as E2F2, PTTG1, Twist-1, and transcriptional cofactor LDB2 (Menicanin et al., 2010). For tissue engineering purposes, the isolation of high proliferative MSCs may be advantageous for culture expansion when used in cell-based therapies. Likewise, these may also be the cell population to target when using bioactive matrices to stimulate the resident MSC towards repair. However, which high proliferative clones provide for the ideal cells in producing functional reparative tissue has yet to be elucidated.

A high proportion of *in vitro* and *in vivo* transplantation studies utilise heterogeneous cell populations of MSCs. Cells would therefore be expected to contain high and low proliferative populations with variable differentiation capacity. However, it is perhaps these cell populations that provide the most consistent results in terms of demonstrating initial high proliferation rates and tri-potentiality. This is perhaps because all required cell populations are present, including the mother stem cell, transit amplifying cells, and pulpal fibroblasts. In addition, MSCs could be providing a direct functional role in the direct synthesis of matrix or an indirect role in providing trophic support to the stem cell niche and its development. However, if these cells are to be used clinically, expansion *in vitro* is a prerequisite in order to achieve sufficient cell numbers. Most studies use early passage cells probably in part because of issue with culture expansion. Studies describe loss of stemness, loss of differentiation capacity, and a slowing of the proliferation rate, purportedly due to cell senescence. It is interesting to note that clonal cell lines can also report a decline in proliferation rate, but with continued culture, higher proliferation rates have been restored (Harrington et al., 2014). However, whether expanding a heterogeneous population or a clonal cell line, prolonged proliferation could induce genetic changes that may affect clinical safety. Minimal studies are available in this area, although successful expansion has been obtained for cells taken from explant culture, where culture for 6 months duration did not affect morphology, expression of MSC markers' differentiation capacity, or karyotypic change, even after cryopreservation. However, cell expansion was noted to decrease with extended culture,

Protocol 3.4 Differentiation protocols to determine multipotency in the characterisation of MSCs.

Confirm cells are free from mycoplasma using mycoplasma detection kit (e.g., VenorGeM, Cambio, Cambridge, UK). Treat positive cells with 10 µg/mL Ciprofloxin antibiotic until test negative.

Osteogenesis

1. Seed cells at $4 \times 10^3/cm^2$ in 6-well culture plates and culture in αMEM (with ribonucleasides and deoxyribonucleosides), 10% fetal bovine serum (FBS) (from an approved source), 100 µM L-ascorbic acid 2-phosphate, 10 µM dexamethasone, 10 mM β-glycerophosphate, 1% antibiotic-antimycotic. Change media every 2–3 days. Include cells cultured in absence of dexamethasone and β-glycerophosphate as a control.
2. Culture cells at 37°C, 5% CO_2. Deposition of a mineralised matrix can take between 21 and 35 days.
3. To assess mineral deposition, wash cells twice adjusted with PBS; fix with 10% formaldehyde for 30 min; wash twice with ddH_2O; incubate with 2% w/v alizarin red S (pH 4.2, adjusted with 0.5% ammonium hydroxide)/ddH_2O for 30 min with gentle agitation. Wash cells thrice with ddH_2O. Visualise cells under light microscope.
4. To quantify alizarin red stain, treat stained cells with 800 µL 10% acetic acid for 30 min with constant agitation; scrape cell layer and collect with acetic acid into an Eppendorf; vortex briefly; heat at 85°C, 10 min, then cool on ice; centrifuge at 17,000 g for 15 min; add 500 µL of supernatant to 10% ammoniumhydroxide. After 5 min measure absorbance at 425 nm.
5. Cells can also be analysed at any time point for gene expression of osteogenic genes RUNX2, Osterix, and bone-specific proteins bone sialoprotein and osteocalcin by qPCR.
6. Cells can also be cultured on 32 mm #1 glass round cover slips for immuno-detection of bone-specific protein synthesised into the matrix, confirming qPCR results.

Adipogenesis

1. Seed cells at $3 \times 10^3/cm^2$ in 8-well chamber slides and culture in αMEM, 10% FBS, 100 µM L-ascorbic acid 2-phosphate, 1% antibiotics-antimycotics (basal media) at 37°C, 5% CO_2 until virtually 100% confluent (*NB* cells need to be tightly packed); replace media with adipogenic induction media (basal media supplemented with 10 µg/mL insulin, 1 µM dexamethasone, 100 µM indomethacin, 100 µM 3-isobutyl-1-methylxanthine [IBMX]) for 3 days, then incubate cells with adipogenic maintenance medium (basal media supplemented with 10 µg/mL insulin) for a further 24 h. Repeat culture in induction and maintenance cycles for a total of 28 days. Prepare fresh media and change media every 2 days.
2. Visualise adipocyte differentiation using LipidTOX™ fluorescent neutral lipid stain as per manufacturer's instruction (Thermofisher). Wash cells thrice with PBS. Remove chamber portion from slide and mount using a fluorescent mounting medium with DAPI. Visualise under fluorescent microscope.
3. Cells can also be analysed at any time point for gene expression of adipogenic genes PPARγ, lipoprotein lipase, FABP4, C/EBPα, and adiponectin using qPCR techniques.

Chondrogenesis

1. Pellet a single-cell suspension at 1,500 rpm in sterile Eppendorf at a concentration of 5×10^5 cells per tube in 1 mL of αMEM, 10% FBS, 100 µM L-ascorbic acid 2-phosphate, 1% antibiotics-antimycotics; incubate overnight, 37°C, 5% CO_2; replace media with chondrogenic induction media (αMEM, 10% FBS, 50 µg/mL L-ascorbate, 1× insulin, transferrin, and selenium (ITS), 5 ng/mL transforming growth factor beta 1 (TGF-β1). Change media every 2 days for up to 24 days.
2. Fix pellet with 4% formaldehyde for 24 h; carefully remove the pellet from Eppendorf and wrap in tissue paper; dehydrate the pellet through increasing concentration of ethanol and then paraffin-embed and cut 5 µm sections. Deparaffinise sections with xylene and rehydrate through a series of decreasing ethanol concentrations.
3. Stain with haematoxylin and eosin to observe cell architecture. Visualise under light microscope.
4. Stain for cartilage matrix mucins with Safranin-O. Stain sections first with 0.001% (w/v) Fast green solution in H_2O for 5 min and wash 1% (v/v) acetic acid. Stain sections with 0.1% (w/v) Safranin-O in H_2O for 5 min. Wash sections with xylene and mount using DPX mounting solution. Visualise under light microscope.
5. Cells can also be analysed at any time point for presence of Type II collagen, aggrecan, and Sox9 within the matrix using immunocytochemistry techniques.

presumably as mature cells reached senescence to leave the continued culture of more immature MSCs or transit amplifying cells more recently derived from the mother stem cell (Lizier et al., 2012). As yet, studies have not looked directly at the impact of long-term culture of DPSCs on other age-related characteristics such as telomere length, morphological changes, and increase in actin stress fibres.

Consideration of the microenvironment during analysis of MSCs

As for MSCs from other tissues, DPSC behaviour is susceptible to the physicochemical nature of the environment, such as oxygen tension and oxidative-reductive balance; pH; ionic concentration of ions such as calcium, sodium, and potassium (in generating membrane potential and localised electric fields, and in influencing cell signalling); and stiffness of the culture surface (including protein matrices in 2D and 3D culture) in imposing compressive and tensile strain on the cell, thereby influencing mechano-transduction and cell signalling. Studies have identified changes in MSC behaviour as a consequence of changes in oxygen tension, which are observed as part of the wound healing process.

Early events during wound repair can lead to a transient period of hypoxia as a consequence of vasoconstriction of the capillaries to decrease bleeding. Hypoxia stimulates neovascularisation along with growth factors present in the clotting tissue, although subsequent normalisation of oxygen tension accelerates vascular growth. In necrotising tissue, the hypoxic status is intensified as a result of continued pathological insult and stymied angiogenesis. *In vitro* studies have indicated increased colony formation and proliferation by DPSCs, including an expansion of the STRO-1 positive cells, when cultured in 3%–5% oxygen compared to the normal culture condition of 21% (Iida et al., 2010; Sakdee et al., 2009). When these cells are cultured in mineralising conditions, increased osteo/odontogenic differentiation has been reported (Lei et al., 2011). Hypoxic conditions increase the expression of the hypoxia-inducible transcription factor 1α (HIF-1α), which regulates over 100 genes, including those associated with angiogenesis and inflammation (Aranha et al., 2010). It is of note that whilst this gene is upregulated in both DPSCs and pulpal fibroblasts, it is only the

conditioned media derived from the differentiated cells that are able to stimulate angiogenesis *in vitro*, indicating different responses dependent upon the differentiation status of the cell. Whilst not an aim of these studies, the control of oxygen tension may provide a route for culture expansion of DPSCs. Definitive evidence is required before translation for clinical practice.

The culture media, which vary with respect to their ionic concentration of salts, amino acids, and vitamin supplementation, can influence cellular behaviour, particularly with respect to cellular expansion. Lizier et al. (2012) have produced a comparative study and demonstrated that alpha minimum essential medium (αMEM) provided an optimised culture media. Cell expansion rapidly reduced with time when cultured in Dulbecco's modified Eagle's medium (low glucose), with cells failing to proceed beyond the seventh passage, although further supplementation with F12 was able to produce growth curves similar to those recorded for DPSC cultured in αMEM.

Epigenetics and posttranslational regulation of DPSC behaviour

An emerging and likely important area for research is the control of stem cell gene expression or cellular phenotype by factors that externally modify the DNA or influence mRNA activity to turn genes on or off. Epigenetic regulation involves changes to the DNA structure such as enzymatic modification of the cytosine nucleotide base to silence promoter sequences or covalent modification of specified lysine residues on histone tails to bring about changes in the chromatin structure to expose or hide specific genes. Modification can be achieved by methylation, acetylation, phosphylation, and ubiquitination. There is increasing recognition that epigenetic mechanisms are involved in the dynamic activation or repression of genes during developmental processes leading right through to terminal differentiation. This is best exemplified following the differentiation of ES cells into the three germ layers, which is accompanied by an increased number of commonly methylated DNA regions (Isagawa et al., 2011). In MSCs histone modification is proposed to play a role in determining differentiation potentiality and lineage specification (Collas, 2010; Noer et al., 2009). Studies comparing histone methyltransferases in MSCs derived from the dental pulp and the dental follicle have indicated differential signature patterns which have been proposed to be responsible for the higher expression of pluripotency associated genes, such as Oct4, Nanog, and Sox2 in DPSCs and the repression of dentine sialophosphoprotein and dentine matrix 1 in dental follicle MSCs. The application of histone deacetylase inhibitors has been shown to increase differentiation potential of primary dental pulp cells towards cells producing mineralised matrix associated proteins, with the study highlighting the potential use of such agents in promoting reparative dentine formation (Duncan et al., 2013). Inflammation in human dental pulp is proposed to be associated with reduced methylation of the promoter region of the IFNγ gene and has been used to explain the increased expression of IFNγ in inflamed pulps (Cardoso et al., 2010). At present, studies in this area are few and far between, and confirmation of these observations and hypotheses are still necessary. Moreover, as the number of histone modification enzymes identified approaches 80-plus, the number of permutations for covalent modification for just the main histone proteins, H3, H4, H2A, and H2B is extremely high, emphasising the complexity in the control mechanisms.

Post-translational modification can also play a role in modifying the functionality of a regulatory protein. An example is the ubiquitination of neural crest specifiers such as Twist, Snai1, and Snai2 proteins, which are proposed to regulate the formation of neural crest stem cells, epithelial mesenchymal transition, and migration of the cells from the neuronal tube (Prasad et al., 2012). Ubiquitination targets the protein for proteasomal degradation, the activation of which may account for their loss from adult stem cells, other than those that retain a neural crest phenotype. The regulation of other embryonic regulatory transcription factors such as SoxE (e.g., Sox9) can also be brought about by either phosphylation or SUMOylation (Small Ubiquitin-like Modifier; does not target protein for degradation), which affect their subcellular localisation, DNA binding, protein-protein interaction, and transcriptional activity (Haung et al., 2011; Gill 2004; Prasad et al., 2012). An increasing list of microRNAs (miRNAs) is also emerging in the literature. miRNAs regulate levels of protein synthesis by repressing mRNA translation or by mRNA cleavage (Mukhopadhyay et al., 2011). These include miR-19a and miR-19b which have been proposed significant roles in neural crest development where in silico analysis predicts targets for TGF-β and Wnt signalling pathways (Mukhopadhyay et al., 2011). Studies on DPSCs are at time of writing limited, but have indicated that mir885-5p, mir586, and mir32 are expressed during differentiation of DPSC to odontoblast cells (Huang et al., 2011).

Pulpal repair and regeneration

The pulp tissue has a rich vasculature and neural plexus, so for pulp regeneration, angiogenesis and reinnervation are critical steps (Nakashima and Akamine, 2005). MSCs have been shown to secrete soluble cytokines/growth factors that function in a paracrine fashion, mediating repair and regeneration of a tissue through stimulation of angiogenesis, neurogenesis, and enhanced cell survivial (Kassis et al., 2011). Isolated subpopulations of DPSCs have been demonstrated as viable cell sources for cell-based therapy of angiogenesis and reinnervation and thus, potentially, pulp regeneration. CD31⁻ side population (SP) cells and CD105⁺ cells isolated from dental pulp induce angiogenesis and neurogenesis in rat cerebral ischemia, mediated by the release of neurotrophic factors such as VEGF, and promote migration and differentiation of the endogenous neuronal progenitor cells to accelerate functional recovery (Sugiyama et al., 2011).

Regeneration of part of a pulp (following pulpal exposure or partial pulpectomy) may provide a realistic translational pathway whereby pulp progenitor cells on an appropriate scaffold or engineered pulp tissue are transplanted into the exposed pulp tissue. Canine autologous CD31⁻ SP cells have been transplanted into a cavity of an amputated pulp following seeding on a collagen scaffold. Results demonstrated that the cavity on the amputated pulp was filled with a newly formed pulp tissue with a well-developed vasculature and innervation (Iohara et al., 2009). The majority of the transplanted CD31⁻ SP cells were observed around the newly formed capillaries and expressed the relevant angiogenic and neurotrophic factors, suggesting positive effects of these trophic effects on neovascularization (Iohara et al., 2009). Interestingly, after transplantation of CD31⁺ SP cells, fewer capillaries and reduced regenerated tissue were observed in the cavity on the amputated pulp compared with transplantation of CD31⁻ SP cells, suggesting different potentiality of subpopulations of isolated DPSCs.

Complete pulp regeneration provides a far greater challenge, and transplantation of DPSCs is required. However, following such transplantation these cells need to survive in the pulpectomized root canals before revascularization can be initiated and where nutrition and oxygen may be in limited supply to maintain cell viability. It would seem unlikely that transplanted DPSCs alone can mediate regeneration of a whole pulp. As highlighted above, subpopulations of DPSCs, SP including the CD105⁺ cells or CD31⁻ SP cells, have been shown to have more regenerative potential and are capable of inducing angiogenesis and reinnervation. Recruitment of MCSs from the surrounding tissues and remaining vasculature in response to migration or homing factors secreted by transplanted DPSCs may facilitate pulp regeneration. One such factor may be SDF-1, a chemokine for CXCR4-positive stem cells. DPSC subpopulations CD31⁻ SP cells and CD105⁺ cells are CXCR4 positive and are responsive to SDF-1 (Iohara et al., 2011; Nakashima et al., 2009). SDF-1 transplanted with DPSCs may provide the ideal signals for homing and proliferation of endogenous stem cells originating from surrounding dental tissues and associated vasculature.

A further challenge surrounds the choice of scaffold to carry the cells for transplantation. Any scaffold has to be biocompatible, with high bioactivity to integrate trophic factors secreted by the DPSC populations. The scaffold must also be biodegradable, thus releasing trophic factors and being replaced by newly regenerated tissue. More challenging is that any scaffold must not stimulate odontoblast differentiation or lead to secretion of a mineralizing matrix within the root canal except at the periphery where the scaffold/regenerated tissue is in contact with the dentinal wall of the pulp cavity.

Pulp regeneration has been demonstrated by using this approach of DPSC transplantation along with cell homing factors and a collagen scaffold in an experimental pulpectomised dog model (Iohara et al., 2011; Ishizaka et al., 2012). Current data suggest that a pulp-like loose connective tissue containing a vasculature and nerve fibres forms in the pulp cavity following transplantation of pulp CD31⁻ SP cells or CD105⁺ cells. Odontoblast-like cells were also observed, attached to the dentinal of the root canal. When a total or mixed DPSC population was transplanted into pulpectomised root canals, significantly less regenerated tissue was

observed, and this tissue appeared to undergo less specific mineralization.

Whilst the above studies are encouraging, is DPSC implantation likely to see clinical translation for pulp regeneration? Can regeneration of the pulp be mediated without the need for DPSC transplantation and rely solely on endogenous cells? Regeneration of pulp-like tissue by cell homing and without the requirement for cell transplantation has been reported. Delivery of bFGF and VEGF to endodontically treated human teeth implanted into a mouse dorsum resulted in a recellularized and revascularized connective tissue that integrated into the root canal walls (Kim et al., 2010).

Concluding remarks

The rapid expansion of published work regarding DPSCs over the past 14 years clearly suggests that these are a population of cells that have potential therapeutic use in translational medicine beyond that of regenerative endodontics and dental tissue repair. Several commercial companies now bank these cells for personalised medicine; however, as further research is undertaken with these cells, it is apparent that there are significant gaps in our knowledge regarding their full characterisation, biological function, and commitment. Is clonal expansion required or should we be utilising a heterogeneic population of cells? What determines the behaviour of different clonal populations? How do these cells behave in more complex extracellular matrix environments? How can these cells be more efficiently expanded in culture for clinical use without loss of potentiality? These are all questions needing to be addressed if these cells are to be used in in any clinical setting. If we are to develop regenerative therapies for dental medicine, then understanding the function of these cells in their own environments, how that environment influences their behaviour, and which population of DPSCs we are influencing is critical to clinical translation.

References

ALKAISI, A., ISMAIL, A. R., MUTUM, S. S., AHMAD, Z. A., MASUDI, S., & ABD RAZAK, N. H. 2013. Transplantation of human dental pulp stem cells: enhance bone consolidation in mandibular distraction osteogenesis. *J Oral Maxillofac Surg*, 71, 1758.e1–13.

ARANHA, A. M., ZHANG, Z., NEIVA, K. G., COSTA, C. A., HEBLING, J., & NÖR, J. E. 2010. Hypoxia enhances the angiogenic potential of human dental pulp cells. *J Endod*, 36, 1633–7.

BAKOPOULOU, A., LEYHAUSEN, G., VOLK, J., TSIFTSOGLOU, A., GAREFIS, P., KOIDIS, P., & GEURTSEN, W. 2011. Assessment of the impact of two different isolation methods on the osteo/odontogenic differentiation potential of human dental stem cells derived from deciduous teeth. *Calcif Tissue Int*, 88, 130–41.

BOLEMAN, A. I., TĂNASIE, G., GĂLUȘCAN, A., CRISTEA, M. I., BOJIN, F. M., PANAITESCU, C., & PĂUNESCU, V. 2012. Studies regarding the in vitro wound healing potential of mouse dental pulp stem-like progenitor cells. *Biotechnol. & Biotechnol. Eq*, 26, 2781–5.

BATOULI, S., MIURA, M., BRAHIM, J., TSUTSUI, T. W., FISHER, L. W., GRONTHOS, S., ROBEY, P. G., & SHI, S. 2003. Comparison of stem-cell-mediated osteogenesis and dentinogenesis. *J Dent Res*, 82, 976–81.

BROHEM, C. A., DE CARVALHO, C. M., RADOSKI CL, SANTI, F. C., BAPTISTA, M. C., SWINKA, B. B., DE A URBAN, C., DE ARAUJO, L. R., GRAF, R. M., FEFERMAN, I. H., & LORENCINI, M. 2013. Comparison between fibroblasts and mesenchymal stem cells derived from dermal and adipose tissue. *Int J Cosmet Sci*, 35, 448–57.

CARDOSO, F. P., VIANA, M. B., SOBRINHO, A. P., DINIZ, M. G., BRITO, J. A., GOMES, C. C., MOREIRA, P. R., & GOMEZ, R. S. 2010. Methylation pattern of the IFN-gamma gene in human dental pulp. *J Endod*, 36, 642–6.

CHAI, Y., JIANG, X., ITO, Y., BRINGAS, P., HAN, J., ROWITCH, D. H., SORIANO, P., MCMAHON, A. P., & SUCOV, H. M. 2000. Fate of the mammalian cranial neural crest during tooth and mandibular morphogenesis. *Development*, 127, 1671–9.

CHAN, R. W., SCHWAB, K. E., & GARGETT, C. E. 2004. Clonogenicity of human endometrial epithelial and stromal cells. *Biol Reprod*, 70, 1738–50.

COLLAS, P. 2010. Programming differentiation potential in mesenchymal stem cells. *Epigenetics*, 5, 476–82.

COLTER, D. C, CLASS, R., DIGIROLAMO, C. M., & PROCKOP, D. J. 2000. Rapid expansion of recycling stem cells in cultures of plastic-adherent cells from human bone marrow. *Proc Natl Acad Sci U S A*, 97, 3213–8.

D'AQUINO, R., DE ROSA, A., LANZA, V., TIRINO, V., LAINO, L., GRAZIANO, A., DESIDERIO, V., LAINO, G., & PAPACCIO, G. 2009. Human mandible bone defect repair by the grafting of dental pulp stem/progenitor cells and collagen sponge biocomplexes. *Cells, & Materials*, 8, 75–83.

D'AQUINO, R., GRAZIANO, A., SAMPAOLESI, M., LAINO, G., PIROZZI, G., DE ROSA, A., & PAPACCIO, G. 2007. Human postnatal dental pulp cells co-differentiate into osteoblasts and endotheliocytes: a pivotal synergy leading to adult bone tissue formation. *Cell Death Differ*, 14, 1162–71.

DIMITRIOU, R., TSIRIDIS, E., & GIANNOUDIS, P. V. 2005. Current concepts of molecular aspects of bone healing. *Injury*, 36, 1392–404.

DOCHEVA, D., HAASTERS, F., & SCHIEKER, M. 2008. Mesenchymal stem cells and their cell surface receptors. *Current Rheumatology Reviews*, 4, 155–60.

DOMINCI, M., LE BLANC, K., MUELLER, I., SLAPER-CORTENBACH, I., MARINI, F., KRAUSE, D., DEANS, R., KEATING, A., PROCKOP, D. J., & HORWITZ, E. 2006. Minimal criteria for defining multipotent mesenchymal stromal cells. *The International Society for Cellular Therapy position statement. Cytotherapy*, 8, 315–7.

DUNCAN, H. F., SMITH, A. J., FLEMING, G. J., & COOPER, P. R. 2013. Histone deacetylase inhibitors epigenetically promote reparative events in primary dental pulp cells. *Exp Cell Res*, 319, 1534–43.

GILL G. 2004. SUMO and ubiquitin in the nucleus: different functions, similar mechanisms? *Genes Dev*, 18, 2046–59.

GRONTHOS, S., ARTHUR, A., BARTOLD, P. M., & SHI, S. 2011. A method to isolate and culture expand human dental pulp stem cells. *Methods Mol Biol*, 698, 107–21.

GRONTHOS, S., BRAHIM, J., LI, W., FISHER, L. W., CHERMAN, N., BOYDE, A., DENBESTEN, P., ROBEY, P. G., & SHI, S. 2002. Stem cell properties of human dental pulp stem cells, *J Dent Res*, 81, 531–5.

GRONTHOS, S., MANKANI, M., BRAHIM, J., ROBEY, P. G., & SHI, S. 2000. Postnatal human dental pulp stem cells (DPSCs) in vitro and in vivo. *Proc Natl Acad Sci U S A*, 97, 13625–30.

HARRINGTON, J., SLOAN, A. J., & WADDINGTON, R. J. 2014. Quantification of clonal heterogeneity of mesenchymal progenitor cells in dental pulp and bone marrow. *Connect Tissue Res*, 55(Suppl 1), 62–7.

HUANG, G.T., GRONTHOS, S., & SHI, S. 2009. Mesenchymal stem cells derived from dental tissues vs. those from other sources: their biology and role in regenerative medicine. *J Dent Res*, 88, 792–806.

HUANG, X., XU, S., GAO, J., LIU, F., YUE, J., CHEN, T., & WU, B. 2011. miRNA expression profiling identifies DSPP regulators in cultured dental pulp cells. *Int J Mol Med*, 28, 659–67.

IIDA, K., TAKEDA-KAWAGUCHI, T., TEZUKA, Y., KUNISADA, T., SHIBATA, T., & TEZUKA, K. 2010. Hypoxia enhances colony formation and proliferation but inhibits differentiation of human dental pulp cells. *Arch Oral Biol*, 55, 648–54.

IOHARA, K., IMABAYASH,I K., ISHIZAKA, R., WATANABE, A., NABEKURA, J., ITO, M., MATSUSHITA, K., NAKAMURA, H, & NAKASHIMA, M. 2011. Complete pulp regeneration after pulpectomy by transplantation of CD105+ stem cells with stromal cell-derived factor-1. *Tissue Eng Part A*, 17, 1911–20.

IOHARA, K., NAKASHIMA, M., ITO, M., ISHIKAWA, M., NAKASIMA, A., & AKAMINE, A. 2004. Dentin regeneration by dental pulp stem cell therapy with recombinant human bone morphogenetic protein 2. *J Dent Res*, 83, 590–5.

IOHARA, K., ZHENG, L., ITO, M.; ISHIZAKA, R., NAKAMURA, H., & INTO T. et al., 2009. Regeneration of dental pulp after pulpotomy by transplantation of CD31-/CD146-side population cells from a canine tooth. *Regen Med*, 4, 377–85.

IOHARA, K., ZHENG, L., ITO, M., TOMOKIYO, A., MATSUSHITA, K. & NAKASHIMA, M. 2006. Side population cells isolated from porcine dental pulp tissue with self-renewal and multipotency for dentinogenesis, chondrogenesis, adipogenesis, and neurogenesis. *Stem Cells*, 24, 2493–503.

ISAGAWA, T., NAGAE, G., SHIRAKI, N., FUJITA, T., SATO, N., ISHIKAWA, S., KUME, S., & ABURATANI, H. 2011. DNA methylation profiling of embryonic stem cell differentiation into the three germ layers. *PLoS One*, 6, e26052.

ISHIKAWA, Y., IDA-YONEMOCHI, H., SUZUKI, H., NAKAKURA-OHSHIMA, K., JUNG, H. S., HONDA, M. J., ISHII, Y., WATANABE, N., & OHSHIMA, H. 2010. Mapping of BrdU label-retaining dental pulp cells in growing teeth and their regenerative capacity after injuries. *Histochem Cell Biol*, 134, 227–41.

ISHIZAKA, R., IOHARA, K., MURAKAMI, M., FUKUTA, O., & NAKASHIMA, M. 2012. Regeneration of dental pulp following pulpectomy by fractionated stem/progenitor cells from bone marrow and adipose tissue. *Biomaterials*, 33, 2109–18.

JANEBODIN, K., HORST, O. V., IERONIMAKIS, N., BALASUNDARAM, G., REESUKUMAL, K., PRATUMVINIT, B., & REYES, M. 2011. Isolation and characterization of neural crest-derived stem cells from dental pulp of neonatal mice. *PloS One*, 6, e27526.

JONES, E. A., KINSEY, S. E., ENGLISH, A., JONES, R. A., STRASZYNSKI, L., MEREDITH, D. M., MARKHAM, A. F., JACK, A., EMERY, P., & MCGONAGLE, D. 2002. Isolation and characterization of bone marrow multipotential mesenchymal progenitor cells. *Arthritis Rheum*, 46, 3349–60.

JONES, P.H., & F.M. WATT. 1993. Separation of human epidermal stem cells from transit amplifying cells on the basis of differences in integrin function and expression. *Cell*, 73, 713–24.

KASSIS, I. VAKNIN-DEMBINSKY, A., & KARUSSIS, D. 2011. Bone marrow mesenchymal stem cells: agents of immunomodulation and neuroprotection. *Curr Stem Cell Res Ther*, 6, 63–8.

KERN, S., EICHLER, H., STOEVE, J., KLUTER, H., & BIEBACK, K. 2006. Comparative analysis of mesenchymal stem cells from bone marrow, umbilical cord blood, or adipose tissue. *Stem Cells*, 24, 1294–1301.

KIM, J. Y., XIN, X., MOIOLI, E.K., CHUNG, J., LEE, C.H., CHEN, M., FU, S. Y, KOCH, P. D., & MAO, J. J. 2010. Regeneration of dental-pulp-like tissue by chemotaxis-induced cell homing. *Tissue Eng Part A*, 16, 3023–31.

KUZNETSOV, S. A., FRIEDENSTEIN, A. J., & ROBEY, P. G. 1997. Factors required for bone marrow stromal fibroblast colony formation in vitro. *Br J Haematol*, 97, 561–70.

LAINO, G., CARINCI, F., GRAZIANO, A., D'AQUINO, R., LANZA, V., DE ROSA, A., GOMBOS, F., CARUSO, F., GUIDA, L., RULLO, R., MENDITTI, D., & PAPACCIO, G. 2006. In vitro bone production using stem cells derived from human dental pulp. *J Craniofac Surg*, 17, 511–5.

LAINO, G., D'AQUINO, R., GRAZIANO, A., LANZA, V., CARINCI, F., NARO, F., PIROZZI, G., & PAPACCIO G. 2005. A new population of human adult dental pulp stem cells: a useful source of living autologous fibrous bone tissue (LAB). *J Bone Miner Res*, 20, 1394–402.

LEI, G., YAN, M., WANG, Z., YU, Y., TANG, C., WANG, Z., YU, J., ZHANG, G. 2011. Dentinogenic capacity: immature root papilla stem cells versus mature root pulp stem cells. *Biol Cell*, 103, 185–96.

LESOT, H., BEGUEKIRN, C., KUBLER, M. D., MEYER, J. M., SMITH, A. J., CASSIDY, N., RUCH, J. V., AUBIN, J. E., GOLDBERG, M., & MAGLOIRE, H. 1993. Experimental induction of odontoblast differentiation and stimulation during reparative processes. *Cells & Materials*, 3, 201–17.

LIZIER, N. F., KERKIS, A., GOMES, C. M., HEBLING, J., OLIVEIRA, C. F., CAPLAN, A.I., & KERKIS, I. 2012. Scaling-up of dental pulp stem cells isolated from multiple niches. *PLoS One*, 7:e39885.

LOVSCHALL, H., MITSIADIS, T. A., POULSEN, K., JENSEN, K. H., KJELDSEN, A. L. 2007. Coexpression of Notch3 and Rgs5 in the pericyte-vascular smooth muscle cell axis in response to pulp injury. *Int J Dev Biol*, 51, 715–21.

LOVSCHALL, H., TUMMERS, M., THESLEFF, I., FUCHTBAUER, E. M., & POULSEN, K. 2005. Activation of the Notch signaling pathway in response to pulp capping of rat molars. *Eur J Oral Sci*, 113, 312–7.

LUISI, S. B., BARBACHAN, J. J., CHIES, J. A., & FILHO, M. S. 2007. Behavior of human dental pulp cells exposed to transforming growth factor-beta1 and acidic fibroblast growth factor in culture. *J Endod*, 33, 833–5.

MENICANIN, D., BARTOLD, P. M., ZANNETTINO, A. C., & GRONTHOS, S. 2010. Identification of a common gene expression signature associated with immature clonal mesenchymal cell populations derived from bone marrow and dental tissues. *Stem Cells Dev*, 19, 1501–10.

MILETICH, I., & SHARPE, P. T. 2004. Neural crest contribution to mammalian tooth formation, *Birth Defects Res C Embryo Today*, 72, 200–12.

MIURA, M., GRONTHOS, S., ZHAO, M., LU, B., FISHER, L. W., ROBEY, P. G., & SHI, S. 2003. SHED: stem cells from human exfoliated deciduous teeth. *Proc Natl Acad Sci U S A*, 100, 5807–12.

MUKHOPADHYAY, P., BROCK, G., APPANA, S., WEBB, C., GREENE, R. M., & PISANO, M. M. 2011. MicroRNA gene expression signatures in the developing neural tube. *Birth Defects Res A Clin Mol Teratol*, 91, 744–62.

NAKASHIMA, M., & AKAMINE, A. 2005. The application of tissue engineering to regeneration of pulp and dentin in endodontics. *J Endod*, 31, 711–8.

NAKASHIMA, M., IOHARA, K., & SUGIYAMA, M. 2009. Human dental pulp stem cells with highly angiogenic and neurogenic potential for possible use in pulp regeneration. *Cytokine & Growth Factor Reviews*, 20, 435–40.

NAKASHIMA, M., & IOHARA, K. 2011. Regeneration of dental pulp by stem cells. *Adv Dent Res*, 23, 313–9.

NOER, A., LINDEMAN, L. C., & COLLAS, P. 2009. Histone H3 modifications associated with differentiation and long-term culture of mesenchymal adipose stem cells. *Stem Cells Dev.* 18, 725–36.

PRASAD, M. S., SAUKA-SPENGLER, T., & LABONNE, C. 2012. Induction of the neural crest state: control of stem cell attributes by gene regulatory, post-transcriptional and epigenetic interactions. *Dev Biol*, 366, 10–21.

REYA, T., MORRISON, S. J, CLARKE, M. F., & WEISSMAN, I. L. 2001. Stem cells, cancer, and cancer stem cells, *Nature*, 414, 105–11.

RIQUELME, P. A., DRAPEAU, E., & DOETSCH, F. 2008. Brain micro-ecologies: neural stem cell niches in the adult mammalian brain. *Philosophical Transactions of the Royal Society B-Biological Sciences*, 363, 123–37.

RUCH, J. V. 1998. Odontoblast commitment and differentiation. *Biochemistry and cell biology = Biochimie et biologie cellulaire*, 76, 923–38.

RUTHERFORD, R. B., & GU, K. 2000. Treatment of inflamed ferret dental pulps with recombinant bone morphogenetic protein-7. *Eur J Oral Sci*, 108, 202–6.

SAKDEE, J. B., WHITE, R. R., PAGONIS, T. C., & HAUSCHKA, P. V. 2009. Hypoxia-amplified proliferation of human dental pulp cells. *J Endod.*, 35, 818–23.

SEO, B. M., MIURA, M., GRONTHOS, S., BARTOLD, P. M., BATOULI, S., BRAHIM, J., YOUNG, M., ROBEY, P. G., WANG, C. Y., & SHI, S. 2004. Investigation of multipotent postnatal stem cells from human periodontal ligament. *Lancet*, 364, 149–55.

SHI, S., & GRONTHOS, S. 2003. Perivascular niche of postnatal mesenchymal stem cells in human bone marrow and dental pulp. *J Bone Miner Res*, 18, 696–704.

SLOAN, A. J., RUTHERFORD, R. B., & SMITH, A. J. 2000. Stimulation of the rat dentine-pulp complex by bone morphogenetic protein-7 in vitro. *Arch Oral Biol*, 45, 173–7.

SLOAN, A. J., & SMITH, A. J. 1999. Stimulation of the dentine-pulp complex of rat incisor teeth by transforming growth factor-beta isoforms 1-3 in vitro. *Arch Oral Biol*, 44, 149–56.

SONOYAMA, W., LIU, Y., YAMAZA, T., TUAN, R. S., WANG, S., SHI, S., & HUANG, G. T. 2008. Characterization of the apical papilla and its residing stem cells from human immature permanent teeth: a pilot study. *J Endod*, 34, 166–71.

SUGIYAMA, M., IOHARA, K., WAKITA, H., HATTORI, H., UEDA, M., MATSUSHITA, K., & NAKASHIMA, M. 2011. Dental pulp-derived CD31(-)/CD146(-) side population stem/progenitor cells enhance recovery of focal cerebral ischemia in rats. *Tissue Eng Part A*, 17, 1303–11.

TECLES, O., LAURENT, P., ZYGOURITSAS, S., BURGER, A. S., CAMPS, J., DEJOU, J., & ABOUT, I. 2005. Activation of human dental pulp progenitor/stem cells in response to odontoblast injury. *Arch Oral Biol*, 50, 103–8.

TUCKER, A. S., & SHARPE, P. T. 1999. Molecular genetics of tooth morphogenesis and patterning: the right shape in the right place. *J Dent Res*, 78, 826–34.

TZIAFAS, D., BELIBASAKIS, G., VEIS, A., & PAPADIMITRIOU, S. 2001. Dentin regeneration in vital pulp therapy: design principles. *Adv Dent Res*, 15, 96–100.

WADDINGTON, R. J., YOUDE, S. J., LEE, C. P., & SLOAN, A. J. 2009. Isolation of distinct progenitor stem cell populations from dental pulp. *Cells Tissues Organs*, 189, 268–74.

WEI, X., LING, J., WU, L., LIU, L., &, XIAO, Y. 2007. Expression of mineralization markers in dental pulp cells. *J Endod*, 33, 703–8.

YANG, X., ZHANG, W., VAN DEN DOLDER, J., WALBOOMERS, X. F., BIAN, Z., FAN, M., & JANSEN, J. A. 2007. Multilineage potential of STRO-1+ rat dental pulp cells in vitro. *J Tissue Eng Regen Med*, 1, 128–35.

YU, J., WANG, Y., DENG, Z., TANG, L., LI, Y., SHI, J., & JIN, Y. 2007. Odontogenic capability: bone marrow stromal stem cells versus dental pulp stem cells *Biol Cell*, 99, 465–74.

ZHANG, W., WALBOOMERS, X. F., SHI, S., FAN, M., & JANSEN, J. A. 2006. Multilineage differentiation potential of stem cells derived from human dental pulp after cryopreservation. *Tissue Eng*, 12, 2813–23.

ZHENG, Y., LIU, Y., ZHANG, C. M., ZHANG, H. Y., LI, W. H., SHI, S., LE, A. D., & WANG, S. L. 2009. Stem cells from deciduous tooth repair mandibular defect in swine. *J Dent Res*, 88, 249–54.

CHAPTER 4

Assessing the potential of mesenchymal stem cells in craniofacial bone repair and regeneration

Rachel J. Waddington, S. Quentin Jones, and Ryan Moseley

School of Dentistry, Cardiff Institute of Tissue Engineering and Repair, Cardiff University, Cardiff, UK

Our ever-increasing knowledge and understanding of the cellular processes of bone repair and regeneration has allowed modern dentistry to come a long way, especially for the specialities of periodontology, implantology, and oral maxillofacial surgery. The greatest achievement is perhaps seen in the placement of implants into the maxilla or mandible driven by effective osseointegration. Success is judged on longevity of the implant, quality of the prosthesis, preservation of the supporting biological tissues in a state of health or some arbitrary weighted balance between all three. Success rates of 93%–98% in providing a 10–15-year lifespan of functionality and patient satisfaction have regularly been quoted in the literature (Roccuzzo et al., 2010; Busenlechner et al., 2014). However, this perceived high success rate is probably because the clinician will only place an implant if a patient has sufficient residual bone, with a high proportion of quality dense cortical bone to provide good integration and biomechanical support, and is systemically healthy to predict longevity (Ayson et al., 2009; Diz et al., 2013). Thus, research within the discipline of bone engineering is still vast in meeting a number of clinical challenges for improving clinical outcomes.

Regeneration of large bone volume

Edentulism very often leads to the loss of mandible jaw bone within a year of the loss of the tooth, leading to debilitation that has a major impact on oral and general heath (Emami et al., 2013). A gradual lowering of the maxillary sinus and an associated loss of bone volume are also often encountered. Bone tissue regeneration is therefore required in clinical procedures such as maxillary sinus floor lift, lateral alveolar augmentation to increase the width of the mandible, and vertical alveolar augmentation to increase the height of the mandible. In addition, bone tissue engineering is required in the replacement of large bone tissue lost due to trauma or tumour resection or in aiding osteogenic distraction processes not only within the craniofacial region, but also the rest of the body (Oryan et al., 2014). For almost all of these procedures, bone autografts still represent the "gold standard" due to their potent osseoinductive activity. Bone grafts contain a reservoir of cells involved in the repair process, including mesenchymal stem cells (MSCs), but also a "cocktail" of growth factors embedded within an extracellular matrix (ECM). These are released during the wound healing process, providing efficient signalling cues to stimulate progenitor cell recruitment and induce osteogenesis. However, harvesting of sufficient tissue and donor site morbidity provides a significant negative clinical side effect. Allografts require the harvest of tissue from a donor (usually cadaveric material), but mediocre osseoinductive properties do not compensate for issues relating to supply and immunological responses experienced on implantation (Shafiei et al., 2009). Xenografts, representing transplant of cells and tissue components from animal bone mainly from porcine and bovine origin, have proven less successful due to the hosts' increased potential for immunological rejection (Oryan et al., 2013).

Tissue Engineering and Regeneration in Dentistry: Current Strategies, First Edition. Edited by Rachel J. Waddington and Alastair J. Sloan.
© 2017 John Wiley & Sons, Ltd. Published 2017 by John Wiley & Sons, Ltd.

Hence, a big challenge for current research is the search for an alternative that will provide equal osseoinductive power of autografts. Demineralised bone matrix derived from allografts, treated to remove the mineral component, often lose osseoinductive potential, with the necessary sterilisation procedure cited as the cause (Sharp et al., 2005). Scaffolds that function as a carrier for a single growth factor have been proposed in encouraging migration, proliferation, and differentiation of the resident host cells, but costly supraphysiologic microgram concentrations of growth factors are required for clinical use (Erben et al., 2014). It is now well recognised that the short biological half-life of the growth factor due to proteolytic degradation in the wound healing site and tissue-selectivity of growth factors, alongside the potential toxicity of the high levels required, represent limitations that currently hamper the full potential of growth factor therapy for clinical success (Rose and Oreffo, 2002). Scaffolds containing adult stem cells have as yet also failed to fully translate into routine use (Erben et al., 2014; Husain et al., 2014). It is now recognised that harvest of MSCs from tissue samples results in a heterogeneous population of cells that represent a variety of subset populations with differing regenerative potentials. The profile of the MSC subsets varies between donor and tissue source, and extensive research has focussed on cell selection, along with manufacturing processes for cell expansion, in maintaining cell survival and the MSC phenotype and increasing cell viability within the transplanted scaffold (Husain et al., 2014; Razzouk and Schoor, 2012).

Accelerating bone regeneration

Within dentistry there is also a need for the regeneration of small bone volumes. For small periodontal defects and where there is a need to improve primary implant stability, resorbable substitutes such as glass/ceramic biomaterials, inorganic bone particles, and collagen sponges have provided reasonable success as osteoconductive scaffolds to support bone formation. However, there is also a desire from both the patient and the clinician to accelerate the osseointegration process to achieve primary stability of the implant sooner. Benefits are to reduce chair time by shortening the implant procedures, possibly allowing for earlier placement and widening loading options for implants (for instance, improving one-stage implant procedures; Álvarez-Camino et al., 2013). In addition, accelerating

osseointgration rates would reduce infection risk, which is higher during early stages of wound repair prior to the deposition of a mineralised tissue. An extensive number of implant surfaces have been proposed where factors such as surface roughness, surface energy, and/or chemistry have all been proposed to directly influence cell activity (Waddington and Sloan, 2012). Unfortunately, due to the wide variety of surface modifications in existence and the methods for determining osseointegration, it has proven difficult to determine the optimal surface conditions, and many of the results are contradictory (Waddington and Sloan, 2012). Many only demonstrate increased bone implant contact with associated increase in removal torque, rather than confirming acceleration of the wound healing events on a temporal scale. On this premise, rough surface implants appear to yield better osseointegration endpoints compared with smooth surfaces, but evidence is not conclusive in terms of accelerating the bone healing process. Small changes in the chemistry, geometry, width, depth, or orientation of surface topography can significantly affect cellular behaviour, and much *in vitro* data is contradictory. Roughened surfaces may therefore be limited to providing better anchorage and hence earlier apparent stability of the implant in the bone. Surfaces may also be made bioactive through the augmentation of specific proteins such as growth factors, but the effects may be confined to the bone healing occurring at the actual implant surface rather than at more distal locations. However, despite contradictions, a consensus opinion is that research that develops biological, chemical, and mechanical changes at the interface between implants could still make an important contribution in improving healing outcomes (Lewallen et al., 2015).

Improving predictability

Another clinical challenge is to improve the predictability of success for patients in all dental, maxillofacial, and orthopaedic procedures. While good metabolic control of these diseases can lead to successful outcomes, poor control negatively affects osseointegration and bone healing. Systemic conditions such as type 1 and type 2 diabetes mellitus, osteoporosis, and ageing impair bone healing. This impairment has partially been attributed to a reduced ability in MSC maturation to form bone-synthesizing osteoblasts due to an altered and inefficient signaling environment. Delay in bone healing leaves the site more prone to infection and hence unsuccessful clinical outcome. Smoking and certain forms of systemic medication, such as nonsteroidal anti-inflammatory drugs (Pountos et al., 2012; Streitzel et al., 2007; Hinode et al., 2006) and long-term immunosuppressive therapy (Ayson et al., 2009), may be considered a risk factor, and our lack of knowledge at the cellular level in this area presents a challenge in predicting success or failure. The translational aim for research in this area will thus be to restore the inefficient signalling environment and hence the bone healing process.

Cellular and molecular events of bone healing

Bone repair is usually an efficient process involving a complex cascade of biological events that involve a multitude of intracellular and extracellular molecular signalling mechanisms, coordinated by several different cell types. If successful, bone regenerates to form a mechanically stable osseous structure with complete restoration of function. The process can, however, be delayed by preexisting diseases such as diabetes, osteoporosis, and general age, which impacts on the signalling events, affecting both revascularisation and the deposition of a mineralised matrix (Armas and Recker, 2012; Borrelli et al., 2012). Rapid bone healing is often the goal for bone healing in craniofacial tissues, and this is ideally achieved by primary bone healing involving predominantly intramembranous ossification where revascularised and bone synthesis facilitate the repair process. Primary bone healing can, however, only be accomplished by rigid fixation of the fractured bone surfaces, as provided in close fit placement of implants, tight packing of the healing site with scaffolds or bone grafts, or with external stabilising fixators to reduce micromotion. Excessive micromotion leads to secondary bone healing, which involves a double process of chondrogenesis through endochondral ossification in regions near the fracture site periosteum (enhanced by soft tissues around the fracture site) and intramembranous ossification in other sites. Secondary bone formation thus involves the additional synthesis of a fibrous and avascular cartilaginous callus stabilising the healing site, which is then resorbed by the action of osteoclasts and endothelial cells to be eventually replaced by vascularised bone.

Although MSCs are critical to the bone repair process in synthesising bone, the process involves signalling interplay with platelets, haemopoietic cells, and endothelial cells. The process of bone repair is now often broadly divided as a sequence of several stages, namely, haematoma formation stimulating an inflammatory phase, a reparative phase ultimately leading to the formation of woven bone either by direct ossification or via a cartilage intermediary stage, and finally a remodelling stage whereby the relatively weak and disordered woven bone is slowly removed by osteoclasts and replaced by new stronger lamella bone deposited by osteoblasts. It is this last stage that allows bone healing to be unique in the body in producing a tissue structurally and functionally equivalent to the bone it is replacing. An understanding of the molecular biology governing these events, defining the role of the various cell types and the signalling molecules in initiating and controlling the cellular process, is important in our therapeutic manipulation of MSCs for several clinical requirements: (1) promoting a rapid repair process, (2) regenerating large bone volume within critical size defects unable to heal naturally, and (3) allowing restoration of the signalling milieu where bone healing is compromised (Table 4.1).

Haematoma formation and the inflammatory phase

The bone healing cascade is initiated by tissue damage. In particular, vascular endothelial damage results in activation of the complement cascade to stem bleeding and promote the accumulation of platelets. Activation of the platelets releases α granules containing bioactive factors. The presence of "foreign" biomaterial, such as an implant surface, also has the potential to activate platelets (Kikuchi et al., 2005). Through the involvement of plasma fibrinogen and thrombin, the platelets aggregate within a stable fibrin clot to provide a provisional matrix. The platelets also represent an important source of signalling factors such as platelet-derived growth factor (PDGF), transforming growth factor β1 and β2 (TGF-β1 and –β2), histamines, and serotonin, triggering chemotactic signalling initially for neutrophils and subsequently for monocytes, lymphocytes, and later, MSCs or osteoprogenitor cells (detailed further by Kuzyk and Schemitsch, 2011). The infiltration of the neutrophils and lymphocytes (T cells) is associated with an increase in inflammatory mediators, including the

Table 4.1 The temporal stages of natural bone healing, providing optimal signalling cues directing cellular migration, proliferation, and differentiation leading to efficient bone regeneration of a fully functional tissue.

	Inflammatory Stage (Days 1–3)		Reparative Stage (Days 3–50)			Late Remodelling (2–9 months)	
Signalling milieu	IL-1, IL-6, IL-8, TNFα, M-CSF, GM-CSF, TGF-ß1, PDGF, FGF, histamines and serotonin		BMP-2, BMP-4, IGF I and II, FGF, VEGF, angiopoietin, TGF-ß1, 2 and 3	BMP-2, BMP-4, BMP-7, IGF I and II, TGF-ß1, 2 and 3, FGF, Wnt		RANKL, OPG, M-CSF, BMP-2, BMP-4, BMP-7, IGF I and II, TGF-ß1, 2 and 3, FGF, Wnt	
Contributing cells	Platelets, lymphocytes, neutrophils, macrophages, osteoclasts	HAEMATOMA	Endothelial cells, MSCs, pericytes	Differentiating osteoblasts	OSTEOID	MSCs, pericytes, osteoblasts, osteoclasts, endothelial cells	WOVEN BONE / LAMELLA BONE
Functional ECM components	Fibrin clot, osteopontin		Collagen, osteopontin, dermatan sulphate conjugated decorin and biglycan, BAG-75, DMP-1, vitronectin, specific MMPs	Collagen, BSP, osteonectin, chondroitin sulphate conjugated decorin and biglycan, osteocalcin, specific MMPs	GRANULATION TISSUE	Continual synthesis and transition of osteoid components into mineralised bone matrix	

proinflammatory cytokines interleukin (IL)-1, IL-6, IL-8, tumour necrosis factor (TNF)α and macrophage colony stimulating factor (M-CSF). Although these inflammatory cytokines have a chemotactic influence for further recruitment of inflammatory cells, thus amplifying further inflammatory signalling events, these factors have all been proposed to be necessary for initiating bone repair. For instance, knockout of TNFα in mice exhibits impaired intramembranous ossification (Gerstenfeld et al., 2001), and TNFα has additionally been shown to promote MSC migration, induce chondrocyte apoptosis, and stimulate osteoclast differentiation and function (Barnes et al., 1999). These proinflammatory cytokines have hence been further attributed to the initiation of ECM synthesis and angiogenesis.

Angiogenesis and the reestablishment of a good vascular supply is a prerequisite condition for normal bone repair in order to restore oxygen tension, neutral pH, and nutrient supply ready for intramembranous ossification during the reparative phase of healing and during the replacement of cartilage by bone matrix during endochondreal ossification. An important mitogen regulating revascularisation is vascular endothelial growth factor (VEGF), which is stored in the mineralised

bone matrix and released by osteoclast activity. Together with PDGF and basic fibroblast growth factor (bFGF), secreted by macrophages, monocytes, MSCs, and later by osteoblasts and chondrocytes, as well as angiopoietin released by endothelial cells, these factors stimulate budding of new endothelial cells from preexisting capillaries for new vessel development (Al-Aql et al., 2008). The ingress of new vessels is facilitated by the degradation of the provisional fibrin matrix (or the cartilage matrix during endochondral ossification), by the release from the endothelial cells of matrix metalloproteinases.

Overall, the fibrin network provides a network for the migration of a range of cells, including endothelial cells, immune cells, and MSCs, to produce a transient granulation tissue. Strong evidence suggests that osteopontin synthesised by macrophages coats the surface of small, particulate, mineralised tissue debris (for example that generated as part of surgical procedures during implant placement) and may act as an opsonin to facilitate adhesion and phagocytosis by macrophages (McKee et al., 2011; Andrews et al., 2012). Disruption to the vascular supply results in hypoxia, acidosis (due to anaerobic cell metabolism), and reduced nutrient supply. Localised to the bone fracture surface, osteocytes die leaving nonvital matrix, which is subsequently degraded by activated osteoclasts. Sclerostin is specifically produced by osteocytes, which is an antagonist of the osteoinductive Wnt-β-catanin signalling pathway; thus, its reduction by apoptosing osteocytes contributes to the stimuli for osteoblast and hence bone formation. The ECM of bone is known to contain a reservoir of growth factors, such as bone morphogenetic proteins (BMPs), VEGF, insulin-like growth factors (IGF), and TGF-ß, bound within it (Frolik et al., 1988; Hauschka et al., 1986; Taipale and Keski-Oja, 1997). The action of the osteoclasts degrading the fractured bone surface is proposed to release these bioactive proteins, initiating optimal bone reparative processes at these sites (Schönherr and Hausser, 2000; Ramirez and Rifkin, 2003).

Reparative phase

Growth factors PDGF and TGF-β1, 2, and 3 present in the provisional fibrin matrix have all been attributed prominent roles associated with the migratory and proliferative responses of the MSCs to the wound healing site. Inflammatory cytokines, particularly TNFα, also appear to assist the process. The MSCs are recruited from the bone marrow tissue located in the cancellous bone and the periosteum. A further major source of MSCs is the pericytes, resident cells associated with the endothelial cells of capillaries and veins and brought to the wound healing site as part of the process of angiogenesis. During intramembranous ossification, high levels of growth factor, such as TGF-β and BMP-2, induce osteogenic differentiation of MSCs, which is characterised by the upregulation of transcription factors RUNX2 and Osterix. Other osteoinductive factors include the Wnt family of ligands, which bind to cell surface receptors (composed of members of the frizzled gene family (Fz) and low-density lipoprotein receptor-related proteins 5 and 6, leading to activation of the canonical β-catenin pathway and osteogenic genes. The importance of Wnt signalling in osteogenesis has been clearly demonstrated by its activation by lithium chloride or strontium, resulting in enhanced bone formation *in vivo* (Clement-Lacroix et al., 2005; Yang et al., 2011). The provisional granulation matrix is replaced by an unmineralised collagenous matrix, termed osteoid, concomitant with angiogenesis and the formation of a Haversian canal system. An essential role of the osteoid is to prevent premature mineralisation prior to the laying down of a collagen-rich scaffold and successful replacement of an efficient vascular network.

Several noncollagenous proteins that have been shown to be synthesised early on during osteoblast differentiation have the potential to inhibit crystal growth, including vitronectin (Rohanizadeh et al., 1998), osteopontin (McKee et al., 2011), bone acidic glycoprotein-75 (BAG-75) (Chen et al., 1992), dentine matrix protein 1 (Gorski, 2011), and the dermatan sulphate-conjugated forms of decorin and biglycan (equivalent to those normally found in nonmineralised tissues such as skin; Waddington et al., 2003). Osteopontin also has a cell binding RGD sequence facilitating the attachment of MSCs/osteoblasts to the bone healing surface (McKee et al., 2011), whilst BAG-75 has also been shown to block the resorptive activity of osteoclasts (Sato et al., 1992). On completion of the osteoid network, the matrix continues to be remodelled with the removal of these inhibitors of mineralisation and the synthesis of noncollagenous proteins by osteoblasts, which facilitate the deposition of amorphous calcium phosphate and subsequently hydroxyapatite along the collagen fibril framework to synthesise bone. The mineralisation stage can be characterised through the appearance in the matrix of bone sialoprotein, chondroitin sulphate-conjugated forms of decorin and biglycan, osteonectin, and osteocalcin. Some osteoblasts become entrapped within the mineralised matrix to form osteocytes, which communicate with one another via a network of cell processes. Alternatively, osteoblasts undergo apoptosis to halt the further synthesis of bone. Critically, growth factors become embedded in the matrix to be released when the bone matrix is resorbed again as part of the remodelling process.

Where endochondral ossification is the route of repair, cartilage is first laid down and MSCs are committed to the chondrocyte lineage, characterised by the expression of the transcription factor SOX9 and the synthesis of a type II collagen-rich matrix. The tissue is avascular and changes in the embedded chondrocytes initiate a signalling cascade, which leads to chondrocyte hypertrophy, tissue invasion by blood vessels from neighbouring bone tissue, and the replacement of the cartilage tissue with woven bone.

Late remodelling of woven bone

The woven bone forms rapidly over an approximate 3-week period. The collagen fibres vary in size and follow a random spatial arrangement with reduced provision for the deposition of hydroxyapatite crystals. Mechanically, the bone is much weaker than the lamellar bone types, where the collagen fibres are much thicker, more highly mineralised, and are orientated to form planes of lamellae that are readily discernable by scanning electron microscopy. Occurring within discrete bone multicellular units of approximately 200 μm in diameter, the remodelling process requires the activation of osteoclasts for the removal of bone (Einhorn, 2005; Kwong and Harris, 2008). This generally noninflammatory process is tightly controlled by the MSCs and osteoblasts that synthesise cytokines RANKL and M-CSF, facilitating the recruitment, differentiation, and fusion of monocytic cells into activated osteoclasts capable of degrading the bone matrix (Edwards and Mundy, 2011). Osteoblasts also halt the process by the synthesis of osteoprotegrin (OPG), which acts as a soluble decoy preventing the binding of RANKL to is cell surface receptor, RANK, on the osteoclast surface. MSCs of pericytic origin and from the marrow spaces subsequently differentiate to produce osteoblasts that replace the lost bone, synthesising first osteoid and then a mineralised bone matrix, similar to the sequence of events witnessed during the reparative stage. This late remodelling process is much slower than the reparative stage, taking from 6 months to up to 4 years to completely replace the woven bone, depending upon the size of the defect (Kwong and Harris, 2008). The formation of the lamella bone is the desired endpoint.

Primary bone healing involving intramembranous ossification can be divided into gap healing and contact healing. The latter requires direct apposition of the fracture ends and lamella bone is able to grow directly across the fracture line. However, for most tissue engineering approaches requiring regeneration of large volumes of bone, contact healing is unlikely to occur, even if the site is packed with bone autograph. Through gap healing (following the sequence of events described above), bone repair is initiated not only on the bone fracture site but also with scaffolds or on implant surfaces. The design of these scaffolds is often to achieve a surface for the attachment of the MSCs that is osteoconductive, or additionally osteoinductive, in enhancing the bone healing process.

Current methods for measuring bone healing

Recognising that bone healing is a continuum of these biological events, assessment should ideally consider a number of stages in order to chronicle the process. Since early stages of the bone repair process lay the foundation for these sequential events, time points of analysis should, as a minimum, capture initial stages characterising cellular infiltration and cellular responses through to woven bone formation. However, woven bone formation is not the final endpoint in the production of functional bone. Consequently, continued analysis through to the later stages of bone remodelling is desirable, although not always practiced. Basic analyses invariably follow tissue formation histologically. Histological analyses (see Protocol 4.1 for detail) require the tissue to be fixed, involving protein cross-linking with paraformaldehyde and subsequent demineralisation with formic acid for 24–48 hours. For a gentler approach, tissue samples should be demineralised with EDTA over 4–7 days and, to minimise shrinkage of soft tissues such as bone marrow, hand processing using methyl salicylate may be employed for better preservation of the marrow–hard tissue interface (Protocol 4.2). Tissue samples are then processed for wax embedding and cut using a microtome to produce approximately 5-μm sections that can be readily stained and viewed by light microscopy. Haematoxylin and Eosin are routinely used to distinguish osseous structures from granulation tissue. Staining with Safranin-O or Fast green will allow identification of cartilage tissue (Protocol 4.1).

Histomorphometric analysis

The 3D architecture of reparative tissue generated will be highly heterogeneous and the wound healing site is unlikely to be geometrically symmetrical. Decisions relating to sectioning of the tissue are therefore paramount. Sectioning of the tissue either in a longitudinal plane or as a cross-section is highly unlikely to capture all potential tissue heterogeneity (reviewed by Gerstenfeld et al., 2005; Allen and Burr, 2014). As an example, this may be demonstrated by the sectioning of bone healing tissue around a titanium implant. Sectioning may be coronal or sagittal, along the length of the implant, and bone healing would be differently influenced by the cortical bone of the lingual and buccal bone plate or the cancellous bone within the alveolar crestal region. Continued sectioning along either plane would therefore see differences between sections. Likewise, cross-sectioning would provide tissue sections that may be

Protocol 4.1 Histological staining procedures for measuring bone healing *in vivo*.

All stains and reagents are best obtained pre-prepared from commercial sources.

1. Dissect out osseous material containing the healing tissue. If containing implants, slowly and carefully remove to preserve surrounding tissue.
2. Using a bone saw, cut the tissue into 2-mm sections, noting orientation and positional location of healing tissue relevant to the original tissue dissection.
3. Chemically fix the tissue to preserve the biological architecture with 10 mL/cm³ 10% neutral buffered formalin (osmotically balanced to minimise shrinkage and swelling) at room temperature for 24 h.
4. Demineralise tissue sections in 10% formic acid for 72 h. If better tissue preservation of antibody epitopes is required, demineralise in 10% EDTA for 1 week. Change demineralising solution daily.
5. If required, confirm demineralisation by assaying demineralising solution for calcium. By dropwise addition of ammonium hydroxide, adjust the pH of 5 mL demineralising solution to neutral, measured using pH paper. Add 5 mL saturated ammonium oxalate, shake well, and allow to stand for 30 min at room temperature. Formation of precipitate indicates the presence of high levels of calcium in solution.
6. For processing of tissue it is best to use an automated processer now found in most pathology laboratories. Place tissue sections in biopsy cassette. Orientate tissue sections correctly so that when the tissue is sectioned the healing tissue is viewed to achieve the optimal plane as a cross, sagittal, or longitudinal section (see histomorphometric analysis). Use tissue paper to help position the tissue specimen in the cassette.
7. Process the tissue sample by first dehydrating. Incubate through a series of 70%, 90%, and 100% ethanol soaks for approximately 2 h each, followed by a further soak for 2 h in xylene.
8. Wax embed the tissue by impregnating with molten paraffin wax and allowing to cool to form the tissue "block."
9. Trim one surface of the wax block close to the tissue section and cool the surface for 10 min in an ice block. Cut 5-μm sections of the tissue sample using a microtome and mount the sections on poly-L-lysine coated glass slides (provides better adherence for repeated incubation required for techniques such as immunohistochemistry) before drying in an oven at 65°C overnight. Store at room temperature.
10. Prior to histological staining or immunohistochemistry, remove wax. Incubate twice in xylene for 30 min each (best achieved if slides are first heated to 65°C in an oven). Rehydrate by incubating through 100%, 90%, 70% ethanol and a final water rinse for 10 min each.

Haematoxylin and eosin (H&E) staining: Remove excess liquid from around the section on the slide by dabbing with tissue paper. Stain the section first with 400 μL haematoxylin solution for 10 min (stains the nucleus of cells blue). Gently rinse with tap water, "blue" in Scott's tap water and "differentiate" in 1% acid alcohol. After a further rinse in tap water, remove excess liquid and stain with 400 μL eosin solution for 30 sec (stains cytoplasmic components red).

Alizarin red staining: Although sections have been demineralised, residual calcium in mineralised tissue areas can still be stained with Alizarin red. Blot excess liquid from rehydrated sections. Stain with 0.1% w/v Alizarin red, adjusted to pH 5.5 with ammonium hydroxide, for approximately 5 min. Gently rinse slides with tap water.

Safranin-O staining: Stains for cartilage matrix mucins. Stain sections first with 0.001% (w/v) Fast green solution in H_2O for 5 min and wash thoroughly with 1% (v/v) acetic acid. Stain sections with 0.1% (w/v) safranin-O in H_2O for 5 min. Gently rinse with tap water.

Toluidine blue staining: Binds to the negatively charged sulphate groups within the glycosaminoglycan chains and thus stains effectively for the cartilage proteoglycan aggrecan. Stain with 0.04% (w/v) toluidine blue, 200 mM sodium acetate buffer for 5 min and immediately wash using tap water.

For all stained sections: Dehydrate section in absolute ethanol for 2 x 5-min rinses followed by 2 x 10-min rinses in xylene. Mount cover slips onto the sections using a DPX mounting medium.

View under a light microscope and capture images using a digital camera with appropriate software.

more uniform in the sequential planes immediately above and below, but sectioning of the tissue may not be perpendicular to the implant surface, producing an elipsoid sample area lengthening or shortening the plane of analysis, thereby affecting the conclusions made. To minimise these features when acquiring histomorphometric data, values such as total osseous tissue, void area, area of cartilage, and area of fibrous or granulation tissue are better expressed as a percentage of the total healing tissue.

Protocol 4.2 Hand processing of tissue sections to minimise shrinkage of soft bone marrow material.

1. Prepare formalin-fixed, EDTA-demineralised tissue sections. Transfer into individual biopsy cassettes and process through the respective graded chemicals, contained in a large beaker, at room temperature, as follows.

2. Place tissue section into 50% ethanol for 2 h, 70% ethanol for 2 h, and 95% ethanol overnight; three incubations in fresh 100% ethanol for 2 h each, 100% ethanol overnight, and finally one further incubation in 100% ethanol for 1 h.

3. Incubate 1 h in methyl salicylate, and incubate for a further 1 h in refreshed methyl salicylate.

4. Incubate for one wash in 0.5% necloidine in methyl salicylate and then two further incubations in 1% necloidine in methyl salicylate for 1 h each.

5. Embed the tissue by hand by incubating in molten paraffin wax at 60°C for 1 h. Replenish the molten wax on two further occasions, 1 h each infusion period. Replace the wax once more and leave overnight at 60°C. Allow the wax to solidify into the process wax block using specified moulds.

Protocol 4.3 TRAP (tartrate-resistant acid phosphatase) staining for osteoclasts in tissue sections.

1. Prepare formalin fixed, demineralized, paraffin-embedded tissue 5-μm sections on poly-L-lysine coated or frosted glass slides as described in Protocol 4.1. Note that the tissue must be demineralised with EDTA because acid demineralisation can inhibit the enzymatic activity detected in the staining process.

2. Rehydrate and deparaffinise sections by rinsing twice with xylene and then through a series of 100%, 90%, 70% ethanol and 2 rinses in water (10 min for each rinse).

3. Prepare the tartrate-containing incubation buffer by dissolving 9.2 g anhydrous sodium acetate, 11.4 g tartaric acid, and 2.8 mL glacial acetic acid in 970 mL of double distilled water. pH to between 4.7 and 5.0 with either sodium hydroxide or glacial acetic acid as required. Adjust volume to 1 L.

4. Dissolve 20 mg naphthol AS-MS phosphate substrate in 1 mL ethylene glycol monoethyl ether (can store for 1 week at 4°C).

5. Freshly prepare the TRAP staining solution; warm to 37°C 200 mL of the tartrate incubation buffer and mix with the 1 mL of naphthol AS-MS phosphate substrate solution and 120 mg Fast Red Violet LB salt.

6. Incubate the section in the TRAP staining solution for 30 min at 37°4C or until colour development is visible. This is best achieved in Coplan jars.

7. Counterstain with 0.001% (w/v) Fast green solution in water for 30 sec and rinse quickly in distilled water.
   Acid phosphatase activity appears as purplish to dark red granules in the cell cytoplasma. TRAP-positive osteoclasts can be distinguished as multinucleated giant cells. Mononuclear preosteoclasts and macrophages can also stain positive for TRAP.

Cellular analysis and immunocytochemistry

Cellular analysis can also be performed on histological sections. Approximate information regarding bone formation and bone resorption can be obtained by counts of osteoblasts lining the bone surfaces on Haematoxylin and Eosin stained sections (Protocol 4.1), or of multinucleated osteoclasts that have been stained with Naphthol AS-MX Phosphate substrate in the presence of tartrate-buffered solution to detect tartrate-resistant acid phosphatase (TRAP), detecting the active cell (Protocol 4.3). Counts are best expressed per unit of area, either within newly synthesised trabecular bone or within late remodelled bone. Analysis can also extend to provide an approximation of new blood vessel formation as a measure of angiogenesis using endothelial cell markers, such as CD31/PECAM-1 or von Willebrand factor.

However, for many of the cell counts obtained for histological stained sections, such as with Haematoxylin and Eosin, problems can be encountered in distinguishing between cell types and their differentiation status. Additional identification can be achieved by immunocytochemical localisation using specific antibodies against cell surface markers to distinguish a specific cell or the stage of bone synthesis (Protocol 4.4). Using this technique, the migration of MSCs, neutrophils, macrophages, and their persistence in the healing tissue can be longitudinally monitored (Table 4.2). The duration of bone synthesis can be described via the cellular expression of bone matrix proteins (Colombo et al., 2011). Due to heterogeneity within the tissue section, the technique is semiquantitative, whereby the counts are obtained of positively expressing cells within several (minimum of five) random fields within an entire section, for at least three serial sections. The information derived by the immuno-detection

Protocol 4.4 Immunocytochmistry for detection of cellular synthesis of osteogenic markers as a semiquantitiative measurement of bone healing.

1. Carefully dissect osseous tissue blocks for 3–5 time points relating to the presumed inflammatory stage (1–3 weeks) and the reparative stage (1–4 months).
2. If necessary, remove nonsectionable biomaterials, such as metallic implants. Take care not to damage adjacent biological tissue. Cut tissue blocks of 2–5 mm length and width.
3. Fix tissue blocks in 10% neutral buffered formalin for 24 h; demineralise in 10% formic acid for 48 h; dehydrate through 70%, 90%, and 100% alcohols and clear with xylene prior to embedding in paraffin wax; cut 5-μm sections with a microtome; mount onto poly-L-lysine coated glass slides (for additional adhesion) and dry overnight at 60°C.
4. For histological examination, deparaffinise with xylene for 10 min; rinse with industrial methylated spirit for 5 min; wash in tap water for 5 min; stain sections with haematoxylin and eosin for 5 min; mount glass coverslip using DPX glue; view using a light microscope at 40x magnification; obtain x300 dpi digital images (TIFF) using imaging software.
5. For immunocytochemical analysis, deparafinise and rehydrate sections as above; quench endogenous peroxidase activity by incubating sections in 3% H_2O_2 for 10 min.
6. Incubate sections with the appropriate 1°antibody, diluted in 1% fetal bovine serum (in Tris buffered saline) for 1 h (determine initial antibody dilution from manufacturer's recommendation, but optimise dilution factor to obtain an ideal staining level without suspician of nonspecific binding of the antibodies). As negative controls, substitute the 1° antibody with a nonimmunogenic IgG control antibody (Sigma Aldrich, UK) (used at the same dilution as the 1° antibody) and/or exclude the 1° antibody. If available, preincubate the 1° antibody with a blocking peptide used to generate the antibodies for 30 min prior to incubation with the section to block antibody epitope interaction and confirm specific antibody interation.
7. Visualise immunoreactivity using the Vectorstain Universal Elite ABC kit (Vector Laboratories, Peterborough, UK) and the DAB peroxidase kit (Vector Laboratories UK) or equivalent; counterstain with 0.1% methyl green for 1 min, with excess stain removed by excessive rinsing with tap water. Soak sections in xylene for 5 min and mount for viewing by light microscopy at x20 magnification.
8. For detection of cell surface proteins and their ligands it may be necessary to retrieve the antigen by treatment with 24 μg/mL proteinase K for 10 min prior to quenching of endogenous peroxidase activity.

Semiquantitative image analysis:

9. Using image analysis package, a minimum of five random view areas of 50 μm^2 are randomly placed over the image (see enclosed figure).
10. Counts of positively staining cells within and on the borders of squares are recorded; cell counts are averaged from a minimum of three images from the same tissue block.
11. To increase statistical validity, cell counts should be averaged with other tissue blocks obtained from the same and experimental repeat sampling sources; note intensity of staining cannot be recorded since level of staining can vary between sections depending upon length of incubation with substrate.

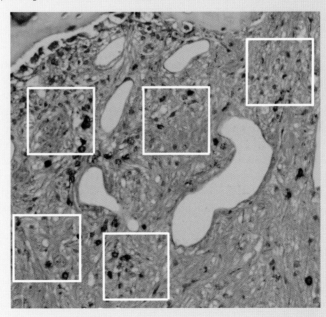

Example of cellular osteo-pontin synthesis detected in healing bone stained black by immunocytochemistry.

Table 4.2 Protein markers for measuring bone healing.

Stro-1	Detection of infiltrating mesenchymal progenitor cells
F4/80	Detection of infiltrating macrophages/eosinophils
CD14	Detection of infiltrating monocytes
Neutrophil elastase	Detection of neutrophil infiltration
IL-1, IL-6, TNFα, TGF-ß	Measurement of the inflammatory response and duration
PCNA	Measurement of cellular proliferation (not cell specific)
CD31, von Willebrand factor	Detection of endothelial cells and angiogenesis
Osteopontin	Assessment of duration of very early reparative stage
Bone sialoprotein	Assessment of duration of mid reparative phase
Osteocalcin	Assessment of for deposition of woven bone

of specific cells is particularly valuable in elucidating potential cellular mechanisms for observed delay in bone healing (Colombo et al., 2011).

Nondestructive imaging

Whilst histological staining and immunocytochemistry provide much detailed data, these techniques are destructive in nature, invariably requiring the sacrifice of animals at several time points during the healing process. Ethical issues and experimental costs result in statistical assessments performed on data with a minimum *n* value. Nondestructive data can be obtained through analysis by radiographic imaging and computed tomography (reviewed by Zhao et al., 2013). The range of imaging data available is more limited to an assessment of mineralised tissue deposition, but a more continued assessment with a greater number of time points is feasible for anaesthetised animals. Carefully calibrated and optimised image analysis for both methodologies can give a quantitative measurement of bone implant contact, total bone volume, and bone mineral density. Computed tomography can provide data relevant to trabecular and cortical bone volume within a 3D field of analysis. The data obtained can be used to support observed biomechanical assessments measuring the strength of the forming bone, as determined by insertion torque, removal torque, and resonance frequency analysis related to implant length (Gerstenfeld

et al., 2005). Biomechanical data in isolation can lead to limited interpretation of the underlying bone repair events.

Role of biomaterials in promoting bone healing

The interaction of cells with a biomaterial, even those described as inert, can affect the behaviour of MSCs. A wealth of peer-reviewed literature has highlighted a combination of factors, including surface topography/roughness, energy, chemistry, and crystallinity, as playing a role in directing bone cell biology, bone formation, and overall implant fixation (Ellingsen et al., 2006; Le Guéhennec et al., 2007). However, differences in surface preparation techniques have led to subtle differences in these interdependent factors and resulted in confusion in our understanding of the precise mechanisms underlying how cellular behaviour is influenced on such surfaces. When a biomaterial is placed into a wound healing site (or within *in vitro* culture conditions), the surface of the biomaterial is immediately coated with proteins derived from the extracellular fluids of the developing haematoma (or the serum supplemented into culture medium). These proteins would include fibronectin and vitronectin, with cell adherent properties, and growth factors such as PDGF, FGF, and TGF-β, which stimulate the cell wound healing responses. Protein composition and architecture will be influenced by factors such as roughness, hydrophobicity/hydrophilicity, and oxide layer formation. The physiochemical properties could also induce conformational changes in the tertiary protein structure and exposure of specific binding ligands on the protein surface. Differences in the architectural arrangement of the adherent proteins will direct the formation of integrin-based cell focal adhesion points, regulating cytoskeletal arrangement and cellular morphology, which, via signalling cascades such as ERK, FAK, and MAPK, in turn affect cell signalling in response to growth factors within the pericellular environment (Sjöström et al., 2009; Lavenus et al., 2011). Consequently, biomaterials possess a substantial ability to influence cell migration, proliferation, and differentiation potential of MSCs. In addition, the material substrate is capable of altering the cellular expression of integrins, which has been eloquently demonstrated for the culture of cells on plastic, titanium, and calcium phosphate surfaces (Colombo et al., 2012).

Surface roughness

Surface roughness is generally regarded as a major influence on MSC behaviour. The influence of increased implant surface roughness at the nano- and micron-scales have been extensively studied, with the proposal that increased surface roughness can influence protein adsorption and cellular responses, in favour of improved bone implant contact and greater implant stability (Wennerberg and Albrektsson, 2009; Anselme et al., 2010). However, certain contradictions in the literature still remain as to how surfaces with contrasting roughness precisely influence cell behaviour. That said, there is general agreement that the degree of roughness and the geometry of the surface are major influential factors, with cells on smooth surfaces exhibiting more spherical or spindle-shaped, flattened morphologies and a well-organised cytoskeleton with clearly defined focal adhesion points (Colombo *et al* 2012; Daw et al., 2013). Similar morphology has been identified on surfaces with a regular nano-scale roughness (15–30 nm) (Sjöström et al., 2009; Lavenus et al., 2011), and it has been proposed that this cell morphology correlates well to cells with high osteogenic potential.

In contrast, further increases in surface roughness of ≥100 nm induce cytoskeletal disorganisation, resulting in more irregular and polygonal cellular morphologies, particularly at levels >2 μm (Sjöström et al., 2009; Wennerberg and Albrektsson, 2009; Lavenus et al., 2011). Such high roughness levels further influence other cellular functions, such as extending the cell proliferation period (Ter Brugge et al., 2002; Colombo et al., 2012), in addition to decreasing adherence, spreading, and enhancing osteogenic differentiation/activity on roughened surfaces (Wennerberg and Albrektsson, 2009; Daw et al., 2013). Of note, these findings are in line with the consensus of opinion that cell proliferation, differentiation, and maturation are, in principle, independent, as actively dividing MSCs do not appear to enter differentiation/maturation pathways, while cells close to functional maturity do not divide (Song et al., 2006). These reports also highlight the existence of an optimal surface roughness range that dictates the extent of cellular activities, such as adherence, spreading, proliferation, and differentiation, on implant surfaces.

However, despite such relatively consistent trends between surface roughness and cellular behaviour, the optimal surface roughness range that induces these effects is yet to be established, as many published papers present inadequate surface characterisation, whilst roughness parameters can vary depending on the method of analysis, such as atomic force microscopy, confocal laser scattering, or contact profilometry, reinforcing the need for the standardisation of measurement and evaluation techniques (Nagassa et al., 2008; Wennerberg and Albrektsson, 2009).

Nonetheless, such findings have led to implant surfaces with hierarchical structures being advocated, which combine both nano- and micron-scale features to preferentially induce alterations in cell-surface interaction and cell behaviour at the nano-scale, and improved implant fixation and biomechanical stability at the micron-scale (Gittens et al., 2011; Daw et al., 2013). Alternatively, whilst ultra-rough surfaces may not provide a surface completely conducive to ostogenesis, nano-patterning does appear to provide the potential to stimulate MSCs to produce bone mineral *in vitro*, in the absence of osteogenic supplements (Dalby et al., 2007, 2014). Such nano-etched surfaces are proposed to guide cell alignment, which has the potential to yield a more uniform direction for the collagen fibrils synthesised in the osteoid and hence provide a higher organisation of the mineral deposited in the woven bone, with higher initial mechanical strength (Dalby et al., 2007, 2014). Within the context of nano-texturing, smooth faceted "dome" patterning and sharp edged "hut" patterning do not appear to influence cell behaviour differently (Dolatshahi-Pirouz et al., 2010), suggesting that it is more the depth of valley to peak that dictates the osteogenic differentiation of MSCs.

3D scaffold support

When considering the natural healing process, the haematoma, granulation tissue, and the osteoid all support the cells within a 3D ECM structure. These natural matrix scaffolds provide a spatial arrangement for facilitating cell focal contacts and the delivery of growth factors to cell surface receptors. Cells form transient focal contacts with multiple surfaces within this 3D environment, which has been proposed to enable better migration, proliferation, and controlled secretion of the osteoid matrix components by mimicking the natural tissue environment (Fraley et al., 2010).

Table 4.3 Key research considerations in the design of therapeutic approaches for the repair and regeneration of bone. Similar issues are relevant for cell-based and acellular-based therapies.

Scaffold Design

- Protection of cells from excessive biomechanical and shear forces that would be detrimental to cell viability.
- Adequate nutritional and oxygen supply
- Biodegradability for release of bioactive factors or replacement by newly formed bone tissue
- Development of smart biomaterials for recapitulating the natural repair process

Enhancement of Signalling Cues

- Ensuring adequate angiogenesis
- Tempered stimulation of cell proliferation that is not counterproductive to cell differentiation or tumour genesis
- Provision of cell survival factors
- Delivery of nontoxic levels of growth factors
- Temporal provision of differentiation cues—tracking of cell behaviour
- Better understanding of the role of stem cell niches in delivering function, and the promotion of cell maturation

Influence on the Wound Healing Environment

- Prevention of an inappropriate immune response leading to prolongation of the inflammatory stage to impairing bone repair
- Prevention of rejection or hypersensitivity reactions of cellular transplants or acellular interventions
- Encompassing immune suppression, immunological tolerance, and immune privilege
- Reducing fibrosis and scar formation

Delivery of MSCs

- Appropriate chemotactic cues for cell infiltration as necessary
- Defined and stringent culture expansion conditions for cell expansion
- Genotypic and phenotypic changes
- Cell heterogeneity and cell selection/sorting
- Damage caused by mass transport injection of cells into scaffolds
- Redistribution of cells outside of the scaffold-cell tracking

Hence, it has been long established that cells behave very differently in 3D cultures, compared with 2D monolayer cultures. The development of biomaterials for tissue engineering purposes endeavors to reproduce this 3D environment via a plethora of synthetic, semisynthetic, or naturally derived scaffolds, existing as hydrogels and more mechanically rigid foams and porous scaffolds (Khan et al., 2008; Kosuge et al., 2013). Current research has yet to identify the ideal biomaterial scaffold(s) for bone tissue engineering. Mechanical properties and surface stiffness will further direct cell behaviour and, similar to implant surfaces, the biomaterials will absorb proteins from the healing wound site (Sachlos and Czernuszka, 2003).

The aim of this chapter is not to review the various methods for synthesizing the array of biomaterials currently available but to outline the justifying principles behind biomaterial constructs (Table 4.3). One method used for scaffold production is to mimic the natural fibrous structures of collagen in the ECM. Natural collagen scaffolds have been generated *in vitro*, and electrospinning techniques have recreated fibres with diameter size in the range of 50–500 nm, matching those of collagen *in vivo*. However, recapitulating the natural environment has currently led to the generation of scaffold with "best fit", probably because research has not provided a definitive answer as to

how the various scaffolds mechanistically influence cell behaviour and their osteogenic potential (Mafi et al., 2012). A general aim is to allow the cells to penetrate the scaffold. When assessing scaffolds, pore sizes in the order of hundreds of microns have the potential to lead to cells stretching along the wall of the pore, adopting a flat and curved morphology, undoubtedly affecting differentiation potential. Larger pores allow for better nutrient diffusion and space for ECM deposition. However, the cells cannot bridge between surfaces and thus line the biomaterial with focal adhesion contact remaining in one plane, akin to cell morphology in monolayer cultures. Most scaffolds are designed to be degraded with time, to be replaced by the newly synthesised natural bone, but questions still remain as to the optimal speed for biomaterial degradation, while still providing a functional role in supporting cellular activity.

MSC-based therapies

One approach for bone regeneration currently under research is stem cell–based therapies, involving the seeding of MSC populations into scaffolds. The transplantation of MSCs offers the replenishment of an MSC population, where surrounding bone quality and quantity is inadequate for the rapid regeneration of bone. MSCs have been sourced from autologous and allogenic preparations of tissues, including bone marrow, dental pulp, periodontal ligament, adipose tissue, and umbilical cord (Grayson et al., 2015). Stem cell therapy is now emerging as a potential therapeutic proposition, with the establishment of a high number of commercial companies offering cell isolation, expansion, and banking services. Consequently, the high therapeutic expectations for stem cell therapy have nicely forced the development of processes that concur with good manufacturing practice (GMP) guidelines (Sensebé et al., 2013). However, despite a significant amount of published research in this area, a large number of challenges remain.

Cell expansion

A major challenge for stem cell therapy is to obtain sufficient numbers of cells to achieve bone healing (reviewed by Razzouk and Schoor, 2012). The number of cells is, of course, dependent upon the volume of bone regeneration required. It has been suggested that transplantation of a minimum of 1,500 MSCs/ cm^3 is required (Hernigou et al., 2005). Within bone marrow, MSC populations represent only 0.001%– 0.01% of total nucleated cells (Pittenger et al., 1999), indicating that once MSCs have been isolated, cells will subsequently require expansion in culture. MSCs within dental pulp tissues are present at higher concentrations, representing approximately 1% of total cell population (Gronthos et al., 2002; Lizier et al., 2012), but retrieval of small tissue samples limits the overall cell number supply. Moreover, as patient donor age increases, the number of MSCs and their regenerative capabilities decrease (Fehrer and Lepperdinger, 2005; Asumda, 2013). Furthermore, although *in vitro* culture allows for the expansion of MSCs through successive passages, excessive MSC culture expansion is associated with decreased proliferation and a gradual loss of stem cell characteristics and differentiation potential as a consequence of telomere shortening and the onset of cellular senescence (Roobrouck et al., 2008). Several studies have suggested that culture expansion should not exceed five passages (Banfi et al., 2000; Bonab et al., 2006), although evidence suggests that dental pulp stem cells can be expanded slightly beyond this (Gronthos et al., 2002, Harrington et al., 2014).

Following GMP guidelines, the culture medium should be clinically safe. High serum concentrations of 10%–20% are often required for effective cell proliferation, but serum source needs to be carefully selected for safety whilst not compromising on preserving stem cell characteristics and function. Further, due to safety and disease transmittance issues surrounding the use of animal serum, alternatives to animal serum have now been developed for cell therapy development under GMP for clinical application, namely, defined growth factors (i.e., "synthetic" serum replacements and natural human blood–derived products (Kinzebach and Bieback, 2013). Minor changes to culture conditions can also greatly influence cell behaviour. For example, changes in oxygen tension leading to a more hypoxic culture environment can increase cell proliferation (Sakdee et al., 2009; Iida et al., 2010). Following passage and during subsequent culture, MSCs will synthesise an extracellular niche that has the potential to alter cellular signalling and expression of cell surface markers (Harrington et al., 2014). Thus, inconsistencies in the frequency of media changes and subculture can result in the harvest of MSCs with unknown phenotypic differences, affecting differentiation potential (Sharma et al., 2014). In addition, genomic instability during culture expansion is a much-discussed factor, with the potential of spontaneous immortalisation and malignant transformations and major safety issues for transplantation. The process leading to chromosomal instability is poorly understood, complicated by a lack of knowledge relevant to cellular control at epigenetic and proteomic levels (Ferreira et al., 2012).

Cell selection and cell survival

Research questions still remain relating to the role of the transplanted MSC within the wound healing site. The number of cells surviving transplantation is currently indeterminate, although it is accepted that retention is relatively poor. Mass injection of the cells into the scaffold and unfavourable biomechanics acting on the cells in poorly defined scaffolds could lead to extensive loss of transplanted cells. Of the cells surviving, it is still not known how many of the transplanted cells fully differentiate to form bone synthesising osteoblasts. MSC populations may provide only "supportive osteogenic cells" that function in the synthesis of trophic factors to aid in the osteogenic process. The transplantation of cells into the wound healing site would be influenced by the signalling factors of the inflammatory stage, which in turn would affect the expression of trophic factors by the MSCs. How the signalling environment is altered is unknown. Are the signals produced by either the transplanted MSCs or the host cells in the wound environment adequate to stimulate angiogenesis and osteoblast differentiation? Moreover, MSCs represent a heterogeneous population with both MSCs of high proliferative capacity and MSCs that are more lineage restricted in terms of their regenerative capacity (see Chapter 3). Which MSC population has the greatest osteogenic potential is also unclear and begs the question whether a specific cell population or populations can be selected to provide a more rapid healing response. Subpopulations rich for a particular cell protein marker have been identified as providing a better osteogenic potential, such as CD105$^+$ Thy$^-$ cells from mouse foetal bone (Chan et al., 2009) and nestin$^+$ (Méndez-Ferrer et al., 2010) and Msx1$^+$ cells (Park et al., 2012) from bone marrow, which appear to show a preference for bone formation. However, it is recognised that within each of these populations, further MSC heterogeneity is evident. This represents the beginning of significant research undertaken in this area, although it is still unclear if in isolating these subpopulations, other supporting or ancillary cells are discarded that are required to provide trophic support for events such as resolving the inflammatory phase or promoting angiogenesis, a prerequisite for bone healing.

Cell tracking

In order to address these questions, many new approaches to cell imaging and tracking are currently under development. It is now possible to commercially obtain transgenic mice that constitutively express the green fluorescent protein (GFP) under the direction of promoter sequences to, for example, ubiquitin C and β-actin. From these GFP-cells, subpopulations enriched for a nominated cell surface marker can be obtained, providing a better understanding of their function and dynamics obtained by study *in vivo* following cell transplantation, *in vitro* as monolayer cell cultures or in 3D scaffolds, or by using *ex vivo* organ culture models (Sloan et al., 2013). In such model systems, the image signal of GFP-cells is continually present even after cell proliferation, which offers a great advantage for long-term tracking of cells compared with other cell labelling methods, such as loading cells with Q dots.

These cells are usually monitored using confocal microscopy, which can provide information regarding cell migration, particularly in response to a wound healing event. Loss of signals in cells loaded with Q dots, however, can give information regarding cellular proliferation, monitored using imaging systems such as second-harmonic generation microscopy. Gene reporter systems, attached to promoter sequences for osteogenic markers, such as Osterix, osteopontin, osteocalcin, and type I collagen, are able to provide event-specific information about the rate of MSC osteogenic differentiation towards osteoblasts. Alkaline phosphatase has also historically been proposed as a marker of osteoblast differentiation, but caution should be taken when using as a sole marker since high alkaline phosphatase activity is also noted in some MSCs, particularly iPS cells (Bassaneze et al., 2013; Zhang et al., 2014a). A variety of gene reporter systems have been utilised, including luciferase or red fluorescent protein (de Almeida et al., 2011).

Currently, noninvasive, real-time, and longitudinal imaging is available to track bone marrow stromal cells in dermal wound healing models. Some of these techniques have been successful in imaging to a depth of 1 mm. Techniques that have been established with detailed methodological protocols for microscopy techniques, including optical coherence tomography, multiphoton microscopy, two-photon excited fluorescence, second-harmonic generation microscopy, and coherent anti-Stokes Raman scattering (CARS). These techniques appear to possess promising applications for *in vitro* and *ex vivo* studies. Certain techniques, such as CARS, have been successfully employed in detecting nonlabelled cells and in identifying molecular vibration of chemical bonds in signature proteins or DNA (Masia et al., 2013). The limited penetration of these techniques through tissues may currently limit similar use of noninvasive techniques for monitoring bone healing *in vivo*. Repeated opening the wound to reveal the healing bone would affect the natural continuum of the process, and thus, analysis using these techniques may for the immediate future require tissue sample collection over specified time points to coincide with the key events of bone wound repair. Their advantage, however, is that they have the capacity to provide data for multiple biomarkers relating to cell behaviour, ECM/osteoid formation, and mineral deposition within a single tissue specimen.

Bioactive factors for promoting bone repair and regeneration

An alternative approach to enhancing bone repair processes is through incorporation of bioactive proteins into natural and synthetic scaffolds (Cartmell, 2009). Numerous scaffolds for the purpose of the delivery of growth factors have been described in the published literature, and in general their principle aim is to encourage the migration of MSCs and stimulate their proliferation and subsequent osteogenic differentiation. Initial studies investigated exogenous application of single growth factors, with TGF-β1 and the BMPs commanding significant research in line with their prominent roles in regulating the osteogenic pathway. TGF-β1 has been proposed in cellular functions in the recruitment and proliferation of MSCs, pre-osteoblasts, chondrocytes, and osteoblasts in wound healing sites (Liebermann et al., 2002; Janssens et al., 2005) and it has been used with partial success for enhancing osseointegration (Smith, 1995). It has also been shown to increase cellular expression of BMP-2 by MSCs, thereby initiating osteoblast differentiation and enhancing collagen production and bone matrix synthesis (Bostrom, 1998). Recognised as potent osseoinductive factors, BMP-2 and BMP-7 have been shown in preclinical trials to stimulate bone formation (reviewed by Ali and Brazil, 2014; Sánchez-Duffhues et al., 2015) and have been clinically approved as a therapy for nonunion fractures. *In vivo* studies, where BMP-2 is impregnated into collagen scaffolds or absorbed onto implant surfaces, have demonstrated accelerated bone repair during osseointegration and vertical augmentation of the alveolar ridge (Wikesjö et al., 2008; Lee et al., 2010; Wang et al., 2012). However, one of the biggest drawbacks for the therapeutic use of recombinant growth factors is that massive supra-physiological microgram and sometimes milligram concentrations and/or multiple doses are required to elicit a biological response (Kofron and Laurencin, 2006). It is also well recognised that growth factors are unstable and exhibit a short half-life in wound healing sites, due to extracellular proteolytic degradation in the wound healing site. Further, the high initial concentrations of growth factor can lead to cytotoxicity issues, with clinical studies describing the potential for ectopic bone formation in adjacent tissues, local bone resorption, and osteolysis due to inappropriate signalling by the BMPs.

Autologous bone grafts remain the gold standard bioactive matrix for augmenting bone repair. Within this natural tissue, growth factors are present in the nanomolar range, a concentration many thousand times less than that required for current therapeutic approaches that utilise the delivery of endogenous single-growth factors (García-Gareta et al., 2015). Although morbidity at the donor site represents a major disadvantage, we can take lessons from the high efficiency of autologous bone grafts as a naturally successful augmentation therapy. The most significant observation is that growth factors do not work efficiently as single supplementations to promote osteogenesis. Studies have indicated that greater synergistic effects are achieved by the combined application of growth factors such as recombinant human forms of BMP-2 with BMP-7, FGF, IGF, or VEGF (Wang et al., 2012; Lee et al., 2015). Combinations of TGF-β1 with IGF-1 and PDGF with IGF-1 have also shown a positive effect on the efficiency of bone repair (Lamberg et al., 2009). Platelet-rich plasma has been clinically advocated in the promotion of bone healing of maxillofacial bone defects and in orthopaedics (Rodriguez et al., 2014). Prepared from blood plasma to produce a concentrated source of platelets, it naturally contains the near optimal concentration of growth factors including PDGF, TGF-β1, and VEGF. Significantly, these are the growth factor required to initiate the early stages of the wound healing process, such as the promotion of angiogenesis, chemotaxis, cell proliferation, and the deposition of a collagenous granulation or osteoid matrix. Mixed success has been observed in reporting the efficacy of platelet-rich plasma, but this may be as a consequence of the preparation methods leading to changes in the composition of the growth factor "cocktail" (Kushida et al., 2014).

Recapitulating the natural scenario

The bone matrix itself is a natural reservoir of growth factors. Osteoclastic activity during the inflammatory stage of wound healing is proposed to lead to the release of matrix-bound growth factors, stimulating osteogenesis. Low concentrations of growth factors, such as TGF-β1, have been extracted from mineralised bone using chemical treatments, such as calcium hydroxide and EDTA (Smith et al., 2011). Significantly, the release of growth factors from the bone matrix results in a bone surface with increased osteogenic potential. Similarly, the demineralisation of bone tissue has been shown to increase the osseoinductive power compared with bone allografts, providing a more accessible reservoir for growth factors (Drososa et al., 2007). Demineralised bone matrix products have received approval for clinical use by the Food and Drug Administration, although these products often lose osseoinductive potential due to prerequisite rigorous processing and terminal sterilisation to prevent disease transmission or an immunological response (Russell and Block, 1999). Continuing this theme, dentine matrix has also been shown to be a rich reservoir of growth factors with osteogenic potential (Graham et al., 2006). A recent *in vivo* study has also demonstrated that demineralised dentine matrix considerably stimulates bone repair in a rabbit critical-size defect and rat tooth socket models (Gomes et al., 2008; Reis-Filho et al., 2012). Moreover, these results also indicate that demineralised dentine matrix is able to ameliorate delayed diabetic bone healing, probably by restoring the signalling environment (Gomes et al., 2008). Of note, commercially available deproteinised bone tissue grafts, which supposedly only contain osseoconductive bone mineral elements, sometimes embedded within porcine collagen matrix, have also been suggested to be osseoinductive in nature, due to the residual presence of bioactive proteins identifiable following their preparation (Schwartz et al., 2000).

These natural bioactive scaffolds described above are all able to facilitate osseogenesis by the provision of growth factors at physiologically relevant nanogram concentrations. However, there is increasing recognition in the literature that specific proteins, not assigned as growth factors but present within the ECM, can modulate growth factor delivery and either directly or indirectly influence signal transduction networks within cells (Chen et al., 2004). Biglycan and decorin have been shown to bind to growth factors and cytokines, including TGF-β1 (Kresse and Schönherr, 2001; Baker et al., 2009) and BMP-2 (Mochida et al., 2006). In regulating growth factor activity, both decorin and biglycan have been proposed to play major roles in sequestering growth factors to the matrix, protecting them from proteolysis, extending their extracellular half-life, and regulating release to the cell (Baker et al., 2009). Biglycan has also been proposed to exert a direct signalling role, and *in vitro* studies have demonstrated that biglycan enhances BMP-2-induced osteoblast differentiation, by direct interaction with cell surface receptors (Mochida et al., 2006). Biglycan has particularly been implicated in the induction of MSC proliferative and during early cell differentiation

(Waddington et al., 2003), whilst decorin has also been ascribed direct cell signalling roles to promote endothelial adhesion and motility (Fiedler et al., 2008).

Delivery systems

In an alternative approach to reduce the delivery of supraphysiological doses of growth factors, recent research has also focused on the development of biomaterial systems that regulate release and at the same time provide growth factor protection from the extracellular environment. Growth factors such as TGF-β1, BMP-2, BMP-4, PDGF, VEGF, IGF-1 (Ferreira et al., 2013), and Wnt3a (Popelut et al., 2010) have been encapsulated into liposomes, microspheres, films, scaffolds, and hydrogels (Lochmann et al., 2010; Ferreira et al., 2013; Farokhi et al., 2013; Lu et al., 2014; Reyes et al., 2014). The slow release of the growth factors protects these bioactives from environmental proteolysis, extending their half-life and enabling delivery at subtoxic and physiologically effective levels. Dual-release encapsulation systems have also been reported, where recombinant VEGF/TGF-β3 are rapidly released from larger $P_{DL}LGA$ microparticles, whilst BMP-2 is slowly released from smaller manufactured $P_{DL}LGA$ microparticles (Smith et al., 2014). Such dual delivery systems enable growth factors to act synergistically, thereby enhancing the extent of bone formation versus individual growth factor responses (Lu et al., 2014). Thus, the timed release of growth factors can recapitulate better and preferentially stimulate normal bone healing cascades, promoting essential angiogenesis and cell proliferation prior to inducing osteoblast differentiation. Polymer-protein conjugates have also recently been designed to be bioresponsive, allowing for the controlled release of a range of growth factors through a process of polymer-masking-unmasking protein therapy (PUMPT; Duncan and Vicent, 2013). Current success has been achieved in the conjugation of recombinant EGF to a biodegradable dextrin polymer for application in the treatment of dermal wound sites (Hardwicke et al., 2010). The principle of therapeutic action is mediated through growth factor released from the conjugate via the localised action of α-amylase, causing dextrin polymer degradation and the release of the bioactive protein. The degree of dextrin polymer cross-linking can be tailored, so that degradation rates can be optimised to best suit the conjugated protein, their susceptibility to degradation, cellular targets, and mechanisms of action, and the clinical environments into which the conjugates are delivered.

Bioelectrical stimulation of bone repair processes

In contrast to exogenous growth factor and other more traditional pharmaceutical approaches to bone repair, there has also been a long-standing interest in the concept of electrically stimulating bone healing (Aaron et al., 2004; Griffin and Bayat, 2011; Griffin et al., 2011). The rationale behind this approach is that during wounding, electric fields are disturbed due to ion fluxes across leaky cell membranes or disrupted tissue barriers, interfering with normal regenerative mechanisms. A number of electrical signalling modalities have been assessed as stimulators of cellular activity *in vitro* and *in vivo*, including direct currents, inductive fields, capacitive coupling, biphasic electrical currents, and pulsed electromagnetic fields (PEMFs; Griffin and Bayat, 2011; Balint et al., 2013). Consequently, the application of exogenous electrical fields at physiologically relevant voltages and/or frequencies enhances impaired repair processes, via the stimulation of signals responsible for cellular proliferation, migration, and differentiation, leading to repair and regeneration. Indeed, although the precise mechanisms underlying these stimulatory effects remain to be fully understood, exogenously applied electrical fields have been shown to play critical roles in wound healing, leading to positive effects on repair in numerous tissues, including skin, cornea, and the central nervous system (Tator et al., 2012; Zhao et al., 2012; Kawasaki et al., 2014).

Specifically relating to bone repair, directed bioelectric strategies have been proposed to aid the treatment of delayed union or nonunion fractures, periodontal repair, and during bone-implant osseointegration, either alone or when used in conjunction with more conventional therapies (Dimitriou and Babis, 2007; Griffin and Bayat, 2011; Griffin et al., 2011; Tomofuji et al., 2013). Research suggests that applied electrical fields influence both mineralisation and angiogenesis during bone repair. *In vitro* studies have shown that bioelectrical stimulation acts as a guidance cue for the migration of bone marrow–derived MSCs (Zhao et al., 2011), in addition to stimulating the proliferation, differentiation, and ECM synthetic capabilities of osteoprogenitor cells and osteoblasts, leading to enhanced mineral deposition through increased intracellular calcium levels and calmodulin signalling, ERK/p38 MAPK signalling, and the production of pro-osteogenic growth factors such as TGF-β1 and BMPs (Tsai et al., 2009; Balint et al., 2013; Griffin et al., 2013; Clark et al., 2014). The positive effects of electrical stimulation on angiogenesis include the reorientation, elongation, and migration of endothelial cells, secondary to the release of angiogenic factors, such as VEGF, IL-8, and bFGF, and related receptor signalling pathways (Kim et al., 2006, Dimitriou and Babis, 2007). Studies also suggest that applied electrical fields can increase osteoclast apoptosis and decrease osteoclastogenesis and overall bone resorption, in an intensity-dependent manner (Chang et al., 2005, 2006). However, despite these positive responses, several other *in vitro* studies have reported inconsistent cell proliferation and differentiation findings following cellular exposure to electrical and electromagnetic fields (Schwartz et al., 2008; Jansen et al., 2010); although such conflicting reports may be a consequence of differences in the cell types employed, their respective stages of maturation and the characteristics of the bioelectric fields applied.

2D models for analysis

Much of the research undertaken to evaluate the effects and mechanisms by which the bioelectrical stimulation of osteogenesis is promoted has been based upon 2D *in vitro* osteogenic culture models (Tsai et al., 2009; Griffin et al., 2013; Clark et al., 2014) and *in vivo* animal model evaluation (Mills and Simpson, 2012). However, due to major differences in the clinical situations being targeted, experimental designs, the respective signal sources and parameters applied, and the underlying cellular mechanisms of action, it is extremely difficult to compare the advantages and disadvantages of each different electrical signalling modality currently available. Similarly, a further challenge has been the ability to extrapolate *in vitro* model findings to those of *in vivo* animal model studies and subsequently to clinical studies. This has been due to the limitations of the *in vitro/in vivo* models used, further confounded by the variability in the optimal durations of stimulation and subsequent responses to each electrical field, related to the respective amplitudes, frequencies, and cycles parameters administered. Therefore, the optimal dosing regimens for each electric treatment modality and the underlying mechanisms of action for the positive clinical responses reported remain poorly understood.

3D models of analysis

In order to better understand the bioelectric regulation and stimulation of bone repair processes, newer 3D models for the *in vitro* assessment of both endogenous and exogenously applied electric field effects on bone healing have been developed. These are based on human-derived cells and capture the 3D nature of cell-cell/cell-matrix interactions, as well as soluble factors and physical factors that exist and mediate the complex and highly regulated process of bone repair *in vivo*. Therefore, such model development increasingly integrates these factors to create an engineered cellular construct with near-native tissue properties, which overcomes the limitations of 2D monolayer cell cultures. Such approaches consequently provide superior *in vitro* mimics to *in vivo* conditions with relevant 3D features, allowing more control of the system than can be achieved *in vivo* and providing options for reproducible and viable experimental conclusions. These include studies that have developed a 3D bone tissue construct model of osteoblast healing, ultimately to serve as a pre-clinical experimental screening platform for studying the electrophysiological regulation of bone healing. This model involves human MSC differentiation into osteoblasts on porous silk fibroin scaffolds, with cellular, electrophysiological, and biomechanical responses examined during bone regeneration following bioelectrical stimulation (Sundelacruz et al., 2013). Other 3D models have included the design of artificial extracellular matrices (aECMs), containing type I collagen and glycosaminoglycans, such as chondroitin sulphate or a high-sulphated hyaluronan derivative, formulated as coatings on 3D poly(caprolactone-co-lactide) scaffolds (Hess et al., 2012). Through the manipulation of the microenvironment within aECMs, this approach was able to identify that pulsed electric field delivery did not influence cell proliferation but enhanced osteogenic differentiation in aECMs containing sulphated hyaluronan or when osteogenic supplements were available. Alternatively, bioelectrical stimulation of human osteoblasts on different 3D calcium phosphate/collagen scaffolds has also been established for the assessment of effectiveness of electroinductive implants, in terms of their ability to promote (Grunert et al., 2014). Therefore, these models aid our understanding of the bone regeneration processes and the development of more relevant and effective biomaterial and tissue-engineered therapies for bone repair.

In vivo models of analysis

However, despite recent advances in 3D *in vitro* model system development, as bone repair in animal models may not be entirely representative of healing events and the clinical scenarios we wish to treat in humans, the design of animal models that adequately replicate human bone repair has been far more challenging. Indeed, it has been suggested that despite the varied *in vivo* fracture models currently available in numerous animal species, these may not adequately reflect the anatomy, physiology, biochemistry, healing, or biomechanical nature of these parameters in humans (Mills and Simpson, 2012). Similar conclusions have also been made on the validity of existing experimental models for bone regeneration in oral and maxillofacial surgery, in terms of the need for more appropriate and standardised models dedicated to specific clinical conditions, which would greatly improve the consistency and reliability of *in vivo* study findings (Gomes and Fernandes, 2011; Mardas et al., 2014).

Piezoelectric materials

Nonetheless, despite issues with *in vitro*/*in vivo* model validity and the identification of the optimal conditions necessary for the successful translation of bioelectrical approaches to the clinical treatment of bone defects in patients, research in this field has led to significant advances in the development of piezoelectric materials for tissue regeneration applications (Rajabi et al., 2015; Ribeiro et al., 2015). Piezoelectric materials are smart materials capable of generating electrical activity in response to minute deformations, such as the asymmetric shift of ions or charges that induce changes in electric polarisation and subsequent electric generation. For tissue engineering applications, piezoelectric materials allow the delivery of an electric stimulus via their introduction into scaffolds, which induce cellular responses required for tissue repair, such as proliferation, migration, and differentiation. Various piezoelectric materials have been employed for tissue repair purposes, particularly in relation to bone healing. Indeed, numerous piezoceramics (e.g., barium titanate and potassium sodium niobate–containing materials), piezopolymers (e.g., poly[vinylidenefluoride-co-trifluoroethylene] [PVDF-TrFE], polypyrrole, and polyaniline–containing scaffolds), carbon nanotubes, and more established biomaterials with piezo-related properties (e.g., type I collagen), have been shown in numerous studies to promote bone repair *in vitro* and *in vivo* (Shao et al., 2011; Cui et al., 2012; Ciofani et al., 2013; Liu et al., 2013; Hu et al., 2014; Zhang et al., 2014b). Similarly, piezoelectric and nanotechnology developments have further enhanced cellular responses and titanium implant osseointegration, through the coupling of electroconducive titanium surfaces topographies with electrical stimulation (Gittens et al., 2013; Nozaki et al., 2014; Shim et al., 2014).

Influence of loading and biomechanical forces

One important factor that significantly influences bone repair is the mechanical environment within which MSCs, osteoprogenitor cells, and osteoblasts reside. The induction of mechanical forces and the overall physical properties of the local tissue environment are critical in dictating stem cell fate and cellular functions, which subsequently regulate normal bone tissue homeostasis and overall bone quality/strength (Hao et al., 2015; Wang and Chen, 2013). The ECM provides the mechanical stability, which subsequently serves as a regulator of cellular activities, such as proliferation, migration, and differentiation, via the transduction of biomechanical cues through cell surface receptor–ECM interactions and/or the induction of growth factor release from cells within the local environment and the subsequent induction of cell signalling cascades (Ko and McCullough, 2001). From a clinical dentistry viewpoint, the dental tissue environment is regarded as being highly mechanoactive, being exposed to load-derived, tensile, compressive, and torsional forces and intestinal flow–derived, shear stresses, of varying magnitudes and frequencies. Indeed, bone-related treatment strategies involving orthodontic tooth movement, implant surgery, and craniofacial procedures rely upon such bone tissue modalities and adaptations to mechanical loads to promote favourable clinical outcomes (Meeran, 2012; Duyck and Vandamme, 2014). Consequently, there is immense interest in assessing the effects of applied mechanical forces on bone cell signalling and behaviour, in order to understand and identify the optimal mechanical load conditions necessary to manipulate cellular functions towards enhanced bone repair.

2D models for analysis

Bone cell responses to mechanical loading depend upon whether the loading modality is tensile, compressive, or shear in nature. This is in addition to the specific parameters of the applied loads, such as strain, stress, static versus dynamic, frequency, cycle number, and resting periods. Hence, in order to evaluate cellular responses to these various mechanical load conditions experimentally, it would appear rational that loads be applied under conditions that replicate bone tissue repair processes *in vivo*. As it is difficult to fully assess and elucidate the precise cellular and molecular events underlying mechanotransduction using *in vivo* models, due to the added complexity surrounding the presence of multiple cell types in bone and at various stages of differentiation, this becomes a particularly prudent consideration. Consequently, much of the research undertaken to evaluate the effects and mechanisms by which mechanical loads influence osteogenesis has been performed using 2D and 3D *in vitro* osteogenic culture model systems, which aim to replicate the forces found within bone microenvironments whilst allowing the mechanotransductive mechanisms involved to be delineated more readily (Delaine-Smith et al., 2015). It is generally accepted that 2D monolayer mechanical load models have paved the way to our initial understanding of cellular responses to specifically applied parameters and the mechanotransduction signalling pathways involved, as exogenous mechanical stimuli can be routinely applied directly to cultures using low-magnitude/high-frequency loading rigs, the application of fluid shear by maintaining cell culture plates and flasks on rocking platforms, or the application of strain via a vacuum-drive, FlexCell system, or four-point, bending models (Zhou et al., 2010; Uzer et al., 2012; Tucker et al., 2014). However, 2D mechanotransduction culture systems are acknowledged to have many drawbacks associated with their relevance to the bone microenvironment.

3D models of analysis

Aided by advances in biomaterials and tissue engineering, a host of 3D bone cell culture/scaffold material models have been developed with superior properties to 2D cultures, providing a more realistic spatial environment for cells to offer behavioural cues and form bone tissue architectures more reminiscent of those *in vivo*, although they may be subjected to the same mechanical load modalities as with the 2D cultures. Numerous biomaterials have been used for the seeding of MSCs and mature osteoblasts for the assessment of mechanotransductive responsiveness to various external loading modalities in 3D culture, including type I collagen, type I collagen-glycosaminoglycan, hydroxyapatite, tricalcium phosphate, ceramics, and polyurethane (Jaasma and O'Brien, 2008; Dumas et al., 2009; Kim et al., 2012; Sittichockechaiwut et al., 2009). Further studies have introduced these 3D constructs into various bioreactor systems capable of introducing mechanical loads to the constructs within (Kimelman-Bleich et al., 2011; Bouet et al., 2015; Hoffmann et al., 2015), whilst an alternative strategy has been to assess mechanoresponsiveness utilising various multicellular 3D explant approaches, including rat bone marrow explants, porcine/bovine trabecular bone explant, and rabbit cancellous bone explant culture models for the assessment of mechanical load responses (Gurkan et al., 2011; Ming et al., 2013; Birmingham et al., 2015).

Based on these initial 3D model validation successes, further more sophisticated 3D coculture systems have also been developed, which more closely resemble and replicate the *in vivo* bone microenvironment, which can be employed to study the responses and interactions of several cell types to the loads applied. These particularly include the introduction of a novel osteoblast-osteocyte coculture system, using seeded osteocytes and osteoblasts in a type I collagen scaffold at a ratio mimicking the *in vivo* bone environment (Vazquez et al., 2014). As osteocytes are the principle mechanosensors in bone, this model for the first time has permitted the elucidation of osteocyte-controlled, osteoblastic bone formation to be collectively assessed in response to mechanical loading. The findings of such 3D studies have greatly expanded the original work using 2D culture model systems, although further studies are still required to establish the precise mechanotransduction pathways initiated in 3D systems, which remain unclear compared to our understanding of events in 2D environments.

Concluding remarks

Significant advancements have been made in recent years in basic and applied stem cell biology, biomaterials and implant developments, nanotechnology, bioreactor design, tissue engineering, and in technologies enabling the exogenous electrical and mechanical stimulation of bone repair and regeneration processes, it is evident that such strategies offer huge potential for the future treatment of clinical conditions associated with craniofacial bone loss, where issues with existing therapies have led to the search for alternative cellular and acellular approaches to bone repair enhancement. Within the varied treatment strategies currently under investigation, MSCs are pivotal to the success of these treatments, either by the enhancement of bone healing through the restoration of normal endogenous MSC molecular signalling events and bone repair responses, or via the delivery of exogenously-derived MSCs to contribute to bone repair processes where endogenous MSC responses are impaired or inadequate for the replacement of larger craniofacial defects. However, despite advances in key areas, fundamental questions and challenges still remain. This is particularly true in terms of the research areas where our knowledge remains insufficient, partly due to inconsistencies in experimental approaches leading to variable findings and conclusions preventing the confirmation of optimal treatment parameters for the promotion of bone repair. Such scenarios are confounded by issues surrounding the validity of certain *in vitro* and *in vivo* experimental models, which has hindered the attainment of consistent and reliable findings, thereby limiting successful therapy translation towards clinical application. Nonetheless, addressing these existing inadequacies in preclinical research methodologies will undoubtedly help facilitate the progression of these potentially viable treatment options through translational development and ultimately, to their exploitation for improved clinical outcomes in craniofacial bone repair.

References

AARON, R. K., CIOMBOR, D. M., & SIMON, B. J. 2004. Treatment of nonunions with electric and electromagnetic fields. *Clin Orthop Relat Res*, 419, 21–29.

AI-AQL, Z. S., ALAGL, A. S., GRAVES, D. T., GERSTENFELD, L. C., & EINHORN, T. A. 2008. Molecular mechanisms controlling bone formation during fracture healing and distraction osteogenesis. *J Dent Res* 87, 107–18.

ALI, I. H., & BRAZIL, D. P. 2014. Bone morphogenetic proteins and their antagonists: current and emerging clinical uses. *Br J Pharmacol*, 171, 3620–32.

ALLEN, M. R., & BURR, D. B. 2014. Techniques in histomorphometry. In: Burr, D. B., and Allen, M. R. (eds.), *Basic and applied bone biology*. Elsevier, pp. 131–48.

ÁLVAREZ-CAMINO, J. C., VALMASEDA-CASTELLÓN, E., & GAY-ESCODA, C. 2013. Immediate implants placed in fresh sockets associated with periapical infectious process: A systematic review. *Med Oral Patol Cir Buccal*, 18, 780–85.

ANDREWS, S., FORD, D., & MARTIN, P. 2012. Knockdown of osteopontin reduces the inflammatory response and subsequent size of post-surgical adhesions in a murine model. *Am J Pathol*, 181, 1165–72.

ANSELME, K., DAVIDSON, P., POPA, A. M., GIAZZON, M., LILEY, M., & PLOUX, L. 2010. The interaction of cells and bacteria with surfaces structured at the nanometre scale. *Acta Biomater* 6, 3824–46.

ARMAS, L. A., & RECKER, R. R. 2012. Pathophysiology of osteoporosis: new mechanistic insights. *Endocrinol Metab Clin North A*, 41, 475–86.

ASUMDA, F. Z. 2013. Age-associated changes in the ecological niche: implications for mesenchymal stem cell aging. *Stem Cell Res Ther*, 4, 47–57.

AYSON, M., LEICHTER, J., & LYONS, K. 2009. Dental implant patient selection factors: an evidence based review 2009. University of Otago, New Zealand, publication of the New Zealand Government Department of Health. Available at http://www.acc.co.nz.

BAKER, S. M., SUGARS, R. V., WENDEL, M., SMITH, A. J., WADDINGTON, R. J., COOPER, P. R., & SLOAN, A. J. 2009. TGF-beta/extracellular matrix interactions in dentin matrix: a role in regulating sequestration and protection of bioactivity. *Calcif Tissue Int*, 85, 66–74.

BALINT, R., CASSIDY, N. J., & CARTMELL, S. H. 2013. Electrical stimulation: a novel tool for tissue engineering. *Tissue Eng Part B Rev*, 19, 48–57.

BANFI, A., MURAGLIA, A., DOZIN, B., MASTROGIACOMO, M., CANCEDDA, R., & QUARTO, R. 2000. Proliferation kinetics and differentiation potential of *ex vivo* expanded human bone marrow stromal cells: implications for their use in cell therapy. *Exp Hematol*, 28, 707–15.

BARNES, G. L., KOSTENUIK, P. J., GERSTENFELD, L. C., & EINHORN, T. A. 1999. Growth factor regulation of fracture repair. *J Bone Miner Res*, 14, 1805–15.

BASSANEZE, V., SACRAMENTO, C. B., FREIRE, R., DE ALENCAR, P. F., ORTEGA, N. R., & KRIEGER, J. E. 2013. Development of a new approach to aid in visual identification of murine iPS colonies using a fuzzy logic decision support system. *PLoS One*, 8, e70605.

BIRMINGHAM, E., KREIPKE, T. C., DOLAN, E. B., COUGHLIN, T. R., OWENS, P., MCNAMARA, L. M., et al. 2015. Mechanical stimulation of bone marrow in situ induces bone formation in trabecular explants. *Ann Biomed Eng*, 43, 1036–50.

BONAB, M. M., ALIMOGHADDAM, K., TALEBIAN, F., GHAFFARI, S. H., GHAVAMZADEH, A., & NIKBIN, B. 2006. Aging of mesenchymal stem cell *in vitro*. *BMC Cell Biol*, 10(7), 14.

BORRELLI, J., PAPE, C., HAK, D., HSU, J., LIN, S., GIANNOUDIS, P., & LANE, J. 2012. Physiological challenges of bone repair. *J Orthop Trauma*, 26, 708–11.

BOSTROM, M. P. 1998. Expression of bone morphogenetic proteins in fracture healing. *Clin Orthopead Rel Res*, 355, S116–23.

BOUET, G., CRUEL, M., LAURENT, C., VICO, L., MALAVAL, L., & MARCHAT, D. 2015. Validation of an *in vitro* 3D bone culture model with perfused and mechanically stressed ceramic scaffold. *Eur Cell Mater*, 29, 250–66.

BUSENLECHNER, D., FÜRHAUSER, R., HAAS, R., WATZEK, G., MAILATH, G., & POMMER, B. 2014. Long term implant success at the Academy for Oral Implantology: 8 year follow-up and risk factor analysis. *J Periodontal Implant Sci*, 44, 102–108.

CARTMELL, S. 2009. Controlled release scaffolds for bone tissue engineering. *J Pharm Sci*, 98, 430–41.

CHAN, C. K., CHEN, C. C. LUPPEN, C. A., KIM, J. B., DEBOER, A. T., WIE, K., et al. 2009. Endochondral ossification is required for haematopoietic stem-cell niche formation. *Nature*, 457(7228), 490–4.

CHANG, K., CHANG, W. H., HUANG, S., HUANG, S., & SHIH, C. 2005. Pulsed electromagnetic fields stimulation affects osteoclast formation by modulation of osteoprotegerin, RANK ligand and macrophage colony-stimulating factor. *J Orthop Res*, 23, 1308–14.

CHANG, K., CHANG, W. H., TSAI, M. T., & SHIH, C. 2006. Pulsed electromagnetic fields accelerate apoptotic rate in osteoclasts. *Conn Tiss Res*, 47, 222–8.

CHEN, X. D., FISHER, L. W., ROBEY, P. G., & YOUNG, M. F. 2004. The small leucine-rich proteoglycan biglycan modulates BMP-4-induced osteoblast differentiation. *FASEB J*, 18, 948–58.

CHEN, Y., BAL, B. S., & GORSKI, J. P. 1992. Calcium and collagen binding properties of osteopontin, bone sialoprotein, and bone acidic glycoprotein-75 from bone. *J Biol Chem*, 267, 24871–8.

CIOFANI, G., RICOTTI, L., CANALE, C., D'ALESSANDRO, D., BERRETTINI, S., MAZZOLAI, B., & MATTOLI, V. 2013. Effects of barium titanate nanoparticles on proliferation and differentiation of rat mesenchymal stem cells. *Colloids Surf B Biointerfaces*, 102, 312–20.

CLARK, C. C., WANG, W., & BRIGHTON, C. T. 2014. Upregulation of expression of selected genes in human bone cells with specific capacitively coupled electric fields. *J Orthop Res*, 32, 894–903.

CLÉMENT-LACROIX, P., AI, M., MORVAN, F., ROMAN-ROMAN, S., VAYSSIÈRE, B., BELLEVILLE, C., et al. 2005. Lrp5-independent activation of Wnt signaling by lithium chloride increases bone formation and bone mass in mice. *Proc Natl Acad Sci U S A*, 102, 17406–11.

COLOMBO, J. S., BALANI, D., SLOAN, A. J., CREAN, StJ., OKAZAKI, J., & WADDINGTON, R. J. 2011. Delayed osteoblast differentiation and altered inflammatory response around implants placed in incisor sockets of type 2 diabetic rats. *Clin Oral Impl Res*, 22, 578–86.

COLOMBO, J. S., CARLEY, A., FLEMING, G. J. P., CREAN, StJ., SLOAN, A. J., & WADDINGTON, R. J. 2012. Monitoring the osteogenic potential of bone marrow stromal cells on smooth, roughened and tricalcium phosphate modified Ti6Al4V surfaces. *Int J Oral Maxillofac Impl*, 27, 1029–42.

CUI, H., LIU, Y., DENG, M., PANG, X., ZHANG, P., WANG, X., et al. 2012. Synthesis of biodegradable and electroactive tetraaniline grafted poly(ester amide) copolymers for bone tissue engineering. *Biomacromolecules*, 13, 2881–9.

DALBY, M. J., GADEGAARD, N., & OREFFO, R. O. C. 2014. Harnessing nanotopography and integrin–matrix interactions to influence stem cell fate. *Nature Materials*, 13, 558–69.

DALBY, M. J., GADEGAARD, N., TARE, R., ANDAR, A., RIEHLE, M. O., HERZYK, P., et al. 2007. The control of human mesenchymal cell differentiation using nanoscale symmetry and disorder. *Nature Materials*, 6, 997–1003.

DAW, A. E., KAZI, H. A., COLOMBO, J. S., ROWE, W. G., WILLIAMS, D. W., WADDINGTON, R. J., et al. 2013. Differential cellular and microbial responses to nano-/micron-scale titanium surface roughness induced by hydrogen peroxide treatment. *J Biomater Appls*, 28, 144–60.

DE ALMEIDA, P. E., VAN RAPPARD, J. R., & WU, J. C. 2011. *In vivo* bioluminescence for tracking cell fate and function. *Am J Physiol Heart Circ Physiol*, 301, H663–71.

DELAINE-SMITH, R. M., JAVAHERI, B., EDWARDS, J. H., VAZQUEZ, M., & RUMNEY, R. M. H. 2015. Preclinical models for *in vitro* mechanical loading of bone-derived cells. *BoneKEy Rep*, 4, 728.

DIMITRIOU, R., & BABIS, G. C. 2007. Biomaterial osseointegration enhancement with biophysical stimulation. *J Musculoskelet Neuronal Interact*, 7, 253–65.

DIZ, P. SCULLY, C., & SANZ, M. 2013. Dental implants in the medically compromised patient. *J Dent*, 41, 195–206.

DOLATSHAHI-PIROUZ, A., JENSEN, T., KRAFT, D. C., FOSS, M., KINGSHOTT, P., HANSEN, J. L., et al. 2010. Fibronectin adsorption, cell adhesion, and proliferation on nanostructured tantalum surfaces. *ACS Nano*, 4, 2874–82.

DROSOSA, G. I., KAZAKOSA, K. I., KOUZOUMPASISB, P., & VERETTASA, D-A. 2007. Safety and efficacy of commercially available demineralised bone matrix preparations: a critical review of clinical studies. *Injury*, 38, S13–21.

DUMAS, V., PERRIER, A., MALAVAL, L., LAROCHE, N., GUIGNANDON, A., VICO, L., & RATTNER, A. 2009. The effect of dual frequency cyclic compression on matrix deposition by osteoblast-like cells grown in 3D scaffolds and on modulation of VEGF variant expression. *Biomaterials*, 30, 3279–88.

DUNCAN, R., & VICENT, M. J. 2013. Polymer therapeutics prospects for 21st century: the end of the beginning. *Adv Drug Deliv Rev*, 65, 60–70.

DUYCK, J., & VANDAMME, K. 2014. The effect of loading on peri-implant bone: a critical review of the literature. *J Oral Rehabil*, 41, 783–94.

EDWARDS, J. R., & MUNDY, G. R. 2011. Advances in osteoclast biology: old findings and new insights from mouse models. *Nat Rev Rheumatol*, 7, 235–43.

EINHORN, T. A. 2005. The science of fracture healing. *J Orthop Trauma*, 19, S4–6.

ELLINGSEN, J. E., THOMSEN, P., & LYNGSTADAAS, S. P. 2006. Advances in dental implant materials and tissue regeneration. *Periodont 2000*, 41, 136–56.

EMAMI, E., DE SOUZA, R. F., KABAWAT, M., & FEINE, J. S. 2013. The impact of edentulism on oral and general health. *Int J Dent*, 2013, 498305.

ERBEN, R. G, SILVA-LIMA, B., REISCHL, I., STEINHOFF, G., TIEDEMANN, G., DALEMANS, W., et al. 2014. White paper on how to go forward with cell-based advanced therapies in Europe. Advanced Therapies in Europe. *Tissue Eng Part A*, 20, 13–14.

FAROKHI, M., MOTTAGHITALAB, F., AI, J., & SHOKRGOZAR, M. A 2013. Sustained release of platelet-derived growth factor and vascular endothelial growth factor from silk/calcium phosphate/PLGA based nanocomposite scaffold. *Int J Pharm*, 454, 216–25.

FEHRER, C., & LEPPERDINGER, G. 2005. Mesenchymal stem cell aging. *Exp Gerontol* 40, 926–30.

ROSE, F. R. A. J., & OREFFO R. O. C. 2002. Bone Tissue Engineering: Hope vs Hype. *Biochem Biophys Res Comms* 292, 1–7.

FERREIRA, C. L., ABREU, F. A., SILVA, G. A., SILVEIRA, F. F., BARRETO, L. B., PAULINO, TDE, P., et al. 2013. TGF-β1 and BMP-4 carried by liposomes enhance the healing process in alveolar bone. *Arch Oral Biol*, 58, 646–56.

FERREIRA, R. J., IRIODA, A. C., CUNHA, R. C., FRANCISCO, J. C., GUARITA-SOUSA, L. C., SRIKANTH, G. V., et al. 2012. Controversies about the chromosomal stability of cultivated mesenchymal stem cells: their clinical use is it safe? *Curr Stem Cell Res Ther* 7, 356–63.

FIEDLER, L. R., SCHONHERR, E., WADDINGTON, R., NILAND, S., SEIDLER, D. G., AESCHLIMANN, D., EBLE, J. A. 2008. Decorin regulates endothelial cell motility on collagen I through activation of insulin-like growth factor I receptor and modulation of α2β1 integrin activity. *J Biol Chem* 283, 17406–15.

FRALEY, S. I., FENG, Y., KRISHNAMURTHY, R., KIM, D-H., CELEDON, A., LONGMORE, G. D., WIRTZ, D. 2010. A distinctive role for focal adhesion proteins in three-dimensional cell motility. *Nature Cell Biol*, 12, 598–604.

FROLIK, C. A., ELLIS, L. F., & WILLIAMS, D. C. 1988. Isolation and characterization of insulin-like growth factor-II from human bone. *Biochem Biophys Res Comms*, 151, 1011–8.

GARCÍA-GARETA, E., COATHUP, M. J., & BLUNN, G. W. 2015. Osteoinduction of bone grafting materials for bone repair and regeneration. *Bone*, 81, 112–21.

GERSTENFELD, L. C., CHO, T. J., KON, T., AIZAWA, T., CRUCETA, J., GRAVES, B. D., & EINHORN, T. A. 2001. Impaired intramembranous bone formation during bone repair in the absence of tumor necrosis factor-alpha signaling. *Cells Tissues Organs*, 169, 285–94.

GERSTENFELD, L. C., WRONSKI, T. J., HOLLINGER, J. O., & EINHORN, T. A. 2005. Application of histomorphometric methods to the study of bone repair. *J Bone Miner Res*, 10, 1715–22.

GITTENS, R. A., MCLACHLAN, T., OLIVARES-NAVARRETE, R., CAI, Y., BERNER, S., TANNENBAUM, R., et al. 2011. The effects of combined micron-/submicron-scale surface roughness and nanoscale features on cell proliferation and differentiation. Biomaterialsi, 32, 3395–403.

GITTENS, R. A., OLIVARES-NAVARRETE, R., RETTEW, R., BUTERA, R. J., ALAMGIR, F. M., BOYAN, B. D., & SCHWARTZ, Z. 2013. Electrical polarization of titanium surfaces for the enhancement of osteoblast differentiation. Bioelectromagnetics, 34, 599–612.

GOMES, M. F., DESTRO, M. F., BANZI, E. C., VIEIRA, E. M., MOROSOLLI, A. R., & GOULART, M. D. 2008. Optical density of bone repair after implantation of homogenous demineralized dentin matrix in diabetic rabbits. Braz Oral Res, 22(3), 275–80.

GOMES, P. S., & FERNANDES, M. H. 2011. Rodent models in bone-related research: the relevance of calvarial defects in the assessment of bone regeneration strategies. Lab Anim, 45, 14–24.

GORSKI, J. P. 2011. Biomineralization of bone: a fresh view of the roles of non-collagenous proteins. Front Biosci, 17, 2598–621.

GRAHAM, L., COOPER, P. R., CASSIDY, N., NOR, J. E., SLOAN, A. J., & SMITH, A. J. 2006. Effect of calcium hydroxide on solubilisation of bio-active dentine matrix components. Biomaterials, 27, 2865–73.

GRAYSON, W. L., BUNNELL, B. A., MARTIN, E., FRAZIER, T., HUNG, B. P., & GIMBLE, J. M. 2015. Stromal cells and stem cells in clinical bone regeneration. Nat Rev Endocrinol, 11, 140–50.

GRIFFIN M, & BAYAT, A. 2011. Electrical stimulation in bone healing: critical analysis by evaluating levels of evidence. Eplasty, 11, e34.

GRIFFIN, M., SEBASTIAN, A., COLTHURST, J., & BAYAT, A. 2013. Enhancement of differentiation and mineralisation of osteoblast-like cells by degenerate electrical waveform in an in vitro electrical stimulation model compared to capacitive coupling. PLoS One, 8, e72978

GRIFFIN, X. L., COSTA, M. L., PARSONS, N., & SMITH, N. 2011. Electromagnetic field stimulation for treating delayed union or non-union of long bone fractures in adults. Cochrane Database Syst Rev, 4, CD008471.

GRONTHOS, S., BRAHIM, J., LI, W., FISHER, L. W., CHERMAN, N., BOYDE, A., et al. 2002. Stem cell properties of human dental pulp stem cells, J Dent Res, 81, 531–5.

GRUNERT, P. C., JONITZ-HEINCKE, A., SU, Y., SOUFFRANT, R., HANSMANN, D., EWALD, H., et al. 2014. Establishment of a novel in vitro test setup for electric and magnetic stimulation of human osteoblasts. Cell Biochem Biophys, 70, 805–17.

GURKAN. U. A., KRUEGER, A., & AKKUS, O. 2011. Ossifying bone marrow explant culture as a three-dimensional mechanoresponsive in vitro model of osteogenesis. Tissue Eng Part A, 17, 417–28.

HAO, J., ZHANG, Y., JING, D., SHEN, Y., TANG, G., HUANG, S., & ZHAO, Z. 2015. Mechanobiology of mesenchymal stem cells: perspective into mechanical induction of MSC fate. Acta Biomater, 20, 1–9.

HARDWICKE, J., MOSELEY, R., STEPHENS, P., HARDING, K., DUNCAN, R., & THOMAS, D. W. 2010. Bioresponsive dextrin-rhEGF conjugates: in vitro evaluation in models relevant to its proposed use as a treatment for chronic wounds. Mol Pharm, 7, 699–707.

HARRINGTON, J., SLOAN, A. J., & WADDINGTON, R. J. 2014. Quantification of clonal heterogeneity of mesenchymal progenitor cells in dental pulp and bone marrow. Connect Tissue Res, 55(Suppl 1), 62–7.

HAUSCHKA, P. V., MAVRAKOS, A. E., IAFRATI, M. D., DOLEMAN, S. E., & KLAGSBRUN, M. 1986. Growth factors in bone matrix. Isolation of multiple types by affinity chromatography on heparin-Sepharose. J Biol Chem, 261, 12665–74.

HERNIGOU, P., POIGNARD, A., BEAUJEAN, F., & ROUARD, H. 2005. Percutaneous autologous bone-marrow grafting for nonunions. Influence of the number and concentration of progenitor cells. J Bone Joint Surg Am, 87, 1430–7.

HESS, R., JAESCHKE, A., NEUBERT, H., HINTZE, V., MOELLER, S., SCHNABELRAUCH, M., et al. 2012. Synergistic effect of defined artificial extracellular matrices and pulsed electric fields on osteogenic differentiation of human MSCs. Biomaterials, 33, 8975–85.

HINODE, D., TANABE, S., YOKOYAMA, M., FUJISAWA, K., YAMAUCHI, E., & MIYAMOTO, Y. 2006. Influence of smoking on osseointegrated implant failure: a meta-analysis. Clin Oral Implants Res, 17, 473–8.

HOFFMANN, W., FELICIANO, S., MARTIN, I., DE WILD, M., & WENDT, D. 2015. Novel perfused compression bioreactor system as an in vitro model to investigate fracture healing. Front Bioeng Biotechnol, 3, 10.

HU, W. W., HSU, Y. T., CHENG, Y. C., LI, C., RUAAN, R. C., CHIEN, C. C., et al. 2014. Electrical stimulation to promote osteogenesis using conductive polypyrrole films. Mater Sci Eng C Mater Biol Appl, 37, 28–36.

HUSAIN, S. R., OHYA, Y., TOGUCHIDA, J., & PURI, R. K. 2014. Current status of multipotent mesenchymal stromal cells. Tissue Eng Part B, 20, 189.

IIDA, K., TAKEDA-KAWAGUCHI, T., TEZUKA, Y., KUNISADA, T., SHIBATA, T., & TEZUKA, K. 2010. Hypoxia enhances colony formation and proliferation but inhibits differentiation of human dental pulp cells. Arch Oral Biol, 55, 648–54.

JAASMA, M. J., & O'BRIEN, F. J. 2008. Mechanical stimulation of osteoblasts using steady and dynamic fluid flow. Tissue Eng Part A, 14, 1213–23.

JANSEN, J. H., VAN DER JAGT, O. P., PUNT, B. J., VERHAAR, J. A., VAN LEEUWEN, J. P., WEINANS, H., & JAHR H. 2010. Stimulation of osteogenic differentiation in human osteoprogenitor cells by pulsed electromagnetic fields: An in vitro study. BMC Musculoskelet Disord, 11, 188.

JANSSENS, K., TEN DIJKE, P., JANSSENS, S., & VAN HUL, W. 2005. Transforming growth factor-β_1 to the bone. Endocr Rev, 26, 743–74.

JUNGREUTHMAYER, C., DONAHUE, S. W., JAASMA, M. J., AL-MUNAJJED, A. A., ZANGHELLINI, J., KELLY, D. J., O'BRIEN, F. J. 2009. A comparative study of shear stresses in collagen-glycosaminoglycan and calcium phosphate scaffolds in bone tissue-engineering bioreactors. *Tissue Eng Part A*, 15, 1141–9.

KAWASAKI, L., MUSHAHWAR, V. K., HO, C., DUKELOW, S. P., CHAN, L. L., & CHAN, K. M. 2014. The mechanisms and evidence of efficacy of electrical stimulation for healing of pressure ulcer: a systematic review. *Wound Rep Regen*, 22, 161–73.

KHAN, Y., YASZEMSKI, M. J., MIKOS, A. G., & LAURENCIN, C. T. 2008. Tissue engineering of bone: material and matrix considerations. *J Bone Joint Surg Am*, 90, 36–42.

KIKUCHI, L., PARK, J. Y., VICTOR, C., & DAVIES, J. E. 2005. Platelet interactions with calcium-phosphate-coated surfaces. *Biomaterials*, 26, 5285–95.

KIM, I. S., SONG, J. K., ZHANG, Y. L., LEE, T. H., CHO, T. H., et al. 2006. Biphasic electric current stimulates proliferation and induces VEGF production in osteoblasts. *Biochim Biophys Acta*, 1763, 907–16.

KIM, I. S., SONG, Y. M., LEE, B., & HWANG, S. J. 2012. Human mesenchymal stromal cells are mechanosensitive to vibration stimuli. *J Dent Res*, 91, 1135–40.

KIMELMAN-BLEICH, N., SELIKTAR, D., KALLAI, I., HELM, G. A., GAZIT, Z., GAZIT, D., & PELLED, G. 2011. The effect of *ex vivo* dynamic loading on the osteogenic differentiation of genetically engineered mesenchymal stem cell model. *J Tissue Eng Regen Med*, 5, 384–93.

KINZEBACH, S., & BIEBACK, K. 2013. Expansion of mesenchymal stem/stromal cells under xenogenic-free culture conditions. *Adv Biochem Eng Biotechnol*, 129, 33–57.

KO, K. S., & MCCULLOCH, C. A. 2001. Intercellular mechanotransduction: cellular circuits that coordinate tissue responses to mechanical loading. *Biochem Biophys Res Commun*, 285, 1077–83.

KOFRON, M. D., &, LAURENCIN, C. T. 2006. Bone tissue engineering by gene delivery. *Adv Drug Deliv Rev*, 58, 555–76.

KOSUGE, D., KHAN, W. S., HADDAD, B., & MARSH, D. 2013. Biomaterials and scaffolds in bone and musculoskeletal engineering. *Curr Stem Cell Res Ther*, 8, 185–91.

KRESSE, H., & SCHÖNHERR, E. 2001. Proteoglycans of the extracellular matrix and growth control. *J Cell Physiol*, 189, 266–74.

KUSHIDA, S., KAKUDO, N., MORIMOTO, N., HARA, T., OGAWA, T., MITSUI, T., & KUSUMOTO, K. 2014. Platelet and growth factor concentrations in activated platelet-rich plasma: a comparison of seven commercial separation systems. *J Artif Organs*, 17, 186–92.

KUZYK, P. R., & SCHEMITSCH, E. H. 2011. The basic science of peri-implant bone healing. *Indian J Orthop*, 45, 108–15.

KWONG, F. N., & HARRIS, M. B. 2008. Recent developments in the biology of fracture repair. *J Am Acad Orthop Surg*, 16, 619–25.

LAMBERG, A., BECHTOLD, J. E., BAAS, J., SØBALLE, K., & ELMENGAARD, B. 2009. Effect of local TGF-beta1 and IGF-1 release on implant fixation: comparison with hydroxyapatite coating: a paired study in dogs. *Acta Orthop*, 80, 499–504.

LAVENUS, S., BERREUR, M., TRICHET, V., LOUARN, G., & LAYROLLE, P. 2011. Adhesion and osteogenic differentiation of human mesenchymal stem cells on titanium nanopores. *Eur Cells Mater*, 22, 84–96.

LEE, J., DECKER, J. F., POLIMENI, G., CORTELLA, C.A,, ROHRER, M. D., WOZNEY, J. M. *et al.* 2010. Evaluation of implants coated with rhBMP-2 using two different coating strategies: a critical-size supra-alveolar peri-implant defect study in dogs. *J Clin Periodontol*, 37, 582–90.

LEE, J. H., JANG, S. J., BAEK, H. R., LEE, K. M., CHANG, B. S., & LEE, C. K. 2015. Synergistic induction of early stage of bone formation by combination of recombinant human bone morphogenetic protein-2 and epidermal growth factor. *J Tissue Eng Regen Med*, 9, 447–59.

LE GUÉHENNEC, L., SOUEIDAN, A., LAYROLLE, P., & AMOURIQ, Y. 2007. Surface treatments of titanium dental implants for rapid osseointegration. *Dent Mats*, 23, 844–54.

LEWALLEN, E. A., RIESTER, S. M., BONIN, C. A., KREMERS, H. M., DUDAKOVIC, A., KAKAR, S., et al. 2015. Biological strategies for improved osseointegration and oseoinduction of porus metal orthopedic implants. *Tissue Eng Part B Rev*, 21, 218–30.

LIEBERMAN, J. R., DALUISKI, A., & EINHORN, T. A. 2002. The role of growth factors in the repair of bone. Biology and clinical applications. *J Bone Joint Surg Am*, 84-A, 1032–44.

LIU, L., LI, P., ZHOU, G., WANG, M., JIA, X., LIU, M., et al. 2013. Increased proliferation and differentiation of pre-osteoblasts MC3T3-E1 cells on nanostructured polypyrrole membrane under combined electrical and mechanical stimulation. *J Biomed Nanotechnol*, 9, 1532–9.

LIZIER, N. F., KERKIS, A., GOMES, C. M., HEBLING, J., OLIVEIRA, C. F., CAPLAN, A. I., & KERKIS, I. 2012. Scaling-up of dental pulp stem cells isolated from multiple niches. *PLoS One*, 7, e39885.

LOCHMANN, A., NITZSCHE, H., VON EINEM, S., SCHWARZ, E., & MÄDER, K. 2010. The influence of covalently linked and free polyethylene glycol on the structural and release properties of rhBMP-2 loaded microspheres. *J Control Rel*, 147, 92–100.

LU, S., LAM, J., TRACHTENBERG, J. E., LEE, E. J,, SEYEDNEJAD, H,, VAN DEN BEUCKEN, J. J. 2014. Dual growth factor delivery from bilayered, biodegradable hydrogel composites for spatially-guided osteochondral tissue repair. *Biomaterials*, 35, 8829–39.

MAFI, P., HINDOCHA, S., MAFI, R., & KHAN, W. S. 2012. Evaluation of biological protein-based collagen scaffolds in cartilage and musculoskeletal tissue engineering: a systematic review of the literature. *Curr Stem Cell Res Ther*, 7, 302–9.

MARDAS, N., DEREKA, X., DONOS, N., & DARD, M. 2014. Experimental model for bone regeneration in oral and cranio-maxillo-facial surgery. *J Invest Surg*, 27, 32–49.

MASIA, F., GLEN, A., STEPHENS, P., BORRI, P., & LANGBEIN, W. 2013. Quantitative chemical imaging and unsupervised analysis using hyperspectral coherent anti-Stokes Raman scattering microscopy. *Anal Chem*, 85, 10820–8.

MCKEE, M. D., PEDRAZA, C. E., & KAARTINEN, M. T. 2011. Osteopontin and wound healing in bone. *Cells Tissues Organs*, 194, 313–9.

MEERAN, N. A. 2012. Biological response at the cellular level within the periodontal ligament on application of orthodontic force: an update. *J Orthod Sci*, 1, 2–10.

MÉNDEZ-FERRER, S., MICHURINA, T. V., FERRARO, F., MAZLOOM, A. R., MACARTHUR, B. D., LIRA, S. A., et al. 2010. Mesenchymal and haematopoietic stem cells form a unique bone marrow niche. *Nature*, 466(7308), 829–34.

MILLS, L. A., SIMPSON, A. H. 2012. *In vivo* models of bone repair. *J Bone Joint Surg Br*, 94, 865–74.

MING, W. Z., YU, L. J., XIN, L. R., HAO, L., YONG, G., LU, L., et al. 2013. Bone formation in rabbit cancellous bone explant culture model is enhanced by mechanical load. *Biomed Eng Online*, 12, 35.

MOCHIDA, Y., PARISUTHIMAN, D., & YAMAUCHI, M. 2006. Biglycan is a positive modulator of BMP-2 induced osteoblast differentiation. *Adv Exp Med Biol*, 585, 101–13.

NAGASSA, M. E., DAW, A. E., ROWE, W. G., CARLEY, A., THOMAS, D. W., & MOSELEY, R. 2008. Optimisation of the hydrogen peroxide pre-treatment of titanium: surface characterisation and protein adsorption. *Clin Oral Implants Res*, 19, 1317–26.

NOZAKI, K., WANG, W., HORIUCHI, N., NAKAMURA, M., TAKAKUDA, K., YAMASHITA, K., & NAGAI, A. 2014. Enhanced osteoconductivity of titanium implant by polarization-induced surface charges. *J Biomed Mater Res A*, 102, 3077–86.

ORYAN, A., ALIDADI, S., & MOSHIRI A. 2013. Current concerns regarding healing of bone defects. *Hard Tissue*, 2, 13.

ORYAN, A., ALIDADI, S., MOSHIRI, A., & MAFFULLI, N. 2014. Bone regenerative medicine: classic options, novel strategies, and future directions. *J Orthop Surg Res*, 9, 18.

PARK, D., SPENCER, J. A., KOH, B. I., KOBAYASHI, T., FUJISAKI, J., CLEMENS, T. L., et al. 2012. Endogenous bone marrow MSCs are dynamic, fate-restricted participants in bone maintenance and regeneration. *Cell Stem Cell*, 10, 259–72.

PITTENGER, M. F., MACKAY, A. M., BECK, S. C., JAISWAL, R. K., DOUGLAS, R., MOSCA, J. D. *et al.* 1999. Multilineage potential of adult human mesenchymal stem cells. *Science*, 284, 143–7.

POPELUT, A., ROOKER, S. M., LEUCHT, P., MEDIO, M., BRUNSKI, J. B., & HELMS, J. A. 2010. The acceleration of implant osseointegration by liposomal Wnt3a. *Biomaterials*, 31, 9173–81.

POUNTOS, I., GEORGOULI, T., CALORI, G. M., & GIANNOUDIS, P. V. 2012. Do nonsteroidal anti-inflammatory drugs affect bone healing? a critical analysis. *The ScientificWorld Journal*, 2012, 606404.

RAJABI, A. H., JAFFE, M., & ARINZEH, T. L. 2015. Piezoelectric materials for tissue regeneration: a review. *Acta Biomater*, 24, 12–23.

RAMIREZ, F., & RIFKIN, D. B. 2003. Cell signalling events: a view from the matrix. *Matrix Biol*, 22, 101–7.

RAZZOUK, S., & SCHOOR, R. 2012. Mesenchymal stem cells and their challenges for bone regeneration and osseointegration. *J Periodontol* 83, 547–50.

REIS-FILHO, C. R., SILVA, E. R., MARTINS, A. B., PESSOA, F. F., GOMES, P. V., DE ARAÚJO, M. S. et al. 2012. Demineralised human dentine matrix stimulates the expression of VEGF and accelerates the bone repair in tooth sockets of rats. *Arch Oral Biol*, 57, 469–76.

REYES, R., DELGADO, A., SÁNCHEZ, E., FERNÁNDEZ, A., HERNÁNDEZ, A., & EVORA, C. 2014. Repair of an osteochondral defect by sustained delivery of BMP-2 or TGFβ$_1$ from a bilayered alginate-PLGA scaffold. *J Tissue Eng Regen Med*, 8, 521–33.

RIBEIRO, C., SENCADAS, V., CORREIA, D. M., & LANCEROS-MÉNDEZ, S. 2015. Piezoelectric polymers as biomaterials for tissue engineering applications. *Colloids Surf B Biointerfaces*, 136, 46–55.

ROCCUZZO, M., DE ANGELIS, N., BONINO, L., & AGLIETTA, M. 2010. Ten-year results of a three-arm prospective cohort study on implants in periodontally compromised patients. Part 1: implant loss and radiographic bone loss. *Clin Oral Implants Res*, 21, 490–6.

RODRIGUEZ, I. A., GROWNEY KALAF, E. A., BOWLIN, G. L., & SELL, S. A. 2014. Platelet-rich plasma in bone regeneration: engineering the delivery for improved clinical efficacy. *Biomed Res Int*, 2014, 392398.

ROHANIZADEH, R., PADRINES, M., BOULER, J. M., COUCHOUREL, D., FORTUN, Y., & DACULSI, G. 1998. Apatite precipitation after incubation of biphasic calcium-phosphate ceramic in various solutions: influence of seed species and proteins. *J Biomed Mater Res*, 42, 530–9.

ROOBROUCK, V. D., ULLOA-MONTOYA, F., & VERFAILLIE, C. M. 2008. Self-renewal and differentiation capacity of young and aged stem cells. *Exp Cell Res*, 314, 1937–44.

RUSSELL, J. L., & BLOCK, J. E. 1999. Clinical utility of demineralized bone matrix for osseous defects, arthrodesis, and reconstruction: impact of processing techniques and study methodology. *Orthopedics*, 22, 524–31.

SACHLOS, E., & CZERNUSZKA, J. T. 2003. Making tissue engineering scaffolds work. Review on the application of solid freeform fabrication technology to the production of tissue engineering scaffolds. *Eur Cells Mater*, 5, 29–40.

SAKDEE, J. B., WHITE, R. R., PAGONIS, T. C., & HAUSCHKA, P. V. 2009. Hypoxia-amplified proliferation of human dental pulp cells. *J Endod*, 35, 818–23.

SÁNCHEZ-DUFFHUES, G., HIEPEN, C., KNAUS, P., & TEN DIJKE, P. 2015. Bone morphogenetic protein signaling in bone homeostasis. *Bone*, 80, 43–59.

SATO, M., GRASSER, W., HARM, S., FULLENKAMP, C., & GORSKI, J. P. 1992. Bone acidic glycoprotein 75 inhibits resorption activity of isolated rat and chicken osteoclasts. *FASEB J*, 6, 2966–76.

SCHÖNHERR, E., & HAUSSER, H. J. 2000. Extracellular matrix and cytokines: a functional unit. *Devel. Immunol*, 7, 89–101.

SCHWARTZ, Z., SIMON, B. J., DURAN, M. A., BARABINO, G., CHAUDHRI, R., & BOYAN, B. D. 2008. Pulsed electromagnetic fields enhance BMP-2 dependent osteoblastic differentiation of human mesenchymal stem cells. *J Orthop Res*, 26, 1250–5.

SCHWARTZ, Z., WEESNER, T., VAN DIJK, S., COCHRAN, D. L, MELLONIG, J. T., LOHMANN, C. H., et al. 2000. Ability of deproteinized cancellous bovine bone to induce new bone formation. *J Periodontol*, 71, 1258–69.

SENSEBÉ, L., GADELORGE, M., & FLEURY-CAPPELLESSO, S. 2013. Production of mesenchymal stromal/stem cells according to good manufacturing practices: a review. *Curr Stem Cell Res Ther*, 4, 66.

SHAFIEI, Z., BIGHAM, A. S., DEHGHANI, S. N., & NEZHAD, S. T. 2009. Fresh cortical autograft versus fresh cortical allograft effects on experimental bone healing in rabbits: radiological, histopathological and biomechanical evaluation. *Cell Tissue Bank*. 10, 19–26.

SHAO, S., ZHOU, S., LI, L., LI, J., LUO, C., WANG, J., LI, X., & WENG, J. 2011. Osteoblast function on electrically conductive electrospun PLA/MWCNTs nanofibers. *Biomaterials*, 32, 2821–33.

SHARMA, R. R., POLLOCK, K., HUBEL, A., & MCKENNA, D. 2014. Mesenchymal stem or stromal cells: a review of clinical applications and manufacturing practices. *Transfusion*, 54, 1418–37.

SHARP, J. G., MURPHY, B. O., JACKSON, J. D., BRUSNAHAN, S. K., KESSINGER, A., & NEFF, J. R. 2005. Promises and pitfalls of stem cell therapy for the promotion of healing. *Clin Orthop Relat Res*, 435, 52–61.

SHIM, I. K., CHUNG, H. J., JUNG, M. R., NAM, S. Y., LEE, S. Y., LEE, H., et al. 2014. Biofunctional porous anodized titanium implants for enhanced bone regeneration. *J Biomed Mater Res A*, 102, 3639–48.

SITTICHOCKECHAIWUT, A., SCUTT, A. M., RYAN, A. J., BONEWALD, L. F., & REILLY, G. C. 2009. Use of rapidly mineralising osteoblasts and short periods of mechanical loading to accelerate matrix maturation in 3D scaffolds. *Bone*, 44, 822–9.

SJÖSTRÖM, T., DALBY, M. J., HART, A., TARE, R., OREFFO, R. O., & SU, B. 2009. Fabrication of pillar-like titania nanostructures on titanium and their interactions with human skeletal stem cells. *Acta Biomater*, 5, 1433–41.

SLOAN, A. J., TAYLOR, S. Y., SMITH, E. L., ROBERTS, J. L., CHEN, L., WEI, X. Q., & WADDINGTON, R. J. 2013. A novel *ex vivo* culture model for inflammatory bone destruction. *J Dent Res*, 92, 728–34.

SMITH, E. L., COLOMBO, J. S., SLOAN, A. J., & WADDINGTON, R. J. 2011. TGF ß1 exposure from bone surfaces treated by chemical treatment modalities. *Eur Cells Mater*, 21, 193–201.

SMITH, E. L., KANCZLER, J. M., GOTHARD, D., ROBERTS, C. A., WELLS, J. A., WHITE, L. J. et al. 2014. Evaluation of skeletal tissue repair. Part 2: enhancement of skeletal tissue repair through dual-growth-factor-releasing hydrogels within an *ex vivo* chick femur defect model. *Acta Biomater*, 10, 4197–205.

SMITH, R. A. 1995. The effect on TGF-beta 1 on osseointegration. *J Calif Dent Assoc*, 23, 49–53.

SONG, L., WEBB, N. E., SONG, Y., & TUAN, R. S. 2006. Identification and functional analysis of candidate genes regulating mesenchymal stem cells self-renewal and multipotency. *Stem Cells*, 24, 707–1718.

STRIETZEL, F. P., REICHART, P. A., KALE, A., KULKARNI, M., WEGNER, B., & KÜCHLER, I. 2007. Smoking interferes with the prognosis of dental implant treatment: a systematic review and meta-analysis. *J Clin Peridontol*, 34, 523–44.

SUNDELACRUZ, S., LI, C., CHOI, Y. J., LEVIN, M., & KAPLAN, D. L. 2013. Bioelectric modulation of wound healing in a 3D *in vitro* model of tissue-engineered bone. *Biomaterials*, 34, 6695–705.

TAIPALE, J., & KESKI-OJA, J. 1997. Growth factors in the extracellular matrix. *FASEB J*, 11, 51–9.

TATOR, C. H., MINASSIAN, K., & MUSHAHWAR, V. K. 2012. Spinal cord stimulation: therapeutic benefits and movement generation after spinal cord injury. *Handb Clin Neurol*, 109, 283–96.

TER BRUGGE, P. J., WOLKE, J. G., & JANSEN, J. A. 2002. Effect of calcium phosphate coating crystallinity and implant surface roughness on differentiation of rat bone marrow cells. *J Biomed Mater Res*, 60, 70–78.

TOMOFUJI, T., EKUNI, D., AZUMA, T, IRIE, K., ENDO, Y., KASUYAMA, K., et al. 2013. Effects of electrical stimulation on periodontal tissue remodeling in rats. *J Periodontal Res*, 48, 177–183.

TSAI, M. T., LI, W. J., TUAN, R. S., & CHANG, W. H. 2009. Modulation of osteogenesis in human mesenchymal stem cells by specific pulsed electromagnetic field stimulation. *J Orthop Res*, 27, 1169–74.

TUCKER, R. P., HENNINGSSON, P., FRANKLIN, S. L., CHEN, D., VENTIKOS, Y., BOMPHREY, R. J., & THOMPSON, M. S. 2014. See-saw rocking: An *in vitro* model for mechanotransduction research. *J R Soc Interface*, 11, 20140330.

UZER, G., MANSKE, S. L., CHAN, M. E., CHIANG, F. P., RUBIN, C. T., FRAME, M. D., & JUDEX, S. 2012. Separating fluid shear stress from acceleration during vibrations in vitro: Identification of mechanical signals modulating the cellular response. *Cell Mol Bioeng*, 5, 266–76.

VAZQUEZ, M., EVANS, B. A., RICCARDI, D., EVANS, S. L., RALPHS, J. R., DILLINGHAM, C. M., MASON, D. J. 2014. A new method to investigate how mechanical loading of osteocytes controls osteoblasts. *Front Endocrinol (Lausanne)*, 5, 208.

WADDINGTON, R. J., ROBERTS, H. C., SUGARS, R. V., & SCHÖNHERR, E. 2003. Differential roles for small leucine-rich proteoglycans in bone formation. *Eur Cells Mater*, 6, 12–21.

WADDINGTON, R. J., & SLOAN, A. J. 2012. Is there anything to be gained by augmenting the implant surface? *Faculty Dental Journal*, 3, 28–33.

WANG, J., ZHENG, Y., ZHAO, J., LIU, T., GAO, L., GU, Z., & WU, G. 2012. Low-dose rhBMP2/7 heterodimer to reconstruct peri-implant bone defects: a micro-CT evaluation. *J Clin Periodontol*, 39, 98–105.

WANG, Y. K., & CHEN, C. S. 2013. Cell adhesion and mechanical stimulation in the regulation of mesenchymal stem cell differentiation. *J Cell Mol Med*, 17, 823–32.

WENNERBERG, A., & ALBREKTSSON, T. 2009. Effects of titanium surface topography on bone integration: a systematic review. *Clin Oral Implants Res*, 4, 172–84.

WIKESJÖ, U. M., QAHASH, M., POLIMENI, G., SUSIN, C., SHANAMAN, R. H., ROHRER, M. D., et al. 2008. Alveolar ridge augmentation using implants coated with recombinant human bone morphogenetic protein-2: histologic observations. *J Clin Periodontol*, 35,1001–10.

YANG, Y., YANG, J., LIU, R., LI, H., LUO, X., & YANG, G. 2011. Accumulation of β-catenin by lithium chloride in porcine myoblast cultures accelerates cell differentiation. *Mol Biol Rep*, 38, 2043–9.

ZHANG, Y., WEI, C., ZHANG, P., LI, X., LIU, T., PU, Y., et al. 2014a. Efficient reprogramming of naïve-like induced pluripotent stem cells from porcine adipose-derived stem cells with a feeder-independent and serum-free system. *PLoS One*, 9, e85089.

ZHANG, Y., CHEN, L., ZENG, J., ZHOU, K., & ZHANG, D. 2014b. Aligned porous barium titanate/hydroxyapatite composites with high piezoelectric coefficients for bone tissue engineering. *Mater Sci Eng C Mater Biol Appl*, 39, 143–9.

ZHAO, M., CHALMERS, L., CAO, L., VIEIRA, A. C., MANNIS, M., & REID, B. 2012. Electrical signaling in control of ocular cell behaviors. *Prog Retin Eye Res*, 31, 65–88.

ZHAO, Y., BOWER, A. J., GRAF, B. W., BOPPART, M. D., & BOPPART, S. A. 2013. Imaging and tracking of bone marrow-derived immune and stem cells. *Methods Mol Biol*, 1052, 57–76.

ZHAO, Z., WATT, C., KARYSTINOU, A., ROELOFS, A. J., MCCAIG, C. D., GIBSON, I. R., & DE BARI, C. 2011. Directed migration of human bone marrow mesenchymal stem cells in a physiological direct current electric field. *Eur Cell Mater*, 22, 344–58.

ZHOU, X., LIU, D., YOU, L., & WANG, L. 2010. Quantifying fluid shear stress in a rocking culture dish. *J Biomech*, 43, 1598–602.

CHAPTER 5

Tissue culture models and approaches for dental tissue regeneration

Alastair J. Sloan[1], John Colombo[2], Jessica Roberts[3], Rachel J. Waddington[1], and Wayne Nishio Ayre[1]

[1] School of Dentistry, Cardiff Institute of Tissue Engineering and Repair, Cardiff University, Cardiff, UK

[2] School of Dentistry, University of Utah, Salt Lake City, UT, USA

[3] North Wales Centre for Primary Care Research, Bangor University, Wrexham, UK

The development of alternative treatment modalities for the management of significant dental tissue disease or trauma, such as caries, dentinal fractures, periodontal disease or obtaining biological evidence to support current clinical treatment regimes is hampered by the limitations of laboratory model systems currently available for the study of dental tissue repair. At present this routinely involves the use of animal models (*in vivo*) or simpler *in vitro* models to investigate the dentine, periodontal ligament (PDL), and bone repair process. The problems associated with *in vitro* (oversimplified representation of the multicellular complex using a single-cell system or, at the most, two cell types in the case of co-cultures and 3D organoid cultures) models do not account for the important cellular interactions that occur *in vivo* and they are unable to recapitulate the spatial arrangement of cells *in vivo* and as such can be severely limiting. In addition, it does not take into account any possible altered cell behaviour when cells are cultured on two dimensions on tissue culture plastic or glass that may limit the relevance of the data obtained.

In vivo experimentation is always the gold standard in elucidating tissue regenerative processes that occur during dental tissue and bone repair, or tissue responses to new interventions. However, such animal models have significant cost implications and usually require large numbers of animals for each study, which impacts on the ethical standing of such studies. It can be difficult to obtain clear data in these *in vivo* experiments due to systemic influences, which make investigation of specific cellular and tissue responses difficult. *Ex vivo* culture models have been developed to overcome these issues and to study a wide variety of developmental, physiological, and pathological conditions. These *ex vivo* models have the advantage over simple cell culture protocols in that the cells and tissue are cultured in the same spatial arrangement as would be found in the *in vivo* situation, and unlike whole animal studies, the systemic influences, which often hinder *in vivo* work, are removed. This has led to the development of a number of *ex vivo* models (Sloan et al., 1998; Sloan and Smith, 1999; Dhopatkar et al., 2005 Ong et al., 2013; Roberts et al., 2013). Such *ex vivo* culture systems are not uncommon and find use within the tissue engineering and regenerative medicine community. These models allow cells to be cultured in the spatial arrangement they would be found *in vivo* but enable multiple experiments to be performed using the tissue from a single animal providing an ideal system for investigating specific biological processes, as well as a promising alternative to *in vivo* testing of novel clinical therapeutics (Turner et al., 2002; Graichen et al., 2005). The organ culture of cartilage has facilitated the understanding of cartilage repair (Graichen et al., 2005) and with respect to mineralised tissues the development of a tooth slice *ex vivo* culture system (Sloan et al., 1998; Sloan and Smith, 1999; Magloire et al., 1996) has greatly enhanced the understanding of dental tissue repair processes.

An important application of such models is in the development and understanding of clinical dental

---

Tissue Engineering and Regeneration in Dentistry: Current Strategies, First Edition. Edited by Rachel J. Waddington and Alastair J. Sloan.

techniques, the effect of new tissue repair therapies, and the effect of new bioactive agents (such as antimicrobial agents or anti-inflammatory agents). Many popular composite placement techniques, particularly in relation to operatively exposed dentine, are not evidence based and defy common sense. These are mainly "hang overs" from previous amalgam placement techniques. An important example of such confusion in contemporary clinical dentistry is the dilemma of "bonding" or "basing" composite restorations. Following a technique used with amalgam placement, many practitioners choose to place a "base" cement under a composite restoration to "protect" operatively exposed dentin at the expense of the mechanical properties of the completed restoration. However, a growing number of practitioners choose not to use a "base" cement and instead simply "bond" the composite in place without using a cement base. There is no real reliable evidence, biological or clinical, to support the merit of either technique. Therefore, patients are potentially exposed to risk. Clear elucidation of the biological effects of such materials via appropriate model systems is required for proper investigation. The opportunity also exists to explore the development and selection of materials, which can drive dental tissue repair via studying material/dentine interactions in appropriate dentine/pulp complex models. The ultimate aim of such an approach is to improve treatment outcomes for patients and retain tooth viability.

Models for dental tissue regeneration

In vivo, the mineralised dentine, the odontoblast cells, and the pulpal soft connective tissue are considered a cooperative functional complex. Various attempts have been made to culture odontoblasts and other cells of the pulp *in vitro* (Nakashima et al., 1991; Bègue-Kirn et al., 1992, 1994), but these and other previous attempts to culture odontoblasts *in vitro* have demonstrated the need to maintain direct contact between those cells and the dentine to preserve the cell's phenotypic morphology (Munksgaard et al., 1978; Heywood and Appleton, 1984). The importance of the dentine, especially the bioactive proteins contained within it, was clearly demonstrated by the successful culture of mouse dental papillae with a dentine matrix extract (Bègue-Kirn et al., 1992, 1994). Contact between the papillae

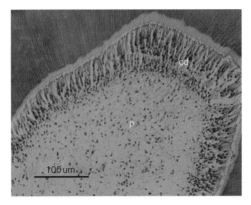

Figure 5.1 Histological appearance of a rodent tooth slice cultured for 14 days demonstrating maintenance of cell and tissue architecture and viability. Pulpal cells (p) and the odontoblast cell layer (od) remain viable during culture.

and the dentine matrix extract led to differentiation of an odontoblast cell population from the papillae cells that were in contact with the dentine extract. These cells were also able to synthesise a new dentine matrix. In those culture systems, the papillae was embedded in a semisolid agar-based medium prior to being cultured at the liquid-gas interface, and it was this successful organ culture method that was modified to develop a culture model system for the mature dentine-pulp complex.

The culture of the dentine-pulp complex of 28-day-old male Wister rat incisor teeth (Sloan et al., 1998) when embedded in a semisolid agar-based medium and cultured in Trowel-type cultures at the liquid-gas interface allowed for culture of the tissue successfully for up to 14 days with maintenance of the tissue architecture of the entire tissue complex during culture period (Figure 5.1). An *in vitro* model of human dental tissue repair has also been developed, whereby thick tooth slices have been cultured in liquid media (Magloire et al., 1996; Melin et al., 2000). Such tissue organotypic culture models now facilitate the investigation of dentinogenesis and tissue repair mechanisms, as the odontoblasts can be examined within the normal environment of the dentine-pulp complex, but in the absence of the normal inflammatory processes that occur *in vivo*. This tooth slice culture system (Protocol 5.1) has been pivotal in understanding the bioactive nature of the dentine matrix and the role of TGF-β1, BMP-7, and other growth factors in directing reparative events in dental tissue repair (Sloan and Smith, 1999;

Protocol 5.1 Rodent tooth slice culture.

1. Prepare supplemented culture media: Dulbecco's modified Eagle's medium (DMEM, with ribonucleosides, deoxyribonucleosides), supplemented with 10% heat-inactivated fetal calf serum, 0.15 mg/mL vitamin C, 200 mmol/L L-glutamine and 1,000 U/mL penicillin G sodium, 10 µg/mL streptomycin sulfate, and 25 µg/mL amphotericin B.
2. Extract upper and lower incisors of sacrificed 28-day-old male Wistar rats, removing soft tissue and bone from outer surface using a sterile scalpel.
3. Temporarily store the incisors in prepared culture media prior to sectioning.
4. Using a diamond-edged rotary bone saw, cut 2-mm-thick transverse sections and transfer into a 12-well plate in 2 mL supplemented DMEM at 37°C, 5% CO_2 for 4 days, changing the media every 24 h.
5. Wash tooth slices in phosphate-buffered saline (PBS), then transfer tooth slices to a fresh sterile washing media at 37°C.
6. Prepare embedding medium consisting of 4 mL of supplemented DMEM culture media and 5 mL of sterile 1% low melting point agar and warm to 45°C until molten. Place 100 µL of embedding media into individual wells of a 96-well plate. Place one tooth slice into each well and allow the embedding medium to gel by gently cooling to room temperature in a tissue culture hood.
7. When semisolid, remove embedded slices from the wells and transfer to a sterile 0.8-µm pore-sized Millipore filter and float the filter at the liquid-gas interface (surface) of supplemented media in a 24-well dish, creating a Trowel-type culture. The floating filter can be supported with the aid of a plastic support.
8. Slices are cultured at 37°C in a humidified incubator in an atmosphere of 5% CO_2 in air, in DMEM culture medium containing all supplements. Medium is changed every 48 h. Mandibles can be cultured in 12-or 24-well plates in 2 mL of culture media. They may also be cultured in larger 6-well plates or 35-mm culture dishes, where 4 mL of culture can be used.
9. After the desired culture time point is reached (e.g., 72 h), fix tooth slices in 2 mL of 10% (w/v) neutral-buffered formalin at room temperature in the dark for 24 h.
10. Following fixation, tooth slices are demineralised in 10% (w/v) formic acid at room temperature in the dark for up to 72 h.
11. Manually dehydrate slices through a series of 50%, 70%, 95%, and 100% alcohols, followed by xylene, prior to embedding vertically in paraffin wax.
12. Cut 5-µm sections and stain sections with haematoxylin/eosin (H&E) and view under a light microscope to capture images for histomorphometry.
13. Cell numbers can be counted using image analysis software or by manually counting cells in a given area (e.g., 50 µm x 50 µm square box).

Sloan et al., 2000; Melin et al., 2000). Since the first publications in the late 1990s, this tooth slice culture system has been further developed for use as a reproducible method for assessing biocompatibility and cytotoxicity of novel and existing dental materials (Murray et al., 2000) and advancing the field of regenerative endodontics. It has also been essential as an experimental system to investigate the effects of fluoride on dentine extracellular matrix (ECM) alterations and subsequent mineralisation (Moseley et al., 2003a, 2003b; Waddington et al., 2004). It is now accepted that the ECM plays a critical role in mediating the induction of odontoblast differentiation during tooth development (reviewed by Smith and Lesot, 2001; Smith et al., 2012) and also mediates similar processes in dental tissue repair in the mature tooth.

After injury, the process of reparative dentinogenesis leads to the differentiation of a new generation of odontoblast-like cells, which are recruited and differentiated from a progenitor cell population from within the pulp. These newly differentiated cells secrete a tertiary dentin matrix, and many of these events recapitulate, to a certain extent, those seen during tooth development (Smith and Lesot, 2001). The dentine matrix contains a reservoir of bioactive growth factors that can mediate these processes, and the functional roles of members of the TGF-β super-family in reparative dentinogenesis suggests a possible role in novel therapeutic mediators or tissue engineering solutions to dental regeneration. During dental disease or trauma, tissue damage and inflammation at sites of injury may compromise the ability of the pulpal ECM to mediate reparative events, and there may be advantages to providing a suitable matrix to encourage cell migration and differentiation at such sites. Recent studies using the tooth slice *ex vivo* culture system and a similar human tooth slice system (using 500-µm-thick longitudinal sections of extracted human teeth) have demonstrated the ability of the bioactive growth factors BMP-7 and TGF-ß1 when added to the slices in solution, or when contained within alginate hydrogels, to induce odontoblast-like cell differentiation within the dentin-pulp complex, with subsequent upregulation of dentine matrix secretion (Sloan and Smith, 1999; Sloan et al., 2000; Dobie et al., 2002). Our knowledge of dentine regeneration has improved significantly in recent times. For example, it was previously thought that pulp capping (application of a calcium hydroxide–based material to exposed dental pulp tissue) could stimulate "dentine bridge" formation, secretion of new calcified tissue. The nature of this process was unclear and it was thought that "irritation" of the dental pulp by calcium hydroxide–containing cements caused recruitment of calcium ions from pulpal vasculature to help generate this calcified barrier. Using information gleaned from *in vitro* tooth development models (Bègue-Kirn et al., 1992, 1994) and 3D tooth slice tissue culture models (including from human tissue), we now know that the increased pH of certain pulp capping agents results in the liberation of bioactive molecules, such as TGF-β, amongst others, sequestered within dentin, and/or recruitment of dental pulp stem cells, which lead to the formation of new dentin or dentinlike material (Graham et al., 2006; Tomson et al., 2007; Smith et al., 2012).

Tissue culture models for periodontal disease and bone destruction

Novel models are required to mimic and advance our understanding of inflammatory bone destruction during periodontal disease, as well as provide adequate and reproducible clinical systems to investigate biological effects of new therapeutics. Currently, *in vivo* models using significant numbers of rodents and primates, along with *in vitro* cell culture systems using rodent cells and genetic knockout mice models are used to investigate inflammatory disease, inflammatory mediated bone loss, and periodontal disease in particular. Bone destruction is modelled and investigated using the *in vivo* rodent and primate models of experimental periodontitis. The understanding of the role of proinflammatory cytokines and bone loss has been modelled extensively using a primate ligature model to induce periodontitis and injections of various cytokines delivered to examine their influence of osteoclastogenesis

and bone resorption (Assuma et al., 1998). This well-established system of inducing clinical periodontitis has provided evidence of how administration of IL-1α accelerates ligature bone resorption in rats (Koide et al., 1995). Other studies have used similarly well-established murine models of bone resorption, which is induced by delivery of high doses of bacterial lipopolysaccharide (LPS) (Chiang et al., 1999). It is clear that the practice of infecting and/or immunizing rodents and primates with potential periodontal pathogens has been a useful tool to investigate disease progression, inflammatory cell activity, and tissue destruction.

The different *in vivo* models available are used to investigate certain aspects of periodontal disease progression and associated bone loss. For example, the rat feeding model is particularly useful when examining aspects of bacterial behaviour that promote colonisation and the initiation of periodontal disease (Graves et al., 2008). The mouse oral gavage model allows administration of human strains of bacteria in a viscous suspension to induce reproducible alveolar bone loss. The use of *Aggregatibacter actinomycetemcomitans* (feeding model) and *Porphyromonas gingivalis* (in oral gavage) to induce proinflammatory cytokine production and bone resorption in rats and mice has also been reported (Baker et al., 2001; Graves et al., 2008), and such models have been useful in understanding the role of immune cells in the progression of disease (Kawai et al., 2000). Similar studies have also been performed in nonhuman primates (Persson et al., 1994) and with experimental periodontitis in a humanised diabetic SCID mouse model (Graves et al., 2008). Coupled with these specific examples are the numerous genetic knockout mice that are used to investigate roles for various cytokines and receptors in inflammatory diseases. Studies using such *in vivo* models are numerous (Taubman and Kawai, 2001) and have been used over many years. Even though such animal models have limitations, they are still considered superior to *in vitro* or clinical studies for addressing mechanistic questions, and all are currently used in preference to other models. Current studies investigating the efficacy of the proresolving lipid molecules for resolving periodontal inflammation use the *in vivo* induced experimental models of periodontitis described above. Studies using the *P. gingivalis* induced experimental rabbit model have demonstrated that the resolvin RvE1 prevents inflammation and bone loss in these animals when applied topically (Hasturk et al., 2006, 2007).

The same rabbit model has also been used to investigate the efficacy of lipoxins to resolve periodontal inflammation and associated bone loss (Serhan, 2004). Similar studies using rats where LPS has been used to induce periodontitis also suggests that polyunsaturated fatty acid derivatives inhibit disease progression (Vardar et al., 2005). In addition to these studies, it has also been suggested that overexpression of the 15-LOX type I lipoxygenase pathway in transgenic rabbits reduces the inflammatory phenotype in periodontitis (Van Dyke, 2008). Looking at both of the *in vivo* models to understand molecular and cellular progression of the disease or to trial new actives, it is clear that the cost of running such experiments, the difficulty in obtaining clear data, and the ethical implications regarding the number of animals that must be used to look at the many variables associated with such experiments (time points, dose points, 'n' numbers) suggests that we should be looking at using more novel, laboratory-based systems in our investigations and as high-throughput testing systems. This means we require more appropriate laboratory-based systems to assess new actives prior to trials for novel treatments in a living system.

Although there are many *in vitro* studies of the effects of cytokines or proresolving molecules on osteoclast differentiation, results from such studies can be far removed from the *in vivo* situation as cell-cell interaction between differing cell types may influence behaviour. The use of *in vitro* assays for rodent primary alveolar bone cells (Roberts et al., 2008) and PDL cells allows us to investigate the behaviour of specific cells and reduces the number of animals being used for experimentation. However, these cells are difficult to extract and culture due to the very small area of tissue being dissected, along with the difficulty in obtaining a sufficient quantity of cells for culture.

Several *ex vivo* culture models have been developed to study a wide variety of developmental, physiological, and pathological conditions. The development and use of such models not only provides the ability to carefully manipulate cells and tissue to fully understand the biological response, but also addresses the importance of the three *R*s (refinement, reduction, and replacement) in animal studies as they significantly reduce the number of animals required for *in vivo* experimentation. The organ culture of cartilage has facilitated the understanding of cartilage repair and determination of defects (Graichen et al., 2005) and has potential for use in

toxicological research and drug activity (Turner et al., 2002). Based on the successful culture of rodent tooth slices, further development of a mandibular slice culture system (Smith et al., 2010) to investigate periodontal inflammation and bone destruction has facilitated the development of an *ex vivo* culture that supports the differentiation, proliferation, and activity of fibroblasts, osteoblasts, osteoclasts, and immune system cells within cultured slices of mouse mandible (Taylor et al., 2008).

The system utilises murine hemi-mandibles from 12-week-old male CD1 mice. Similar cultures can also be created from mandible slices from 4-week-old Wistar rats (Protocol 5.2). As with the tooth slice culture model, here 2-mm-thick slices of rodent mandible are cultured in Trowel-type cultures at the liquid-gas interface, which, as before, allows the culture of cells and tissue *in situ*, providing a natural tissue environment to allow cells to be successfully cultured in 3D for up to 14 days. Although some reduction in cell numbers has been reported, there is good viability and architecture of the cells and tissues within the mandible slice during all culture periods (Figure 5.2), and no significant alterations in the numbers of dividing cells suggests viability is not significantly compromised by extended culture. Expression of bone matrix proteins, including bone sialoprotein and osteopontin, are maintained during culture with no significant alterations in expression within the cells and tissue of the PDL or surrounding alveolar bone (Sloan et al., 2013). Importantly, the system supports the culture of osteoclasts present within the tissue slice, specifically within the PDL. Although the number of tartrate resistant form of acid phosphatase (TRAP) positive osteoclasts was small, numbers did not significantly decrease with extended culture. It was also demonstrated that an inflammatory response can be invoked in the system, when stimulated appropriately with bacterial LPS or proinflammatory cytokines (e.g., IL-1β, TNFα). Such stimulation leads to increases in osteoclast cell numbers within the slice and ultimately loss of tissue architecture and viability of ligament fibroblasts (Figure 5.3). Decreases in bone sialoprotein expression also appeared to be LPS dependent. Increases in monocytes and neutrophils within the system and the synthesis and secretion of inflammatory cytokines by resident cells in response to LPS and proinflammatory cytokine stimulation have also been noted, and such cytokine responses have also shown to have been mediated by the addition of

Protocol 5.2 Mandible slice culture.

Transport and washing media: DMEM, supplemented with 200 mM L-glutamine, 1% penicillin/streptomycin solution (containing 10,000 units penicillin and 10 mg/mL streptomycin) is used for all culture procedures.
Embedding media: A semisolid agarose gel composed of 4 mL DMEM containing all the supplements as above and 5 mL sterile 1% low melting point agar (type VII agarose)
Culture media: DMEM containing all the supplements as above, with 10% heat inactivated fetal calf serum and 0.15 mg/mL ascorbic acid

1. Carefully dissect mandibles from freshly sacrificed 10–12-week-old male CD-1 mice or 28-day-old male Wistar rats and remove all soft tissue (mucosal tissue, muscle) using sterile scalpel and dissection tools. Once free of all soft tissue, place in sterile transport medium.
2. Cut dissected mandibles on a diamond edged rotary bone saw, using washing media as a coolant and a segmented blade (which reduces tearing of tissue at hard/soft tissue interface).
3. First, remove the ramus, coronoid process, and lower molar teeth with the bone saw and discard to create a planar surface. This is achieved by holding the mandible at the incisor end and applying soft pressure to the bone saw to remove the condyle and molars. Holding the incisor end of the mandible, section the remainder of the mandible into transverse slices of between 1 and 1.5 mm thickness. Store freshly cut slices in sterile washing medium.
4. Wash mandible slices several times in washing medium at 37°C.
5. Warm the embedding medium at 45°C until molten and place 100 μL into individual wells of a 96-well plate. One mandible slice is placed into each well and the embedding medium is allowed to gel by gently cooling to room temperature in the tissue culture hood.
6. When semisolid, remove embedded slices from the wells and transfer to a sterile 0.8-μm pore-sized Millipore filter. Place the filter at the liquid-gas interface of 2 mL supplemented DMEM in a 12- or 24-well plate creating a Trowel-type culture. A plastic support can be used to facilitate floating of the filter on the surface of the culture medium.
7. Slices are cultured at 37°C in a humidified incubator in an atmosphere of 5% CO_2 in air, in DMEM culture medium containing all supplements. Medium is changed every 48 h. Mandibles can be cultured in 12-or 24-well plates in 2 mL of culture media. They may also be cultured in larger 6-well plates or 35-mm culture dishes, where 4 mL of culture can be used.
8. Immediately postculture, fix mandibles in 10% (w/v) neutral buffered formalin for 24 h and then demineralise in 10% formic acid (v/v). When demineralising mandible slices, tissues are placed in a universal tube and 10 mL of acid added. Tubes are placed on a shaker and demineralised over a 48–72 h period with acid changed daily.
9. Following demineralisation, process slices for routine histological examination by thorough dehydration through a graded series of alcohols (50%, 70%, 95%, 100%), follow with xylene, and finally embed in paraffin wax. Cut sections of tissue at 5 μm for staining with haematoxylin and eosin.
10. It is possible to cryopreserve the slices of tissue following culture for cryo-sectioning if that method is preferred. Again, 5-μm sections should be prepared using the cryostat.

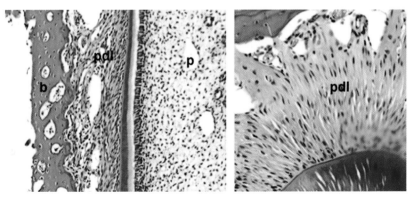

Figure 5.2 A culture rat mandible slice after 14 days in culture. Cells and tissues of the alveolar bone (b), periodontal ligament (pdl), and pulp (p) show good viability following culture.

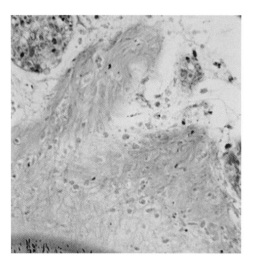

Figure 5.3 Loss of cell viability and tissue structure of the periodontal ligament in a culture mandible slice following stimulation with bacterial lipopolysaccharide.

anti-inflammatory cytokines. The model therefore provides a 3D organotypic tissue slice system, which can be carefully manipulated to induce local inflammatory cytokine-mediated cell responses and thus the potential to understand how the complex multicellular tissue responds to such insults.

The system also provides an environment that supports insertion/transplantation of osteoclasts and cells of the innate immune system into the PDL tissue by microinjection, and allows for differentiation into osteoclasts. These transplanted cells can be observed through long-term culture by tracer fluorescence labelling. Here, preosteoclasts, isolated via nonadherence to tissue culture plastic following bone marrow aspirates and overnight stimulation with M-CSF, were labelled with a cell tracker dye and 100 cells injected into the ligament of a murine mandible slice using a small-gauge needle. Cultures were maintained for 14 and 21 days in media supplemented with RANKL and M-CSF. Following culture, TRAP-positive multinuclear cells could be identified in areas within the mandible slice that correlated with red tracer fluorescence in the same sections examined with fluorescence microscopy. The microinjection of preosteoclasts within this *ex vivo* system may provide a viable model for generating a localised inflammatory response using cells and tissue from the same species and also, if required, the same animal source. Regeneration or engineering of tissues within

compromised or inflamed areas is challenging, and being able to recreate such an environment benefits not only investigations into novel treatment modalities for inflammatory mediated diseases such as periodontal disease, but also the development of new methods to engineer and regenerate tissues *in situ*.

Appropriate culture systems for pulpal infection

The unique nature of the pulpal extracellular matrix is of particular importance when considering models of pulpal infection and disease, as it provides a specific surface for bacterial attachment and acts as a reservoir of growth nutrients. Two-dimensional monolayer culture experiments are often inadequate for endodontic research models, so *in vivo* models are often favoured. Additionally, researchers advocate the use of these models to allow for both development of pathogenesis models and effectiveness of new materials, agents, and surgical procedures. *In vivo* systems usually involve surgical exposure of the dental pulp and inoculation with infective material. This material may be in the form of dental plaque or a bacterial species isolated from the oral cavity and cultured *in vitro* (Friedman et al., 1997; Balto et al., 2002; Tawil et al., 2009; Yildrim et al., 2011). One such model has been presented using baboons (Cleaton-Jones et al., 2004), where occlusal cavities were cut in all 16 primary molars of the animals in order to expose the pulp. They were then covered with human dentine with advanced caries to infect the pulps or inoculated directly with *Streptococcus mutans* grown *in vitro*. The infective material was sealed into the exposed pulp for 14 days before the animals were sacrificed and pulpal histology examined. Although there are a number of primate studies into pulpitis, it is more common for *in vivo* models to utilise dogs and mice (Ribeiro Sobrinho et al., 2002), and similar studies using beagle dogs induce pulpal infection through inoculation of surgically exposed pulp with supragingival plaque. The use of *in vivo* models for the testing of endodontic antimicrobial and filling materials is also widespread. These may be carried out on animals that have not been experimentally infected and are used to assess the effect of the filling material on the success of the restoration (Wälivaara et al., 2012). However, there are also models that have been developed where experimental pulpitis

---

Protocol 5.3 Quantifying cell counts and bacteria on an *ex vivo* rat tooth co-culture infection model.

1. Prepare supplemented culture media: DMEM, with ribonucleosides, deoxyribonucleosides, supplemented with 10% heat inactivated fetal calf serum, 0.15 mg/mL vitamin C, 200 mmol/L L-glutamine and 1,000 U/mL penicillin G sodium, 10 µg/mL streptomycin sulfate, and 25 µg/mL amphotericin B.
2. Extract upper and lower incisors of sacrificed 28-day-old male Wistar rats, removing soft tissue and bone from outer surface using a sterile scalpel.
3. Temporarily store the incisors in prepared culture media prior to sectioning.
4. Using a diamond-edged rotary bone saw, cut 2-mm-thick transverse sections and transfer into a 12-well plate in 2 mL supplemented DMEM at 37°C, 5% CO_2 for 4 days, changing the media every 24 h.
5. Wash tooth slices in PBS then transfer tooth slices to a fresh sterile 12-well plate with 2 mL of supplemented media *without* antibiotics and incubate for a further 24 h.
6. Inoculate bacteria of interest (e.g., *S. anginosus, S. constellatus, E. faecalis*) in Brain Heart Infusion (BHI) broth and incubate at 37°C, 5% CO_2 until the log growth phase is reached (e.g., 4 h).
7. Dilute broth culture to 10^2 colony-forming units (CFUs)/mL (based on optical density measurements and colony counts).
8. For fluorescence visualisation of bacteria, add 20 µL of 1% fluorescein diacetate (FDA) in acetone per milliliter of bacterial suspension and incubate in the dark for 30 minutes at 37°C, 5% CO_2.
9. Pass bacterial suspension through a 0.22-µm filter unit.
10. Resuspend bacteria captured on the filter unit in supplemented media without antibiotics and with 10% BHI.
11. Culture tooth slices in media containing bacteria or sterile supplemented media with 10% BHI as controls in the dark at 37°C, 5% CO_2.
12. After desired time point is reached (e.g., 24 h) fix tooth slices in 2 mL of 10% (w/v) neutral-buffered formalin at room temperature in the dark for 24 h.
13. Demineralise in 10% (w/v) formic acid at room temperature in the dark for 72 h.
14. Dehydrate slices through a series of 50%, 70%, 95%, and 100% alcohols, followed by xylene, prior to embedding vertically in paraffin wax.
15. Cut 5 µm sections and visualise under a fluorescent microscope using a FITC filter to quantify fluorescent bacteria. Alternatively, stain sections with haematoxylin/eosin (H&E) and view under a light microscope to quantify cell numbers.
16. Fluorescent bacteria can be quantified by percentage area coverage using image analysis software (e.g., ImageJ, COMSTAT) and by applying appropriate thresholds. Cell numbers can be counted using image analysis software or by manually counting cells in a given area (e.g., 50 µm x 50 µm square box).

---

is induced prior to treatment with the material being tested (Otani et al., 2011). Despite the severity of such studies, conclusions drawn often do not advance the understanding of the pathological processes involved in pulpitis, and demonstrate only that exposure to infective materials produces abscesses and pulp hyperaemia.

Alternative models employ *in vitro* methods using pulpal fibroblast cells grown in 2D monolayer culture on tissue plastic but are an oversimplified representation of the clinical situation. In addition to lacking the characteristics of the extracellular matrix, they also fail to consider the multicellular dentine-pulp complex and, as has been mentioned previously in this chapter, the interactions that occur *in vivo* between cells.

In an attempt to overcome the limitations associated with these different approaches, a number of *ex vivo* model systems have been introduced, the aim of which is to provide a robust, clinically relevant,

laboratory-based model system. As many of the *in vivo* studies investigate only the local responses of the tissues and not those of the systemic inflammatory response, it is reasonable that they could be replaced by an *ex vivo* tooth slice model. The culture conditions of the tooth slice culture model of Sloan and colleagues (1998) have been modified so that it allows successful culture of both mammalian cells/tissues and *Streptococcus anginosus* spp. and *Enterococcus faecalis,* bacteria that are implicated in purulent pulpal infections. By culturing the tooth slices in a culture medium consisting of DMEM and 10% Brain Heart Infusion broth, bacteria can be inoculated onto the tooth slice prior to culture for up to 48 hours (Protocol 5.3). This unique mix of bacterial culture broth and a standard tissue culture medium demonstrated bacterial growth was maintained under mammalian cell culture conditions and enabled the co-culture of *Streptococcus anginosus* group (SAG) bacteria on tooth

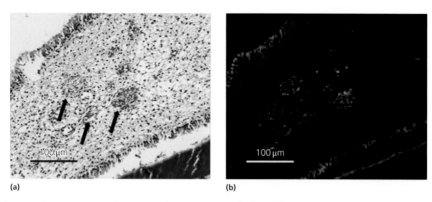

(a)   (b)

Figure 5.4 Attachment of *Streptococcus anginosus* group bacteria to a tooth slice following 24 hours in culture. Histological staining (a) indicates small microcolonies of bacteria adhering to and invading the tissue (arrows), and this is confirmed through observation of fluorescein diacetate positively stained bacteria (b).

slice sections to provide an *ex vivo* model of pulpal infection (Roberts et al., 2013). Histological analysis demonstrated that tooth slices cultured with SAG bacteria showed small concentrated areas of bacterial attachment (Figure 5.4). Incubation of the bacteria prior to inoculation with fluorescein diacetate allowed for further examination of bacterial attachment to the tissues during culture (Figure 5.4). Green fluorescence staining of the bacteria confirmed bacterial attachment to the tooth slice during culture and corresponded with areas of bacteria observed through histological staining. These focal points of attachment were seen to increase in size as the period of incubation with the bacteria was extended, suggesting that, following attachment to the pulp tissue, SAG bacteria were able to divide and reproduce. It is also likely that planktonic bacteria in the medium were able to attach to those bacteria already fixed onto the pulpal matrix, as progressive attachment of *Streptococci* bacteria has been extensively reported. *Streptococci* bacteria have also been previously shown to express multiple adhesins that allow them to attach to other microbial species and host cells. This model is useful for investigating the importance of the ability of SAG bacteria to attach directly to the pulp tissue, which may be the mechanism by which further invasion by other bacteria is mediated. Certain species of bacteria may not directly adhere to the pulpal matrix but are able to attach to the adhesins on the surface of the SAG bacteria.

The model has also demonstrated potential use for investigating host cell/tissue responses to invading bacteria. The small, focussed colonisation of bacteria on the tooth slice seen in the histological examination and fluorescein diacetate staining of the SAG-infected tooth slices appeared to be associated with a breakdown of the pulpal matrix. This loss of matrix was observed as an absence of staining between fibroblasts in the histological sections and was particularly pronounced in the areas immediately surrounding the bacterial infection sites. Such areas of matrix loss suggested that the attached bacteria were having a localised effect on the surrounding tissues. This matrix loss was not observed in nonbacterial control cultures, and it has been postulated that this may be a direct result of the bacterial attachment and growth disrupting the matrix or, more likely, an indirect effect caused by soluble factors such as enzymes that are produced by the attached bacteria and secreted into the surrounding area (Jacobs and Stobberingh, 1995). It has also been possible to quantify host cell viability during the culture period, and a direct effect on viable cell numbers within cultured tissues caused by SAG infection was noted, with cell counts showing that there was a significant decrease in numbers of viable pulpal cells during culture. In addition, real-time polymerase chain reaction demonstrated an increase in proinflammatory cytokine production as a result of SAG inoculation (Roberts et al., 2013; Natarajan et al., 2013), which indicates that cells within the model respond to the introduction of SAG bacteria into the system (Protocol 5.4). This *ex vivo* pulpal infection model therefore can be considered to accurately represent events that occur *in vivo*. This is significant when considering a model to use for testing new antimicrobial or anti-inflammatory treatments. These cytokines are often produced *in vivo* by cells such as macrophages and

---

Protocol 5.4 Assessing gene expression of an *ex vivo* rat tooth co-culture infection model.

1. Perform steps 1–3 in Protocol 5.3.
2. Using a diamond-edged rotary bone saw, cut 4-mm-thick transverse sections and transfer into a 12-well plate in 2 mL supplemented DMEM at 37°C, 5% CO_2 for 4 d, changing the media every 24 h.
3. Wash tooth slices in PBS then transfer tooth slices to a fresh sterile 12-well plate with 2 mL of supplemented media without antibiotics and incubate for a further 24 h.
4. Inoculate bacteria of interest (e.g., *S. anginosus*, *S. constellatus*, *E. faecalis*) in Brain Heart Infusion (BHI) broth and incubate at 37°C, 5% CO_2 until the log growth phase is reached (e.g., 4 h).
5. Dilute broth culture to 10^3 CFUs/mL (based on optical density measurements and colony counts).
6. Add this to supplemented media without antibiotics to produce a final concentration of 10% BHI and 10^2 CFUs/mL of bacteria.
7. Culture tooth slices in media containing bacteria or sterile supplemented media with 10% BHI as controls at 37°C, 5% CO_2.
8. After desired time point is reached (e.g., 24 h), transfer tooth slices to sterile PBS in a fresh 12-well plate.
9. Using a needle and syringe, extirpate the pulp by flushing PBS through the pulpal chamber.
10. Transfer the pulp into appropriate solutions for downstream RNA extraction (e.g., Qiagen kits or Trizol methods).

T-lymphocytes, but due to the lack of a circulatory system in this model they are most likely to be produced by the pulpal fibroblasts themselves, in addition to any immune cells residing within the pulp at the time of culture. The ability to quantify the damage caused to cells in the tooth slice as a result of incubation with SAG bacteria, along with the ability to investigate bacterial adherence to pulpal matrix, provides a model for the study of pulpal infection in a carefully controlled system. The success of creating a culture environment where clinical bacterial isolates can be co-cultured on living mammalian tissues provides an exciting template for further development to investigate periodontal pathogen behaviour on living periodontal tissue cells on the full mandible slice culture system.

Modelling of dental pulp stem cell behaviour in 3D systems

Mesenchymal progenitor cells (MPCs), multipotent cells from which connective tissues arise, are currently the focus of intense scientific interest from the standpoint of regenerative medicine and tissue engineering. Harnessing the MSC population to initiate repair has wide-ranging implications in many tissue types, including teeth, bone, and the cardiovascular system (Richardson et al., 2010; Huang et al., 2010; Hilfiker et al., 2011). There have been many investigations directed at characterising the behaviour of these cells, particularly the ways in which a multipotent population of cells is maintained in fully differentiated tissues, and

how this population can be isolated and directed to differentiate into complex tissues and organs (Arthur et al., 2009; reviewed in Chapter 3). *In vivo* models used to investigate the potential of MPCs for tissue engineering often involve the implantation of progenitor cell–impregnated matrices into animals, primarily rats, mice, and rabbits. The explants are then removed after the animals are sacrificed and the amount of cell differentiation or ectopic tissue development assessed—this is considered to be the "gold standard" approach. Other models of MPC differentiation involve defect-repair models, in which animals are subjected to an injury, which is then treated by injecting of progenitor cells and/or the insertion of an explant. Overall, this is not a satisfactory scientific approach to understanding the mechanisms of mesenchymal progenitor cell biology and their role in tissue engineering. *In vivo* experimentation is widely applied because the surrounding ECM in which MPCs reside is considered critical in the maintenance of their multipotency and in regulating their recruitment and differentiation (Abdallah and Kassem, 2009). Thus, the 2D monolayer cultures could be considered an oversimplification. The understanding of how a complex 3D tissue environment is involved in the maintenance of MPCs in a quiescent progenitor cell state, and at the same time are primed to respond to tissue damage, is crucial to the development of new tissue regeneration treatment modalities. At present, these critical cell/matrix interactions that influence progenitor cell function are not clearly understood, and there remains a need for better cellular model systems that enable careful and systematic examination of MPC niches.

In addition, the possibility for developing more physiologically relevant 3D model systems for use in *in vitro* high-content screening highlights exciting opportunities.

In the context of clinical translation, the *ex vivo* mandible slice organ culture model systems described in this chapter have great application in the area of biomaterial testing. When considering the ability of a given material or population of cells to drive pulpal repair or regeneration, it is advantageous to expose them directly to intact dental pulp tissue, thereby directly modelling both cellular and acellular approaches to oral tissue engineering.

To take a recent example, Colombo and colleagues (2015) used the *ex vivo* mandible slice model to observe the interactions of an enriched population of green fluorescent protein (GFP) expressing rat dental pulp–derived progenitor cells (DPPCs) with the dentine-pulp complex. GFP DPPCs were clonally isolated from "green rats" that ubiquitously express GFP under the control of a chicken β-actin promoter, using the fibronectin-adhesion method. These cells, which were characterised as belonging to a mesenchymal lineage through biomarker expression and population kinetics, continually express GFP throughout culture, allowing them to be tracked in real time, without fixation. This enriched population of GFP DPPCs was injected using a 35-gauge microneedle into the incisor pulp of rat mandible organ culture slices. Over 7 days, injected cells were observed at several time points to spread out, colonise the cut surfaces of the dentine, and begin to exhibit significant changes in morphology, aligning and becoming elongated. By utilizing the rat mandible organ culture model, the movement and interactions of a characterised DPPC population in their native 3D extracellular matrix environment have been observed. Such model systems have the potential to elucidate the mechanisms by which specific populations of cells involved in the repair and regeneration of the dentine-pulp complex migrate and differentiate *in situ*, informing various strategies in regenerative endodontics and oral tissue engineering. Whilst this report is preliminary, it is exciting to speculate that this dynamic organ culture model, where delivery of MPCs can be tracked in terms of their migration and differentiation, may prove to be useful in further exploring MPC biology and function and to address questions that conventional 2D *in vitro* culture systems cannot. This is specifically important regarding the influence of the ECM and growth factors on

maintaining "stem-ness," and determining cell-lineage fates and cell responses to tissue injury.

Similarly, this organ culture approach has been used to observe the interactions between intact pulp tissues and a bioactive tissue engineering scaffold system, allowing the interactions of both primary odontoblasts and other pulp cells with injectable multidomain peptide hydrogels (MDPs) to be observed. Moore and colleagues (2015) injected an MDP hydrogel containing both an RGDS cell adhesion sequence and an MMP-2 vulnerable cleavage site into both the odontoblast space and central pulp of the rat mandible slice model. These scaffolds were delivered by 35-gauge microneedle in a continuous column through the entire 2-mm height of the mandible slice incisor pulp, so as to maximise contact with the relevant pulpal area in a 3-dimensional sense. Over 10 days, standard histological techniques revealed that odontoblasts in contact with the injected scaffold were preserved in terms of their appropriate histological architecture and secretory activity, depositing DSPP into the MDP scaffold, which also showed early signs of partial mineralisation. By contrast, MDP scaffolds injected centrally into the pulp showed partial degradation, with MMP-2 expression at early time points and remodelling, with pulp extracellular matrix markers expressed by invading pulp cells. In controls where either the injection of phosphate-buffered saline or an endodontic file physically ablated comparable portions of the odontoblast layer, widespread pulp cell death was observed, possibly due to alterations in the mechanical support structure of the pulp tissue, which were prevented by the application of the MDP scaffold. Thus, important observations were made about the nature of the reactions of two distinct pulpal regions to the MDP scaffold system. Further information regarding the potential importance of the mechanical support provided by the anatomical arrangement of the dentine-pulp complex on pulp vitality was also gleaned, due to the complexity of this model system over more traditional systems involving the *in vitro* culture of isolated cell populations.

The use of organ culture model systems has therefore opened up a number of exciting possibilities for translational research in pulp repair/regeneration by granting the ability to closely observe the interactions of relatively intact pulp tissue with both enriched dental pulp progenitor cell populations and a sophisticated tissue engineering scaffold system. While *ex vivo* organ culture systems will most likely not serve as perfect alternatives to the traditional *in vivo* experiments associated with translating bioactive materials into clinical practice, they may serve an important role as less costly alternatives, allowing the delivery and observation of potentially regenerative cell populations and matrices into complex native tissue environments.

Acknowledgements

Several of the studies discussed within this chapter were supported by research grants from the NC3Rs, MRC, EPSRC, and Heath and Social Care Wales.

References

ABDALLAH, B. M., & KASSEM, M. 2009. The use of mesenchymal (skeletal) stem cells for treatment of degenerative diseases: current status and future perspectives. *J Cell Physiol*, 218(1), 9–12.

ARTHUR, A., ZANNETTINO, A., & GRONTHOS, S. 2009. The therapeutic applications of multipotential mesenchymal/stromal stem cells in skeletal tissue repair. *J Cell Physiol*, 218(2), 237–45.

ASSUMA, R., OATES, T., COCHRAN, D., AMAR, S., & GRAVES, D. 1998. IL-1 and TNF antagonists inhibit the inflammatory response and bone loss in experimental periodontitis. *J Immunol*, 160, 403–9.

BAKER, P. J., GARNEAU, J., HOWE, L., & ROOPENIAN, D. C. 2001. T-cell contributions to alveolar bone loss in response to oral infection with *Porphyromonas gingivalis. Acta Odontol Scand*, 59, 222–5.

BALTO. H., WHITE, R., MUELLER, R., & STASHENKO, P. 2002. A mouse model of inflammatory root resorption induced by pulpal infection. *Oral Surg Oral Med Oral Pathol Oral Radiol Endod*, 93(4), 461–8.

BEGUE-KIRN, C., SMITH, A. J., RUCH, J. V., et al. 1992. Effects of dentin proteins, transforming growth factor beta 1 (TGF beta 1) and bone morphogenetic protein 2 (BMP2) on the differentiation of odontoblast *in vitro. Int J Dev Biol*, 36, 491–503.

BEGUE-KIRN, C., SMITH, A. J., LORIOT, M., KUPFERLE, C., RUCH, J. V., & LESOT, H. 1994. Comparative analysis of TGF-βs, BMPs, IGF1, msxs, fibronectin, osteonectin and bone sialoprotein gene expression during normal and *in vitro*-induced odontoblast differentiation. *Int J Dev Biol*, 38, 405–20.

CHIANG, C., KYRITSIS, G., GRAVES, D., & AMAR, S. 1999. Interleukin-1 and tumor necrosis factor activities partially account for calvarial bone resorption induced by local injection of lipopolysaccharide. *Infect Immun*, 67, 4231–6.

CLEATON-JONES, P., DUGGAL, M., PARAK, R., WILLIAMS, S., & SETZER, S. 2004. Pulpitis induction in baboon primary teeth using carious dentine or *Streptococcus mutans SADJ*, 59(3), 119–22.

COLOMBO, J. S., HOWARD-JONES, R. A., YOUNG, F. I., WADDINGTON, R. J., ERRINGTON, R. J., & SLOAN, A. J. 2015. A 3D *ex vivo* mandible slice system for longitudinal culturing of transplanted dental pulp progenitor cells. *Cytometry A*, 87(10), 921–8.

DHOPATKAR, A. A., SLOAN, A. J., ROCK, W. P., COOPER, P. R., SMITH, & A. J. 2005. A novel *in vitro* culture model to investigate the reaction of the dentine-pulp complex to orthodontic force. *J Orthod*, 32, 122–32.

DOBIE, K., SMITH, G., SLOAN, A. J., & SMITH, A. J. 2002. Effects of alginate hydrogels and TGF-β1 on human dental pulp repair *in vitro. Conn Tiss Res*, 43, 381–6.

FRIEDMAN, S., TORNECK, C. D., KOMOROWSKI, R., OUZOUNIAN, Z., SYRTASH, P., & KAUFMAN, A. 1997. *In vivo* model for assessing the functional efficacy of endodontic filling materials and techniques. *J Endod*, 23(9), 557–61.

GRAHAM, L., COOPER, P. R., CASSIDY, N., NOR, J. E., SLOAN, A. J., & SMITH, A. J. 2006. The effect of calcium hydroxide on solubilisation of bio-active dentine matrix components. *Biomaterials*, 27(14), 2865–73.

GRAICHEN, H., AL-SHAMARI, D., HINTERWIMMER, S., VON EISENHART-ROTHE, R., VOGL, T., & ECKSTEIN, F. 2005. Accuracy of quantitative magnetic resonance imaging in the detection of *ex vivo* focal cartilage defects. *Am Rheum Dis*, 64, 1120–5.

GRAVES, D. T., FINE, D., TENG YEN-TUNG, A., VAN DYKE, T. E., & HAJISHENGALLIS, G. 2008. The use of rodent models to investigate host-bacteria interactions related to periodontal diseases. *J Clin Periodontol*, 35(2), 89–105.

HASTURK, H., KANTARCI, A., GOGUET-SURMENIAN, E., BLACKWOOD, A., ANDRY, C., SERHAN, C. N., & VAN DYKE, T. E. 2007. Resolvin E1 regulates inflammation at the cellular and tissue level and restores tissue homeostasis *in vivo. J Immunol*, 179, 7021–9.

HASTURK, H., KANTARCI, A., OHIRA, T., ARITA, M., EBRAHIMI, N., CHIANG, N., PETASIS, N. A., LEVY, B. D., SERHAN, C. N., & VAN DYKE, T. E. 2006. RvE1 protects from local inflammation and osteoclast-mediated bone destruction in periodontitis. *FASEB J*, 20, 401–3.

HEYWOOD, B. R., & APPLETON, J. 1984. The ultrastructure of the rat incisor odontoblast in organ culture. *Archs Oral Biol*, 29, 327–9.

HILFIKER, A., KASPER, C., HASS, R., & HAVERICH, A. 2011. Mesenchymal stem cells and progenitor cells in connective tissue engineering and regenerative medicine: is there a future for transplantation? *Langenbeck's Archives of Surgery*, 396(4), 489–97.

HUANG, G. T., YAMAZA, T., SHEA, L. D., DJOUAD, F., KUHN, N. Z., TUAN, R. S., & SHI, S. 2010. Stem/progenitor cell-mediated de novo regeneration of dental pulp with newly deposited continuous layer of dentin in an *in vivo* model. *Tissue Engin Part A*, 16(2), 605–15.

JACOBS, J. A., & STOBBERINGH, E. E. 1995. Hydrolytic enzymes of *Streptococcus anginosus, Streptococcus constellatus* and *Streptococcus intermedius* in relation to infection. *Eur J Clin Microbiol Infect Dis*,14(9), 818–20.

KAWAI, T., EISEN-LEV, R., SEKI, M., EASTCOTT, J. W., WILSON, M. E., & TAUBMAN, M. A. 2000. Requirement of B7 costimulation for Th1-mediated inflammatory bone resorption in experimental periodontal disease. *J Immunol*,164, 2102–9.

KOIDE, M., SUDA, S., SAITOH, S., OFUJI, Y., SUZUKI, T., YOSHIE, H., TAKAI, M., ONO, Y., TANIGUCHI, Y., & HARA, K. 1995. *In vivo* administration of IL-1 beta accelerates silk ligature induced alveolar bone resorption in rats. *J Oral Path Med*, 24, 420–34.

MAGLOIRE, H., JOFFRE, A., & BLEICHER, F. 1996. An *in vitro* model of human dental pulp repair. *J Dent Res*, 75, 1971–8.

MELIN, M., JOFFRE-ROMEAS, A., FARGES, J. C., COUBLE, M. L., MAGLOIRE, H., & BLEICHER, F. 2000. Effects of TGFbeta1 on dental pulp cells in cultured human tooth slices. *J Dent Res*,79(9), 1689–96.

MOORE, A. N., PEREZ, S. C., HARTGERINK, J. D., D'SOUZA, R. N., & COLOMBO, J. C. 2015. *Ex vivo* modeling of multidomain peptide hydrogels with intact dental pulp. *J Dent Res*, 94(12), 1773–81.

MOSELEY, R., SLOAN, A. J., WADDINGTON, R. J., SMITH, A. J., HALL, R. C., & EMBERY, G. 2003a. The influence of fluoride on the cellular morphology and synthetic activity of the rat dentine-pulp complex *in vitro*. *Archs Oral Biol*, 48, 39–46.

MOSELEY, R., WADDINGTON, R. J., SLOAN, A. J., SMITH, A. J., HALL, R. C., & EMBERY, G. 2003b. The influence of fluoride exposure on dentin mineralisation using an *in vitro* organ culture method. *Calcif Tiss Int*, 73, 470–5.

MUNKSGAARD, E. C., RICHARDSON, W. S. III, & BUTLER, W. T. 1978. Biosynthesis of phosphoprotein by rat incisor odontoblast in *in vitro* culture. *Archs Oral Biol*, 23, 583–7.

MURRAY, P. E., LUMLEY, P. J., ROSS, H. F., & SMITH, A. J. 2000. Tooth slice organ culture for cytotoxicity assessment of dental materials. *Biomaterials*, 21, 1711.

NAKASHIMA, M. 1991. Establishment of primary cultures of pulp cells from bovine permanent incisors. *Archs Oral Biol*, 36, 655–63.

NATARAJAN, N., ROBERTS, J., SLOAN, A. J., LYNCH, C., MAILLARD, J. Y., & DENYER, S. P. 2013. Characterisation of pulpal response to *Streptococcus anginosus* group bacterial supernatant *J Dent Res*, 92(Spec Iss B), 88.

ONG, S. L., GRAVANTE, G., METCALFE, M. S., & DENNISON, A. R. 2013. History, ethics, advantages and limitations of experimental models for hepatic ablation. *World J Gastroenterol*, 19(2), 147–54.

OTANI, K., SUGAYA, T., TOMITA, M., HASEGAWA, Y., MIYAJI, H., TENKUMO, T., TANAKA, S., MOTOKI, Y., TAKANAWA, Y., &

KAWANAMI, M. 2011. Healing of experimental apical periodontitis after apicoectomy using different sealing materials on the resected root end. *Dent Mater J*, 30(4), 485–92.

PERSSON, G. R. ENGEL, D., WHITNEY, C., DARVEAU, R., WEINBERG, A., BRUNSVOLD, M., & PAGE, R. C. 1994. Immunization against *Porphyromonas gingivalis* inhibits progression of experimental periodontitis in nonhuman primates. *Infect Immun*, 62, 1026–31.

RIBEIRO SOBRINHO, A. P., DE MELO MALTOS, S. M., FARIAS, L. M., DE CARVALHO, M. A., NICOLI, J. R., DE UZEDA, M., & VIEIRA, L. Q. 2002. Cytokine production in response to endodontic infection in germ-free mice. *Oral Microbiol Immunol*, 17(6), 344–53.

RICHARDSON, S. M., HOYLAND, J. A., MOBASHERI, R., CSAKI, C., SHAKIBAEI, M., & MOBASHERI, A. 2010. Mesenchymal stem cells in regenerative medicine: opportunities and challenges for articular cartilage and intervertebral disc tissue engineering. *J Cell Physiol*, 222(1), 23–32.

ROBERTS, H. C., MOSELEY, R., SLOAN, A. J., YOUDE, S. J., STRINGER, B. M. J., & WADDINGTON, R. J. 2008. Lipopolysaccharide alters decorin and biglycan synthesis in alveolar bone osteoblasts: consequences for bone repair during periodontal disease. *Eur J Oral Sci*, 116, 207.

ROBERTS, J. L., MAILLARD, J. Y., WADDINGTON, R. J., DENYER, S. P., LYNCH, C. D., & SLOAN, A. J. 2013. Development of an *ex vivo* coculture system to model pulpal infection by *Streptococcus anginosus* group bacteria. *J Endod*, 39(1), 49–55.

SERHAN, C. N. 2004. Clues for new therapeutics in osteoporosis and periodontal disease: new roles for lipoxygenases? *Expert Opin Ther Targets*, 8, 643–52.

SLOAN, A. J., SHELTON, R. M., HANN, A. C., MOXHAM, B. J., & SMITH, A. J. 1998. An *in vitro* approach for the study of dentinogenesis by organ culture of the dentine-pulp complex from rat incisor teeth. *Arch Oral Biol*, 43, 421–30.

SLOAN, A. J., & SMITH, A. J. 1999. Stimulation of the dentine-pulp complex of rat incisor teeth by transforming growth factor-beta isoforms 1-3 *in vitro*. *Arch Oral Biol*, 44, 149–56.

SLOAN, A. J., RUTHERFORD, R. B., & SMITH, A. J. 2000. *In vitro* stimulation of the dentine-pulp complex by BMP-7. *Archs Oral Biol*, 45, 173–7.

SLOAN, A. J., TAYLOR, S. Y., SMITH, E. L., ROBERTS, J. L., CHEN, L., WEI, X. Q., & WADDINGTON, R. J. 2013. A novel *ex vivo* culture model for inflammatory bone destruction. *J Dent Res*, 92(8), 728–34.

SMITH, A. J., & LESOT, H. 2001. Induction and regulation of crown dentinogenesis embryonic events as a template for dental tissue repair. *Crit Rev Oral Biol Med*, 12, 425–37.

SMITH, A. J., SCHEVEN, B. A., TAKAHASHI, Y., FERRACANE, J. L., SHELTON, R. M., & COOPER, P. R. 2012. Dentine as a bioactive extracellular matrix. *Arch Oral Biol*, 57(2), 109–21.

SMITH, E. L., LOCKE, M., WADDINGTON, R. J., & SLOAN, A. J. 2010. An ex vivo rodent mandible culture model for bone repair. *Tissue Eng Part C Methods*, 16(6), 1287–96.

TAUBMANN, M., & KAWAI, T. 2001. Involvement of T-lymphocytes in periodontal disease and in direct and indirect bone resorption. *Crit Rev Oral Biol Med*, 12, 125–35.

TAWIL, P. Z., TROPE, M., CURRAN, A. E., CAPLAN, D. J., KIRAKOZOVA, A., DUGGAN, D. J., & TEIXEIRA, F. B. 2009. Periapical microsurgery: an *in vivo* evaluation of endodontic root-end filling materials. *J Endod*, 35(3), 357–62.

TAYLOR, S. Y., SMITH, E. L., WADDINGTON, R. J., WEI, X. Q., & SLOAN, A. J. 2008. Development of an *ex vivo* mandible model of local inflammation. *J Dent Res*, 87(Spec Iss C), 0302.

TOMSON, P. L., GROVER, L. M., LUMLEY, P. J., SLOAN, A. J., SMITH, A. J., & COOPER, P. R. 2007. Dissolution of bio-active dentine matrix components by mineral trioxide aggregate. *J Dent*, 35(8), 636–42.

TURNER, D. J., HOYLE, S. L., SNEWIN, V. A., GARES, M. P., BROWN, I. N., & YOUNG, D. B. 2002. An ex vivo culture model for screening drug activity against in vivo phenotypes of *Mycobacterium tuberculosis*. *Microbiology*, 148, 2929–35.

VAN DYKE, T. E. 2008. The management of inflammation in periodontal disease. *J Periodontol*, 79, 1601–8.

VARDAR, S. BUDUNELI, E., BAYLAS, H., BERDELI, A. H., BUDUNELI, N., & ATILLA, G. 2005. Individual and combined effects of selective cyclooxygenase-2 inhibitor and omega-3 fatty acid on endotoxin-induced periodontitis in rats. *J Periodontol*, 76, 99.

WADDINGTON, R. J., MOSELEY, R., SMITH, A. J., SLOAN, A. J., & EMBERY, G. 2004. Fluroide-induced changes to proteoglycan structure synthesised within the dentine-pulp complex *in vitro*. *Biochem Biophys Acta*, 1689, 142–51.

WÄLIVAARA, Å., ABRAHAMSSON, P., ISAKSSON, S., SALATA, L. A., SENNERBY, L., & DAHLIN, C. 2012. Periapical tissue response after use of intermediate restorative material, gutta-percha, reinforced zinc oxide cement, and mineral trioxide aggregate as retrograde root-end filling materials: a histologic study in dogs. *J Oral Maxillofac Surg*, 70(9), 2041–7.

YILDRIM, S., CAN, A., ARICAN, M., EMBREE, M. C., & MAO, J. J. 2011. Characterization of dental pulp defect and repair in a canine model. *Am J Dent*, 24(6), 331–5.

CHAPTER 6

Industrial translation requirements for manufacture of stem cell–derived and tissue-engineered products

Ivan Wall[1,2], David de Silva Thompson[1], Carlotta Peticone[1], and Roman Perez[2]

[1] University College London, London, United Kingdom

[2] Institute of Tissue Regeneration Engineering (ITREN), Dankook University, Cheonan, Republic of Korea

The emerging regenerative medicine field has significant potential to change health care delivery in the 21st century. A great deal of fundamental work has already delivered proof of concept that tissue engineering and stem cell–derived products can benefit patients with diseases that conventional medicine cannot treat. There are limitations, however. Primarily, stem cell culture methods and tissue engineering approaches typically adopted in biology labs are not scalable, yet scalability is key to ensuring commercial manufacturing success and delivery to clinic.

Biochemical engineering adopts the strapline "translating discovery into reality," drawing on the fact that phenomenal biologic discoveries require industrial translation in order to deliver a consistently high-quality product using scalable and standardised manufacturing tools. More often than not, discovery science is not scalable and so to ensure patients benefit from scientific advances, consideration for manufacturability needs to be considered as early as possible in the product development cycle. This is particularly true for stem cell–based and tissue engineering therapies, which as living products are susceptible to change caused by the impact of manufacturing processes. This chapter will consider the challenges for manufacturing and potential solutions to deliver new tissue-engineered products to the clinic.

The penicillin story…and beyond

An early example of how industrial translation made critical improvements to scalable production and provided near-unlimited access to a medicine is the development of penicillin. Despite penicillin being discovered growing on a petri dish at St Mary's Hospital, London, UK, in 1928, the discovery science for producing penicillin was not scalable. Consequently, more soldiers died in World War II due to infected wounds than were killed directly on the battlefield. Penicillin was not available in the necessary quantities to treat all injured soldiers who required it, and so nurses would collect urine from soldiers who had been treated to harvest nonmetabolised penicillin. Later, in the 1950s and 1960s, key industrial process steps were developed that led to the scalable manufacture of large batches of penicillin, and the manufacturing process transitioned from petri dishes to large stainless steel vessels with advanced downstream purification and formulation.

From the 1970s onwards, similar development hurdles were successfully overcome for other biologic products such as monoclonal antibodies and recombinant therapeutic proteins. In the 21st century, we face the same challenges, this time for stem cell–derived and tissue-engineered products. Again, we start at the lab

Tissue Engineering and Regeneration in Dentistry: Current Strategies, First Edition. Edited by Rachel J. Waddington and Alastair J. Sloan.
© 2017 John Wiley & Sons, Ltd. Published 2017 by John Wiley & Sons, Ltd.

scale, typically growing cells and tissue constructs in small T-flasks and multiwell plates. However, we now face a different type of challenge insomuch as human cells as a product are living rather than chemical-based compounds or protein-based molecular agents. As a living product, all stages of the manufacturing pathway can impact the cell and potentially change important characteristics that define product potency.

What is manufacturing scale?

Manufacturing scale is the appropriate scale to generate the desired amount of clinical-grade product in a cost-effective way. Unfortunately, there is no single defined process to achieve this. There is a big distinction between autologous and allogeneic therapies with respect to manufacturing and quality control requirements (Figure 6.1). It will also depend on multiple other factors such as the type of cells to be used (e.g., adult multipotent versus pluripotent cells) and the disease indication to be treated, and therefore the number of cells required to treat that indication. Many different

clinical indications are currently being investigated with respect to application of cell therapy (including tissue engineering), and the cell quantities required range from 10^5 cells per dose for macular degeneration to potentially 10^9 cells per dose for liver disease and graft versus host disease (clinicaltrials.gov). For tissue engineering to produce dental tissue, the cell quantities needed are less well defined, as they will depend largely on the size of the defect and nature of the biomaterial scaffold used.

The types of cell culture technology used to acquire the necessary cell numbers will change as production scale increases (Figure 6.2). For smaller scale production and autologous therapies, T-flasks (including multilayered flasks) alone may be suitable for cell product manufacture if preparing a relatively small number (~10^8) of cells. For larger quantities (e.g., lots of ~10^{10} cells), hyperflasks and cell factories may have greater application. For larger lot sizes, translation to alternative platform technologies, such as hollow fiber bioreactors or microcarrier-based cell culture in stirred tank bioreactors are predicted to be the most sustainable technology platforms for standardised manufacture of large

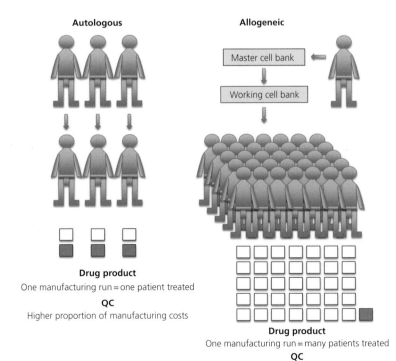

Autologous

Allogeneic

Master cell bank

Working cell bank

Drug product
One manufacturing run = one patient treated
QC
Higher proportion of manufacturing costs

Drug product
One manufacturing run = many patients treated
QC
Significantly lower proportion of manufacturing costs

Figure 6.1 Autologous versus allogeneic manufacture affects the scale and the impact on quality control (QC) requirements and relative cost proportion of the whole manufacturing process. For the cartoon left, there would be three manufacturing "runs" for the autologous therapy and individual QC associated with each. Yet for the allogeneic therapy, potentially only one manufacturing run to produce multiple doses of drug substance. Typically, for a batch of cells derived for allogeneic therapy, the cost of performing QC analysis will be significantly lower than for autologous therapy. (Adapted from Brandenberger et al., 2011.)

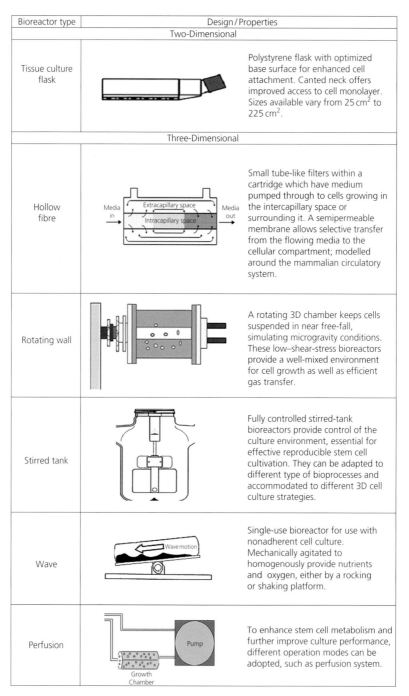

Bioreactor type	Design / Properties
Two-Dimensional	
Tissue culture flask	Polystyrene flask with optimized base surface for enhanced cell attachment. Canted neck offers improved access to cell monolayer. Sizes available vary from 25 cm² to 225 cm².
Three-Dimensional	
Hollow fibre	Small tube-like filters within a cartridge which have medium pumped through to cells growing in the intercapillary space or surrounding it. A semipermeable membrane allows selective transfer from the flowing media to the cellular compartment; modelled around the mammalian circulatory system.
Rotating wall	A rotating 3D chamber keeps cells suspended in near free-fall, simulating microgravity conditions. These low–shear-stress bioreactors provide a well-mixed environment for cell growth as well as efficient gas transfer.
Stirred tank	Fully controlled stirred-tank bioreactors provide control of the culture environment, essential for effective reproducible stem cell cultivation. They can be adapted to different type of bioprocesses and accommodated to different 3D cell culture strategies.
Wave	Single-use bioreactor for use with nonadherent cell culture. Mechanically agitated to homogenously provide nutrients and oxygen, either by a rocking or shaking platform.
Perfusion	To enhance stem cell metabolism and further improve culture performance, different operation modes can be adopted, such as perfusion system.

Figure 6.2 Bioreactor technologies and their utility in cell culture at different scales.

quantities of cell material (Simaria et al., 2014). However, the reality of achieving this scale of cell expansion, whilst retaining desired cell characteristics, is still to be seen. It is likely that automation of processes will play a significant part, due to removal of operator bias and process variability inherent in manual processing (Brindley et al., 2013).

Requirements for manufacture

One of the reasons that manufacture is deemed to be inadequate using bench-scale technologies such as T-flasks hinges on the fact that bench-scale cell culture methods are typically manually intensive and not standardised. On this basis, the cell product itself will potentially exhibit high variability, as product attributes are dictated both by input materials (including the start cell population, culture reagents, etc.) and upstream manufacturing processes. To develop a commercially feasible product, a quality target product profile (QTPP) needs to be defined that characterises the nature of the product in terms of physical and functional characteristics. Defining a QTPP helps to ensure that whatever manufacturing process changes are made, the target product still meets a minimum specification. This is important because cells can be very sensitive to changes in processing platforms, and if the product characteristics change out of specification, then the product will be unusable.

Traditionally, cells used for dental and maxillofacial tissue engineering have been characterised in manual T-flasks processes in static culture conditions. To meet manufacturing demands of protocol standardisation, in-process control, and reduced risk of contamination, all of which are critical to ensure the best chance of commercial success, it will be necessary to translate these manual T-flasks processes to controlled bioreactor systems. Understanding the target product and defining the QTPP will ensure that the cell product specification is within limits after translation. Bioreactor technologies that benefit from control systems and monitoring capabilities will therefore be important for manufacture of clinical-grade material. In the case of generating hard tissue, such as bone for dental and maxillofacial surgery, a significant benefit is that bioreactors would not need to approach the 10s to 1000s of liters scale used for manufacture of biologics such as recombinant proteins

and monoclonal antibodies. They would, however, need to enable perfusion of cell-seeded scaffold structures to promote adequate mass transfer throughout the entire scaffold, as nutrient gradients lead to inconsistent cell growth and differentiation (Volkmer et al., 2008) (see Protocol 6.1, as well as Protocols 3.4 and 4.4 in Chapters 3 and 4, respectively, for methodological protocols).

An argument for bioreactors

Bioreactors have been subject to extensive investigation for bone tissue engineering. By enabling control of oxygen and nutrient supply to cells within scaffolds in the bioreactor, specific environmental conditions can be achieved and maintained (Chao et al., 2007). This is critical for producing cells in a way that minimises the impact of the process environment on product variability as much as is possible. Gradients in nutrients and metabolites that accumulate in static T-flasks create microenvironment fluctuations that exacerbate the intrinsic biologic variability in the source cell material. There are many benefits of using bioreactors in this respect. First, bioreactors generally allow for incorporation of *monitoring* capabilities, so that key physicochemical parameters (temperature, O_2, CO_2, pH) can be measured *in process* by sensors, or at least allow for sampling by the operator to make off-line measurements. Second, and closely linked, is the ability to incorporate *control* technologies. These can enable feedback or feed-forward control of the cell culture through programmable responsiveness to internal disturbances (e.g., nutrient depletion, endogenous protein secretion, etc.) (Kirouac and Zandstra, 2008). For example, a fed-batch stem cell culture process could be designed such that a change in lactate or pH levels detected by the sensor invokes delivery of a defined unit of fresh nutrients. A third significant advantage is the (mostly) reduced need for manual operations during the culture, as these are a major source of failure in cell culture processes due to contamination risk and intra-/inter-operator variability in manual processing. Even subtle differences in pipetting of cell material (rate of flow and number of passes in the pipette) or other minor deviations from the standard operating procedure can culminate in phenotype drift and loss of characteristics, especially with increasing time in culture; such would be the case when expanding larger quantities of cells for allogeneic cell therapy.

Typically, for dental or maxillofacial treatments, the cells will be autologous and used for precision medicine applications tailored to the unique requirements of the individual patient. Therefore, sustained long-term cell expansion will likely not be required, since the cell source will not have to be expanded to produce hundreds or thousands of treatments per lot. However, consideration of how best to incorporate cells with delivery materials (e.g., biomaterial scaffolds) should be considered early in the process, to meet the unique physical dimension specifications of the individual patient defect.

Bioreactors for cell therapy

There are many types of bioreactors that can be applied to the manufacture of cells for dental tissue engineering. When compared with static cell culture processes, it would appear that choosing stirred or perfusion systems that create a homogeneous environment and allow control over critical process parameters would be simple. However, choosing the best bioreactor technology from multiple alternatives is tricky as there are so many different platforms (Table 6.1, modified from Rodrigues et al., 2011). There are also potential compromises due to hydrodynamic shear stress experienced by cells at high media flow rates. Certainly in the case of suspension-adapted cells used in the production of biologics, hydrodynamic shear has been typically reported to be a severe limitation (Garcia-Briones and Chalmers, 1994). For expanding cells in stirred systems, the vortices created at the tips of rotating impellers can create bubbles that are damaging to cell membranes (Papoutsakis, 1991; Garcia-Briones and Chalmers, 1992). The geometry, position, and rotation speed of the impeller are all factors, and other instrumentation such as sensors, probes, spargers, and baffles also disturb flow patterns and can potentially cause damage (Gilbertson et al., 2006). Therefore, understanding the impact of hydrodynamic shear on the cell product and the limits of feasibility in terms of maximal agitation or flow rates can greatly improve manufacturing success by ensuring critical levels of hydrodynamic shear stress are not breached.

Table 6.1 Bioreactor comparisons. Modified from Rodrigues et al. (2011).

Bioreactor Type	Advantages	Disadvantages
Stirred suspension	Homogenous culture conditions and can be used with microcarriers Easily monitored and controlled	Cells subjected to hydrodynamic stress due to agitation Cell/microcarrier agglomeration may occur
Roller bottles	Simple operation protocol Low cost	Complex monitoring and control required Technology suited for anchorage cell cultures Concentration gradients minimised; however, still persist
WAVE Bioreactor ™	Disposable technology that minimises cleaning requirement. Therefore more suitable for GMP manufacture and easier to validate.	Relative difficulty in monitoring and sampling Capital expenditure considerably high
Hollow-fibre	Cells subjected to low levels of shear stress	Monitoring and control not simple Difficult to scale up technology Concentration gradients formed and therefore heterogeneous environment
Rotating wall	Efficient gas transfer Cells subjected to low levels of shear stress	Complex system that is not easy to scale up
Parallel plate	Continuous removal of toxic metabolites High cell yields achieved	Effect of removing secreted factors not fully characterised Hydrodynamic effects of vessel structure unknown
Fixed and fluidised bed	Compatible with 3D scaffolding Cellular interactions exhibit comparability to *in vivo* structure	Scaling up is challenging Shear stress may damage cells Concentration gradients of nutrients and metabolites (fixed bed)

Bioreactors that typically exploit large surface area (e.g., via microcarriers or hollow fibres for cell expansion processes, or biomaterial scaffolds for tissue engineering) can also limit the negative impact of multiple rounds of enzymatic detachment during serial passaging of cells by allowing a longer single expansion phase to achieve high density (Majd et al., 2011) for subsequent production of engineered tissue.

Bioreactors for controlling hard tissue formation

By controlling the rate of flow of nutrient-rich media, development of osteogenic cell characteristics can be improved beyond simple biochemical signaling alone (Marolt et al., 2010). As well as improving mass transport, mechanical stimulation by fluid flow shear stress can activate mechano-transduction pathways by producing tension at the site of integrin binding to extracellular matrix (ECM) ligands (Lee et al., 2008). The integrin-mediated signaling induces downstream activation of ERK1/2 and consequent upregulation of osteogenic gene expression (Weyts et al., 2002; Kapur et al., 2003). Perfusion bioreactor systems consistently yield improved osteogenic induction and maturation in mesenchymal cells (Frohlich et al., 2010; Grayson et al., 2008; Sikavitsas et al., 2003).

Process considerations

Understanding the relationship between process conditions and the final product is important for reducing risk of the product not meeting specification (Ratcliffe et al.,

2011). For a single process or unit operation during manufacture of a cell/tissue-engineered product, there will be multiple different variables in terms of input material (cells, media, growth factors, or serum). Other factors such as operator variability, physicochemical parameters (gradients in nutrients, metabolites, pH, oxygen, etc.) all contribute. Some factors can be controlled (e.g., standardised operator training, automation, etc.), but there are still uncontrolled variables (e.g., variability in biologic material). There will also be inherent statistical variation within the process simply because of the nature of the material you are working with and the fact that there will always be some variation in what is measured. Consequently, the output will be the product of all these different types of variability (Figure 6.3).

Critical process parameters in tissue engineering manufacturing refer to the process conditions that, if not controlled, can result in a deviation of the product away from its approved specification. These can generally be considered as factors determining the quality of the input material and key parameters to be monitored throughout the manufacturing process.

Input material

Tissue engineering typically combines cells with a biomaterial scaffold, supplemented with biologic molecules that can elicit specific biological responses. All these factors represent critical input components.

Cell source

The first critical step will be identifying a suitable cell source to deliver a robust product. Many different candidate cell populations have been identified for

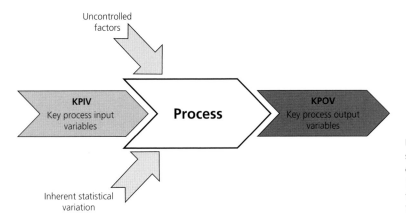

Figure 6.3 Diagram representing, in its simplest form, the inputs to a unit operation that affect the output product. (From Ratcliffe et al., 2011. Reprinted with permission from Oxford University Press.)

dental and craniofacial tissue engineering, as dis-cussed in the accompanying chapters (Inanc and Elcin, 2011). A second consideration is whether autologous or allogeneic material will be used. Autologous cells are advantageous in terms of immu-nocompatibility, yet there are limitations with respect to yield and quality of cells obtained from a biopsy (Sensebe et al., 2011). The interpatient variability in cell material can make manufacturing challenging, because standardised processing and a one-size-fits-all approach will not take into account differences in cell quality that could result in different growth rates, loss of predicted function, and varying sensitivity to pro-cess conditions. With autologous samples, it is also more difficult to predict whether target product spec-ifications will be met. More emphasis is needed to create in-process measurement systems to ensure products will meet specification with reduced risk of failure. Additionally, isolating autologous stem cells requires a source of easily accessible cells, preferably without the need for surgery or at least using mini-mally invasive techniques. On the other hand, alloge-neic therapy using cells from a universal donor could lead to off-the-shelf availability. However, the main drawback with allogeneic tissue is the risk of immune rejection. All things considered, the current preferred choice of source material for dental tissue engineering applications is tissue-specific adult stem cell material from an autologous source (Lymperi et al., 2013; Inanc and Elcin, 2011).

The most easily accessible sources of dental-specific stem cells are those from the adult dental pulp and the periodontal ligament (Lymperi et al., 2013), as discussed in Chapters 1, 3, and 7. Dental stem cells from deciduous teeth, SHEDs, are also easily acces-sible; however, only recently has the practice of iso-lating and banking them for potential therapeutic exploitation been established, while DFSCs (dental follicle stem cells) and SCAPs (stem cells from apical papilla) can only be isolated if the third molar is present (Lymperi et al., 2013). Alternative sources of mesenchymal cells, such as the bone marrow or even oral mucosa, may also have utility for dental tissue engineering applications (Bluteau et al., 2008). Regardless of cell source, the selected population must first be effectively isolated, purified, and characterised, and needs to be free of any contaminants.

Scaffold and signaling molecules

Scaffolds are temporary matrixes that mimic the 3D tissue environment onto which cells are able to attach, proliferate, and differentiate (Hollister, 2005). These are designed to be biocompatible, presenting specific physical and chemical cues to direct cell fate and to migrate throughout the scaffold. Among the physical cues, surface chemistry, topography, or stiffness are known to play a key role in controlling cell fate (Perez et al., 2013). Furthermore, the scaffolds should present a highly porous structure with interconnected pores to allow proper cell penetration and tissue ingrowth and thus enhance the overall regenerating process (Karageorgiou and Kaplan, 2005). While these parame-ters are directed to control the cell fate, the composition and porosity of the scaffolds dictate the degradability, which should be tuned to match the generation of new tissue in the site of implantation (Alsberg et al., 2003). Regarding their composition, scaffolds are mainly com-posed of polymeric and ceramic materials as well as combinations of these two. Typical examples of poly-meric scaffolds are the degradable polylactic and poly-caprolactone scaffolds, whereas calcium phosphate and silica-based materials are examples of their ceramic counterparts (Perez et al., 2013). The versatility of the materials and the increasing numbers of processing techniques, such as electrospinning, 3D printing, salt leaching, or emulsions, allow the production of differ-ent scaffold architectures and morphologies such as nanofibres, microspheres, or 3D plotted scaffolds that may be tuned to match the physical properties of the host tissue (Hollister, 2005).

Besides the physical cues, chemical cues are thought to be an attractive system to control the cell fate through chemical signaling (Perez et al., 2013). This can mainly be achieved through the tethering of molecules on the surface of the scaffold, or by directly incorporating biological molecules in the bulk or surface of the scaf-fold (Perez et al., 2013). Surface tethering is mainly based on the surface modification of scaffolds to expose proteins or their active motifs (e.g., peptides) on the surface. These motifs and proteins are generally designed to allow enhanced cell adhesion through inte-grin recognition, although these can also be designed to enhance cell proliferation or differentiation (Perez et al., 2013). On the other hand, chemical cues may also be delivered in the form of molecules from the scaffold into the cell receptors in order to induce specific cell behavior. For instance, growth factors, drugs, or genes can easily be incorporated in the bulk or the surface of the scaffolds to allow a safe and controlled delivery. Depending on the types of molecules incorporated, these can mainly play a role in controlling cell fate or decreasing inflammation/infection after implantation. Whilst the number of growth factors is very vast and will depend on the target tissue (e.g., fibroblast growth factors or transforming growth factors, among other growth factor families), chemical drugs have shown similar functions regardless of the tissue, mainly decreasing inflammation (e.g., ibuprofen), infection (e.g., gentamicin), or even being able to increase cell differentiation and regeneration (e.g., dexamethasone) (Perez et al., 2013). Recently, ions with therapeutic properties have also been considered a very promising route to direct cell fate or to decrease infection at the site of the defect. For instance, ions such as cobalt and copper have been shown to increase angiogenesis, whereas zinc has been shown to decrease bacterial infection (Mourino et al., 2012). The release of these signaling molecules and ions is therefore of great importance, and designing the scaffolds to allow their delivery at specific time points in a controllable fashion is also likely to be critical.

Finally, the aforementioned characteristics should be in harmony with an efficient and easy fabrication of the material in a cost-effective manner. Of great importance is matrixes that are easy to sterilise and that can be easily implanted in the operating theater. In the presence of biologically active molecules, these processes need to be controlled to maintain the molecules biologically active whilst being fully purified to avoid side effects. Furthermore, the production process should be reproducible and validated (Hutmacher, 2001).

Manufacturing process

Once the input materials have been selected, a robust manufacturing platform needs to be established. Most tissue-engineered products are manufactured at the bench scale, using manual rather than automated methods (Wendt et al., 2009). As sterility plays a key role throughout the manufacturing process, all operations need to be performed under aseptic conditions. Therefore, transition to automated cell-culture platforms would significantly reduce the risk of contamination compared to manual handling. Automation also ensures the establishment of a closed, reproducible, and operator-independent system, thus creating potential for large-scale manufacturing (Wendt et al., 2009).

In tissue engineering manufacturing, the first compositional step requires homogenous seeding of cells onto the 3D scaffold (Wendt et al., 2009). Traditional methods of manually applying cells on top of the scaffold under static conditions are severely limited due to lack of reproducibility and nonuniform distribution of cells throughout the scaffold. Dynamic cell seeding in a bioreactor has consistently proven a more successful and, importantly for commercial manufacture, cost-effective alternative, leading to more homogenous and standardised cell distribution (Wendt et al., 2009). Several bioreactor configurations can be adopted such as spinner flask, rotating wall, and perfusion bioreactors. As an example, since the formation of a bio-tooth requires interactions between multiple cell types, the ratio between epithelial and mesenchymal stem cells (Bluteau et al., 2008), the seeding sequence (Honda et al., 2007), and cell distribution and compartmentalisation within the scaffold are of pivotal importance.

Once the cells are attached to the scaffold, the operating parameters need to be carefully monitored throughout the production phase. The culture media and any additional growth or differentiation factors need to be tested for sterility and ideally should be non-animal derived. Also, the feeding gas mixture and vessel temperature need to be set, monitored, and controlled. Dynamic culture conditions are critical for maintaining 3D engineered tissues. If a uniformly seeded scaffold is then cultivated under static conditions, cells will mainly accumulate at the periphery of the construct, while a necrotic core will form at the center (Partap et al., 2010). Thus, bioreactors play a key role in maintaining mass transfer, in the form of nutrient supply and waste removal throughout the entire construct.

From a commercial manufacturing perspective, understanding and controlling the engineering environment is critical, and process operating parameters typical of any mammalian cell culture that need to be monitored include pH, temperature, pressure, flow rate (and associated shear stress), dissolved oxygen and carbon dioxide, and metabolite levels in the media. However, for engineering human tissues that are more complex and physically sensitive products compared with mammalian cell cultures traditionally used in fermentation processes to make monoclonal antibodies, other more complex measurements need to be made.

Parameters such as cell morphology or phenotype, secreted ECM composition and, in the case of stem cells, potency need to be linked to manufacturing conditions that affect them. For example, hydrodynamic shear stress can stimulate cell differentiation (Brindley et al., 2011). Particularly for dental tissue engineering, it is important to monitor the composition and distribution of secreted ECM through the biomaterial scaffold throughout the culturing period (Wendt et al., 2009), due to the fundamental role of correct deposition and distribution of acellular matrix components in recapitulating odontogenesis.

Monitoring the consequence of culture expansion

As previously discussed, the derivation of a tissue-engineered product has required the development of cell culture technology leading to the production of large cell numbers from a small piece of tissue providing the cell source. As highlighted in Chapter 3, these cells are likely to represent a heterogeneous population of cells relative to their mesenchymal stem cell (MSC) characteristics. Consequently, MSCs with high and low proliferative potential are likely to be present in the same culture, and continued and extensive proliferation of transit amplifying cells will lead to the loss of multipotentiality towards a bi- or unipotent cell. Continued culture may also lead to the development of cell senescence. The change in the characteristics of the MSC population is also highly dependent upon the culture conditions, including fluctuations in oxygen tension, nutrient supply, and pH.

Cellular senescence describes a deteriorative process in which mitotic activity of cells decreases, although cells may still survive (Campisi and d'Adda di Fagagna, 2007). Cellular senescence may also be known as cellular aging or replicative senescence. The reduced proliferative activity of senescent cells is essentially irreversible and often associated with several senescent markers that collectively can indicate the presence of this cell status in at least some of the cell population. Measurement of the proliferative activity and MSC characteristics can be performed through the measurement of colony-forming efficiency and population doublings (see Protocol 6.1). Senescent cells generally fail to form colonies, and population doublings fall to below 0.5 when determined over a week. However, formation of small colonies is also a feature of MSCs that are becoming unipotent. However, it is also now well accepted that there is an inverse relationship where cell proliferation is decreased during maturation of the osteoblast phenotype and synthesis of bone (Malaval et al., 1999), and thus reduced proliferative activity does not necessarily indicate cellular senescence. Here, cellular morphology and size may also be used to assess differentiation status, with differentiated osteoblasts exhibiting a more rounded cell with branched morphology (Sjöström et al., 2009). In addition, increased cell size is also associated with cellular senescence (Campisi and d'Adda di Fagagna, 2007). Continued culture may see the reestablishment within the culture of MSCs with higher proliferative activity, higher in the hierarchical structure of the MSC population (see Chapter 3 for fuller explanation). Equally, senescent-inducing stimuli are potentially oncogenic, and cancer cells can develop if they acquire mutations that facilitate avoidance of the effect of telomere-dependent senescence.

Establishment of differentiation of MSCs towards osteoblast activity can be established through detection of the appropriate differentiation markers at gene and protein level (see Protocols 3.4 and 4.4 for suggested methodological protocols). Cellular senescence can be further inferred through analysis of cells for a broad range of senescent markers, many of which can be analysed through various techniques involving analysis of genes, DNA, and enzymatic activity (see Protocol 6.2 for suggested approaches). A significant feature of senescent cells is the reduction in the telomere length. Located at the termini of chromosomes, telomeres are proposed protect them from degradation or fusion by DNA-repair processes. Shortening of the telomeres leads to malfunction, triggering classical DNA damage response. Human telomeres range from 10 to 15 kb in length, a size that does not indicate cellular senescence (Campisi and d'Adda di Fagagna, 2007). Cellular senescence leads to growth arrest, which can be measured through changes in the expression levels of several cell cycle proteins. Due to the interplay of many of these regulatory factors and signalling pathways, assessments should necessarily focus on a broad range of factors. Other classical features of senescent cells are their resistance to chemically induced apoptosis and the increase in the lysosomal beta-galactosidase in senescent cells, both of which can be measured using commercially available kits.

Protocol 6.1 Determination of proliferative activity and differentiation status of MSCs.

1. Colony-forming efficiency

- Seed cells into 6-well culture plates at a density between 4000 and 2000 cells/cm^2, dependent upon proliferative activity of cells. If colonies are large and merge together after 4 days, reduce seeding density. Culture in media used previously.
- Count colonies at 6, 12, and 14 days. For better viewing, fix cells with 3.7% formaldehyde, wash with PBS (phosphate-buffered saline) and stain with 1% rhodanile blue. Count colonies of greater than 32 cells using a light microscope and calculate as a proportion of the original cell number seeded.
- Count colonies of 32 cells or more; recording cells less than or more than 2 mm in diameter along with the number of days for formation will identify fast-forming colonies.
- Abortive colonies can be determined by counting 2–3 cells, 4–7 cells, 6–15 cells, and 16–31 cells (Jones and Watt, 1993).
- As cells age or become terminally differentiated, the colony-forming efficiency decreases and the number of abortive colonies increases dramatically.

2. Determining the population doublings of cells

- At each passage count the number of viable cells. If necessary, detach cells with Accutase solution (Sigma-Aldrich) following manufacturer's instruction. To a 10-µL aliquot of cell suspension add 30 µL of 0.4% trypan blue stain. Count cells using a Haemocytometer by light microscopy. Calculate the population doubling (PD) using the formula

$$PD = \left(log10\left[total\, cell\, count\, obtained \right] - log10\left[total\, cell\, count\, reseeded \right] \right) / log10(2).$$

- Determine the PD at several passages and plot the cumulative PD against cumulative time in culture. Senescence is proposed to be achieved when PD < 0.5/week. The proliferation of terminally differentiated osteoblasts is also reduced.
- Note that PDs can only be qualitatively compared. Statistical comparison is not possible as each PD is determined for a single population and the date of the culture passage is usually different for each cell population. Multiple PDs can be plotted on the same graph to demonstrate a repeated cumulative PD growth curve.

3. Determination of cell size throughout proliferative lifespan

- Take series of images of the cells throughout their proliferative lifespan using phase contrast microscope attached to a digital camera.
- Using Image J, outline the peripheral borders and perimeter of the cell and calculate their surface area.
- Enlargement of cell area is a possible indication of cell aging. The induction of a branched cell morphology with large focal adhesions and organised actin cytoskelton has been correlated to cells with increased potential for osteogenic differentiation (Malaval et al., 1999, Sjöström et al., 2009).

Final product: critical quality attributes

In manufacturing terms, the product does not just refer to the cells or engineered tissue construct that has been created in the lab. It includes everything that will be implanted into the patient. So as an example, for mesenchymal stromal cells suspended in saline solution and delivered via site-specific injection, the final product includes the saline used for delivery. This is important because critical quality attributes (CQAs) need to take account of potential effects of the delivery vehicle or excipient used in the final formulation, and for a living cell product there can be no negative interactions that will compromise safety or effectiveness of the final

product. CQAs cover four areas: safety, purity, identity, and potency (see Table 6.2). Development of new cell therapy products, including engineered tissue constructs, needs to be guided by an understanding of the product QTPP, including strategies to measure CQAs and define acceptable limits of detection of those measurements. This is particularly important where multiple batches of allogeneic cells will be generated as a universal cell therapy for many patients, as each batch needs to meet a predefined standard for product release.

CQAs are not always an appropriate way of defining products due to inherent heterogeneity, particularly across multiple autologous samples. Differences in start material quantity and quality mean that there needs to be a degree in flexibility in processing to accommodate

---

Protocol 6.2 Markers for determination of senescence of MSCs.

1. β-galactosidase (β-gal) activity

Senescence-associated beta-galactosidase (SA-β-gal or SABG) is a hypothetical hydrolase enzyme that actively hydrolyses β-galactosides only in senescent cells. β-galactosidase activity can readily be detected using a Senescence Cell Histochemical Kit (e.g., Sigma-Aldrich). The assay is based on a histochemical stain for β-galactosidase activity at pH 6. A number of alternative protocols are provided in the literature (Debacq-Chainiaux et al., 2009; Lee et al., 2006).

2. Telomere length

Reduction in the length of telomeres is associated with senescence. First, whole genomic DNA is isolated from the cells using a commercial kit. DNA yields are measured by absorbance at 260 nm. Based on Southern blot techniques, protocols are available to describe the process from first principles (Kimura et al., 2010). Alternatively, kits are available to determine telomere length from whole genomic DNA (for example, Telo TAGGG Telomere Length Assay Kit, Roche, UK). The principle behind both methods relies on the digestion of genomic DNA using a combination of 6 base restriction endonucleases that reduces genomic DNA size to less than 800 bp. Telomeric DNA is not digested due to the lack of restriction enzyme recognition sites within TTAGGG tandem telomeric repeats. Permanent records of the Southern blots are obtained following exposure to x-ray film. Using a scanning densitometer, obtain a digitized image. Mean TRF (telomere restrictive fragment) lengths can be determined using image analysis programmes such as Image J or Image Quant by first measuring pixel OD (adjusted for background readings) versus DNA migration distance. Macro programmes can be created using image analysis to calculate mean TRF length $= \Sigma\,(OD_i)/\Sigma(OD_i/MW_i)$, where OD is the optical density signal at position i and MW_i is the TRF length at that position (graphically described in protocols by Kimura et al., 2010).

3. Increased resistance to chemical-induced apoptosis

Many cells (but not all) develop a resistance to apoptosis and certain apoptotic signals. Apoptosis may be induced by chemicals such as ceramide, DMSO, or increased oxidative stress (hydrogen peroxide) and measured by detection of increased activity of Caspase 3 activity using an immunocytochemical assay (Gown and Willingham, 2002). Fix cells with 2% paraformaldehyde and permeabilised with 3% triton. Block for nonspecific binding of antibodies with 1% bovine serum albumin for 1 h; incubate with rabbit anti-rat cleaved Caspase 3 ASP175 (New England Biolabs; diluted 1:400 in 1% BSA, TBS) overnight at 4°C. Wash cells three times for 5 min with 0.5% Tween 20 in TBS, and then incubate in the dark with goat anti-rabbit FITC (Santa Cruz) for 1 h at 4°C. Wash again with 0.5% Tween 20 in TBS and treat for 1 h with bisbenzimide nuclear counterstain, prior to viewing using fluorescent microscopy.

4. Altered gene expression

Cell senescence is often associated with the repression of genes that facilitate cell-cycle progression such as cFOS, cyclin A, cyclin B, and proliferating cell nuclear antigen and increase in the expression level of genes of known cell-cycle inhibitors, such as the cyclin-dependent kinas inhibitor p21 (also referred to as CDKN1a, P21Cip1, Waf1, or SD11), p16 (also referred as CDKN2a or p16INK4a), and transcriptional regulators p53. Levels can be detected by quantitative PCR techniques. Due to the complex interplay of genes/proteins in regulating the cell cycle processes, analysis should investigate a broad spectrum of genes for better interpretation of results. Changes in gene expression do not always relate to growth arrest, and no one marker identifies a senescent state (Campisi and d'Adda di Fagagna, 2007).

---

these differences. Therefore, critical process parameters need to be understood and a window of operation defined that is permissible for deriving a product that may have some variability.

In terms of safety, probably the main source of concern for autologous therapy is the presence of contaminating microbes introduced in the raw materials or, more typically, by human operators during manual processing. It is also necessary to remove as much residual input material from the process as possible, such as serum components, recombinant growth factors, or harvesting agents such as trypsin.

For identity and potency, the size, integrity, and physical properties of the final construct should also be tested (Lee et al., 2010). Furthermore, postimplantation potency and stability should be predicted, as cells are

Table 6.2 Critical quality attributes and their meanings.

Critical Quality Attribute	Description
Safety	Ensure the material being transplanted is free from contaminating microbes or genetic instability. The latter is particularly important for pluripotent stem cell–derived products and other cell material expanded for extended duration. Moving towards animal-free media to prevent transmission of xenogenic material is desirable.
Purity	Closely linked to safety, it is important to remove residual harvesting agents and other input materials from the manufacturing process that are not a desired part of the product. It is also important to understand what level of purity is acceptable for the final product.
Identity	The physical measurable attributes of the cell or tissue-engineered product define its identity. These include product-specific integral proteins such as cell-surface epitopes or transcription factors. They can include other markers that can be measured using "omics" approaches. Ideally for industrial application, they will be rapid, reliable, and simple measurement tools.
Potency	The biologic activity and magnitude of such activity is referred to as potency. For a tissue-engineered construct the potency may simply be the capacity to fill a defect and provide mechanical strength, whereas for an MSC-based product, the mode of action is often not clear and potency therefore more challenging to define.

likely to migrate out of the scaffold once in the host tissue and due to likely changes in cell/matrix interactions upon resorption of the degradable scaffold (Lee et al., 2010). However, all these tests are difficult and timely to perform, and multiple assays may be required to characterise the product and gain a solid understanding of product attributes. The establishment of a robust and reliable set of tests should occur early in product development.

Conclusions

Translation of lab science to industrial manufacturing platforms is required if dental tissue engineering is to meet widespread clinical demand and achieve commercial success. Application of bioreactor technologies is not a new paradigm, but defining manufacturing parameters that are then controlled in response to monitoring will help to ensure that robust products can be delivered to the patients who need them. Furthermore, defining final product attributes early in the development cycle will ensure that commercial success is most likely achieved, by identifying failures earlier in the cycle.

References

ALSBERG, E., KONG, H. J., HIRANO, Y., SMITH, M. K., ALBEIRUTI, A., & MOONEY, D. J. 2003. Regulating bone formation via controlled scaffold degradation. *J Dent Res*, 82, 903–8.

BLUTEAU, G., LUDER, H. U., DE BARI, C., & MITSIADIS, T. A. 2008. Stem cells for tooth engineering. *Eur Cell Mater*, 16, 1–9.

BRANDENBERGER, R., BURGER, S., CAMPBELL, A., FONG, T., LAPINSKAS, E., & ROWLEY, J. 2011. Cell therapy bioprocessin: Integrating process and product development for the next generation of biotherapeutics. *BioProcess Int*, 9, 30–7.

BRINDLEY, D., MOORTHY, K., LEE, J.-H., MASON, C., KIM, H.-W., & WALL, I. 2011. Bioprocess forces and their impact on cell behavior: implications for bone regeneration therapy. *J Tissue Eng*, 2011, 620247.

BRINDLEY, D., WALL, I., & BURE, K. 2013. Automation of cell therapy biomanufacturing: minimising regulatory risks and maximising return on investment. *BioProcess Int*, 11, 18–25.

CAMPISI, J., & D'ADDA DI FAGAGNA, F. 2007. Cellular senescence: when bad things happen to good cells. *Nat Rev Mol Cell Biol*, 8, 729–40.

CHAO, P. H., GRAYSON, W., & VUNJAK-NOVAKOVIC, G. 2007. Engineering cartilage and bone using human mesenchymal stem cells. *J Orthopaed Sci*, 12, 398–404.

DEBACQ-CHAINIAUX, F., ERUSALIMSKY, J. D., CAMPISI, J., TOUSSAINT, O. 2009. Protocols to detect senescence-associated beta-galactosidase (SA-betagal) activity, a biomarker of senescent cells in culture and in vivo. *Nat Protoc*, 4, 1798–806.

FROHLICH, M., GRAYSON, W. L., MAROLT, D., GIMBLE, J. M., KREGAR-VELIKONJA, N., & VUNJAK-NOVAKOVIC, G. 2010. Bone grafts engineered from human adipose-derived stem cells in perfusion bioreactor culture. *Tissue Eng Part A*, 16, 179–89.

GARCIA-BRIONES, M., & CHALMERS, J. J. 1992. Cell-bubble interactions: mechanisms of suspended cell damage. *Ann N Y Acad Sci*, 665, 219–29.

GARCIA-BRIONES, M. A., & CHALMERS, J. J. 1994. Flow parameters associated with hydrodynamic cell injury. *Biotechnol Bioeng*, 44, 1089–98.

GILBERTSON, J. A., SEN, A., BEHIE, L. A., & KALLOS, M. S. 2006. Scaled-up production of mammalian neural precursor cell aggregates in computer-controlled suspension bioreactors. *Biotechnol Bioeng*, 94, 783–92.

GOWN, A. M., & WILLINGHAM, M. C. 2002. Improved detection of apoptotic cells in archival paraffin sections: immunohistochemistry using antibodies to cleaved caspase 3. *J Histochem Cytochem*, 50, 449–54.

GRAYSON, W. L., BHUMIRATANA, S., CANNIZZARO, C., CHAO, P. H. G., LENNON, D. P., CAPLAN, A. I., & VUNJAK-NOVAKOVIC, G. 2008. Effects of initial seeding density and fluid perfusion rate on formation of tissue-engineered bone. *Tissue Eng Part A*, 14, 1809–20.

HOLLISTER, S. J. 2005. Porous scaffold design for tissue engineering. *Nat Mater*, 4, 518–24.

HONDA, M. J., TSUCHIYA, S., SUMITA, Y., SAGARA, H., & UEDA, M. 2007. The sequential seeding of epithelial and mesenchymal cells for tissue-engineered tooth regeneration. *Biomaterials*, 28, 680–9.

HUTMACHER, D. W. 2001. Scaffold design and fabrication technologies for engineering tissues: state of the art and future perspectives. *J Biomater Sci Polym Ed*, 12, 107–24.

INANC, B., & ELCIN, Y. M. 2011. Stem cells in tooth tissue regeneration: challenges and limitations. *Stem Cell Rev*, 7, 683–92.

JONES, P. H., & WATT, F. M. 1993. Separation of human epidermal stem cells from transit amplifying cells on the basis of differences in integrin function and expression. *Cell*, 73, 713–24.

KAPUR, S., BAYLINK, D. J., & LAU, K. H. 2003. Fluid flow shear stress stimulates human osteoblast proliferation and differentiation through multiple interacting and competing signal transduction pathways. *Bone*, 32, 241–51.

KARAGEORGIOU, V., & KAPLAN, D. 2005. Porosity of 3D biomaterial scaffolds and osteogenesis. *Biomaterials*, 26, 5474–91.

KIMURA, M., STONE, R. C., HUNT, S. C., SKURNICK, J., LU, X., CAO, X., HARLEY, C. B., & AVIV, A. 2010. Measurement of telomere length by the Southern blot analysis of terminal restriction fragment lengths. *Nat Protoc*, 5, 1596–607.

KIROUAC, D. C., & ZANDSTRA, P. W. 2008. The systematic production of cells for cell therapies. *Cell Stem Cell*, 3, 369–81.

LEE, B. Y., HAN, J. A., IM, J. S., MORRONE, A., JOHUNG, K., GOODWIN, E. C., KLEIJER, W. J., DIMAIO, D., & HWANG, E. S. 2006. Senescence-associated beta-galactosidase is lysosomal beta-galactosidase. *Aging Cell*, 5, 187–95.

LEE, D. Y., YEH, C. R., CHANG, S. F., LEE, P. L., CHIEN, S., CHENG, C. K., & CHIU, J. J. 2008. Integrin-mediated expression of bone formation-related genes in osteoblast-like cells in response to fluid shear stress: roles of extracellular matrix, Shc, and mitogen-activated protein kinase. *J Bone Miner Res*, 23, 1140–9.

LEE, M. H., ARCIDIACONO, J. A., BILEK, A. M., WILLE, J. J., HAMILL, C. A., WONNACOTT, K. M., WELLS, M. A., & OH, S. S. 2010. Considerations for tissue-engineered and regenerative medicine product development prior to clinical trials in the United States. *Tissue Eng Part B Rev*, 16, 41–54.

LYMPERI, S., LIGOUDISTIANOU, C., TARASLIA, V., KONTAKIOTIS, E., & ANASTASIADOU, E. 2013. Dental stem cells and their applications in dental tissue engineering. *Open Dent J*, 7, 76–81.

MAJD, H., QUINN, T. M., WIPFF, P. J., & HINZ, B. 2011. Dynamic expansion culture for mesenchymal stem cells. *Methods Mol Biol*, 698, 175–88.

MALAVAL, L., LIU, F., ROCHE, P., & AUBIN, J. E. 1999. Kinetics of osteoprogenitor proliferation and osteoblast differentiation in vitro. *J Cell Biochem*, 74, 616–27.

MAROLT, D., KNEZEVIC, M., & NOVAKOVIC, G. V. 2010. Bone tissue engineering with human stem cells. *Stem Cell Res Ther*, 1.

MOURINO, V., CATTALINI, J. P., & BOCCACCINI, A. R. 2012. Metallic ions as therapeutic agents in tissue engineering scaffolds: an overview of their biological applications and strategies for new developments. *J R Soc Interface*, 9, 401–19.

PAPOUTSAKIS, E. T. 1991. Fluid-mechanical damage of animal cells in bioreactors. *Trends Biotechnol*, 9, 427–37.

PARTAP, S., LYONS, F., & O'BRIEN, F. J. 2010. IV.1. Scaffolds & surfaces. *Stud Health Technol Inform*, 152, 187–201.

PEREZ, R. A., WON, J. E., KNOWLES, J. C., & KIM, H. W. 2013. Naturally and synthetic smart composite biomaterials for tissue regeneration. *Adv Drug Deliv Rev*, 65, 471–96.

RATCLIFFE, E., THOMAS, R. J., & WILLIAMS, D. J. 2011. Current understanding and challenges in bioprocessing of stem cell-based therapies for regenerative medicine. *Br Med Bull*, 100, 137–55.

RODRIGUES, C. A., FERNANDES, T. G., DIOGO, M. M., DA SILVA, C. L., & CABRAL, J. M. 2011. Stem cell cultivation in bioreactors. *Biotechnol Adv*, 29, 815–29.

SENSEBE, L., BOURIN, P., & TARTE, K. 2011. Good manufacturing practices production of mesenchymal stem/stromal cells. *Hum Gene Ther*, 22, 19–26.

SIKAVITSAS, V. I., BANCROFT, G. N., HOLTORF, H. L., JANSEN, J. A., & MIKOS, A. G. 2003. Mineralized matrix deposition by marrow stromal osteoblasts in 3D perfusion culture increases with increasing fluid shear forces. *Proc Natl Acad Sci U S A*, 100, 14683–8.

SIMARIA, A. S., HASSAN, S., VARADARAJU, H., ROWLEY, J., WARREN, K., VANEK, P., & FARID, S. S. 2014. Allogeneic cell therapy bioprocess economics and optimization: single-use cell expansion technologies. *Biotechnol Bioeng*, 111, 69–83.

SJÖSTRÖM, T., DALBY, M.J., HART, A., TARE, R., OREFFO, R.O., & SU B. 2009. Fabrication of pillar-like titania nanostructures on titanium and their interactions with human skeletal stem cells. Acta Biomater, 5,1433–41.

VOLKMER, E., DROSSE, I., OTTO, S., STANGELMAYER, A., STENGELE, M., KALLUKALAM, B. C., MUTSCHLER, W., & SCHIEKER, M. 2008. Hypoxia in static and dynamic 3D culture systems for tissue engineering of bone. *Tissue Eng Part A*, 14, 1331–40.

WENDT, D., RIBOLDI, S. A., CIOFFI, M., & MARTIN, I. 2009. Bioreactors in tissue engineering: scientific challenges and clinical perspectives. *Adv Biochem Eng Biotechnol*, 112, 1–27.

WEYTS, F. A., LI, Y. S., VAN LEEUWEN, J., WEINANS, H., & CHIEN, S. 2002. ERK activation and alpha v beta 3 integrin signaling through Shc recruitment in response to mechanical stimulation in human osteoblasts. *J Cell Biochem*, 87, 85–92.

CHAPTER 7

Periodontal tissue engineering

Saso Ivanovski[1], P. Mark Bartold[2], Stan Gronthos[3], and Dietmar W. Hutmacher[4]

[1] Menzies Health Institute Queensland, School of Dentistry and Oral Health, Griffith University, Gold Coast, Queensland, Australia

[2] Colgate Australian Dental Research Centre, Dental School, University of Adelaide, Adelaide, SA, Australia

[3] School of Medical Sciences, Faculty of Health Sciences, University of Adelaide, Adelaide, SA, Australia, South Australian Health and Medical Research Institute, Adelaide, SA, Australia

[4] Institute of Health and Biomedical Innovation, Queensland University of Technology, Brisbane, Queensland, Australia

The periodontium is composed of the tissues supporting and investing the tooth. It is a complex organ, consisting of soft and mineralised connective tissues that include the gingiva, periodontal ligament, cementum, and alveolar bone, as well as an external epithelial covering. It is between these components that significant interactions occur during the healing process. Periodontal defects resulting from periodontal disease exhibit significant extracellular matrix destruction of alveolar bone, periodontal ligament, and gingiva. Furthermore, the root cementum becomes contaminated by exposure to the oral environment.

It has been recognised for some time that the unique anatomy and composition of the periodontium make periodontal wound healing a more complex process than general soft tissue healing because of the requirement for interaction between hard and soft connective tissues, as well as epithelium (Melcher, 1976). Indeed, at least six tissue types are involved in the repair of a periodontal lesion: the gingival epithelium, gingival connective tissue, periodontal ligament, cementum, alveolar bone, and all the associated vasculature. Nowhere else in the body are epithelium and mineralised and nonmineralised connective tissues juxtaposed in such close anatomic and functional proximity.

Principles of periodontal wound healing and regeneration

One of the major goals of periodontal therapy is to encourage regeneration of tissues that have been destroyed as a result of periodontal disease. Periodontal regeneration is defined as the reproduction or reconstitution of a lost or injured part so that form and function of these structures are restored. However, despite the best that current therapies can offer, the ultimate response of the periodontium depends upon the tissues and cells that participate in the healing process. Periodontal regeneration requires new attachment to the root surface, a process that involves the regeneration of principal fibres and the insertion of these fibres into newly formed cementum on a root surface that has been previously exposed to periodontal pathogens.

It has been shown that cells derived from both gingival connective tissues and alveolar bone lack the ability to form new periodontal attachment (Karring et al., 1980; Nyman et al., 1980), commonly resulting in extensive resorption of root surfaces or ankylosis. On the other hand, if preference is given to repopulation of the root surface by periodontal ligament cells, new connective tissue attachment, including new cementum with inserting collagen fibres, can be formed (Nyman et al., 1982). However, achieving conditions that allow selective repopulation by periodontal ligament cells is difficult to obtain clinically. Following surgical flap procedures, the epithelial cells of the gingival tissues proliferate and migrate at a faster rate than the cells of the underlying connective tissue. This enables them to rapidly establish coverage of the exposed root surface, forming a "long junctional epithelium", which precludes any significant regeneration of the periodontal attachment apparatus (Caton et al., 1980).

Tissue Engineering and Regeneration in Dentistry: Current Strategies, First Edition. Edited by Rachel J. Waddington and Alastair J. Sloan.
© 2017 John Wiley & Sons, Ltd. Published 2017 by John Wiley & Sons, Ltd.

At a cellular level, in order for periodontal regeneration to occur, progenitor periodontal ligament cells must migrate to the denuded root surface, attach to it, proliferate, and mature into an organised and functional fibrous attachment apparatus that inserts into newly formed cementum. Likewise, progenitor bone cells must also migrate, proliferate, and mature in conjunction with the regenerating periodontal ligament. Hence, the concept of periodontal regeneration is based on the principle that remaining healthy cells, and/or cells attracted to the healing site, have the potential to promote regeneration. In this context, there is a requirement for precisely coordinated spatial and temporal events that ensure that the appropriate cells are available within the correct periodontal compartment in order for regeneration to occur. This is difficult to achieve clinically, and hence a tissue engineering approach, whereby the spatial and temporal coordination of different tissue compartments are manipulated *in vitro* prior to insertion *in vivo*, is an attractive strategy for promoting periodontal regeneration.

Overview of past and current clinical periodontal regeneration techniques

The work of Pritchard (1957) provided early evidence that regeneration was not only theoretically possible but also clinically achievable in "ideal" periodontal defects. This work showed that regeneration of the periodontium in the apical aspects of three-wall intrabony defects could be obtained following subgingival debridement through a surgical approach. Regeneration was not achieved in all cases, but this provided the "proof of principle" evidence that if the conditions were optimal, then healing outcomes other than repair could be obtained. Since then, a great deal of research has focused on establishing a clinical technique to achieve these optimal conditions in a variety of clinical situations, not just three-wall defects.

Root surface conditioning

The rationale for root surface conditioning was based on the assumption that a root surface exposed to periodontal pathogens is contaminated with endotoxin and other bacterial components. Therefore, in order to allow reattachment of cells, it was hypothesised that the surface needs to be prepared so as to both remove the contaminants and provide an appropriate environment for cell recolonisation. This preparation has involved the use of a variety of chemical/biological agents, with the rationale being that exposure of the collagen fibrils in the root surface dentine would encourage attachment and differentiation of adjacent mesenchymal cells, and subsequently result in new attachment formation. The agents used have included citric acid, tetracycline, EDTA, or attachment proteins such as fibronectin (Mariotti 2003). Trials of these root conditioning agents in humans, however, have not shown any significant improvement in clinical attachment levels compared to surgical treatment alone, and have often been associated with root resorption or ankylosis (Mariotti 2003). Therefore, it can be concluded that the clinical practice of root surface conditioning is not supported by the available literature. Indeed, even if this practice was shown to be effective, it would only facilitate reattachment of periodontal fibres to the root surface, and hence falls short of achieving regeneration of the original orientation of the periodontium.

Bone grafting materials

Bone grafting materials have been used to replace the alveolar bone lost within the periodontal defect, with the rationale being that this would facilitate new attachment formation to the adjacent root surface. Based on the source of the graft, bone grafting materials can be classified into four categories: autogenous (derived from the same individual), allogenic (derived from a different member of the same species), xenografts (derived from a different species), and alloplastic (synthetic products).

The literature is conflicting on the ability of these grafting materials to promote periodontal regeneration. A review of the use of bone grafting materials in intrabony and furcation defects found that bone grafts increased clinical attachment level and reduced probing depths compared to surgical open flap debridement. For furcation defects, the authors concluded that some benefit could be obtained in mandibular Class 2 furcations, but the lack of consistency among these studies meant that no clear consensus was obtained. Different types of grafting materials produced a similar range of results (Reynolds et al., 2003).

This potential improvement in clinical parameters in some situations, however, does not necessarily reflect true regeneration. The only method to assess whether regeneration has occurred is via histological examination, with conflicting findings reported in the literature as to whether this actually occurs following the use of bone grafting materials. Some studies report the generation of new attachment onto the root surface (Hiatt et al., 1978), whereas others illustrate repair via a long junctional epithelium (Dragoo and Kaldahl, 1983). The general consensus, however, is that bone grafting materials are ineffective at facilitating complete regeneration (Reynolds et al., 2003). Indeed, focusing solely on bone regeneration at the expense of the cementum and periodontal ligament is biologically unsound and hence is unlikely to result in periodontal regeneration.

Guided tissue regeneration (GTR)

Guided tissue regeneration uses biocompatible barrier membranes to enable selective cellular recolonisation of periodontal defects. The principle involves the use of a barrier membrane to exclude tissues that are unable to promote periodontal regeneration, such as the rapidly proliferative epithelium that grows along the root surface and the gingival connective tissues that fill the periodontal defect. Instead, this technique facilitates the repopulation of the defect with cells that have the ability to reestablish the periodontal attachment apparatus, namely those from the periodontal ligament and alveolar bone (Figure 7.1). The concept of GTR is supported by histological evidence of periodontal regeneration following the use of this technique (Gottlow et al., 1986).

The membranes used can be either nonresorbable or resorbable, but due to decreased postoperative complications and reduced number of surgical procedures, resorbable membranes have become more popular. Resorbable membranes come in a variety of materials, with the most common being collagen and copolymers of polylactic/polyglycolic acid.

The benefit of using GTR over the conventional use of open flap debridement has been reviewed in the literature, and the findings support the use of GTR in two clinical situations, Type II mandibular furcations (Jepsen et al., 2002) and intrabony defects (Needleman et al., 2006). However, although GTR is conceptually sound, the clinical results are unreliable and predictable regeneration is elusive in most periodontal defects, with the possible exception of a few "ideal" situations, such as narrow three-wall defects. These ideal clinical scenarios are not frequently encountered in clinical practice.

Growth factors and biologically active regenerative materials

The rationale for the application of growth factors to the periodontal defect is based on their ability to influence key cellular functions such as proliferation, migration, and differentiation. However, their use is not widespread in periodontal regenerative medicine, due to problems with dosage, rapid metabolic clearance, appropriate delivery and carrier systems, and cost (Trombelli and Farina, 2008). The most widely studied biologically active material that has been in widespread clinical use is enamel matrix derivative.

Enamel matrix derivative (EMD)

Enamel matrix proteins (EMPs) are secreted by ameloblasts and play a role in the regulation and growth of hydroxyapatite crystals that comprise enamel (Hammarstrom, 1997). In addition to their well-documented role in enamel biomineralisation, EMPs are

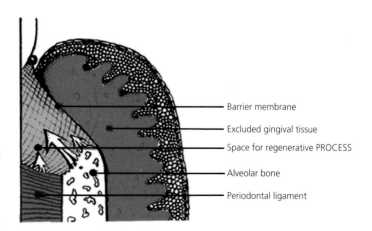

Figure 7.1 Diagrammatic representation of guided tissue regeneration principle involving the use of a barrier membrane to create space and facilitate the selective repopulation of the defect with periodontal ligament cells and osteoblasts at the expense of epithelial cells and gingival fibroblasts.

Barrier membrane

Excluded gingival tissue

Space for regenerative PROCESS

Alveolar bone

Periodontal ligament

considered to be involved in epithelial-mesenchymal interactions at the developing root surface. EMPs exposed on the root surface by the breakdown of Hertwig's epithelial root sheath are thought to play a role in the differentiation of mesenchymal tissues and subsequent formation of the attachment apparatus of the periodontium (Hammarstrom, 1997). The principle behind the use of EMPs in regenerative approaches is therefore that of biomimetics, or mimicking natural biology.

EMP is available commercially as Emdogain (Straumann, Basel, Switzerland). This is an injectable gel solution comprising EMD, water, and a carrier, propylene glycol alginate. The EMD is a cocktail primarily consisting of amelogenin, but it also contains other enamel proteins, such as ameloblastin, amelotin, tuftelin, and enamelin, and is formulated from tooth pouches of porcine origin.

Histological evidence of regeneration following EMD application has been obtained from animal trials, including the treatment of surgically created buccal dehiscence defects in monkeys (Hammarstrom et al., 1997). In humans, histological evidence of regeneration has also been obtained from case reports (Heijl, 1997) and corroborated by clinical outcomes in other studies (Sculean et al., 1999; Heden and Wennstrom, 2006). The findings of large-scale randomised controlled trials and systematic reviews indicate that applications are principally limited to intrabony defects and Grade 2 furcations (Giannobile and Somerman, 2003; Esposito et al., 2005). When compared to GTR, there were no statistically significant differences between the two treatment approaches with respect to key clinical outcomes, especially clinical attachment levels (Sculean et al., 1999).

Platelet-derived growth factor (PDGF)

Platelet-derived growth factor has the potential to enhance wound healing due to its efficient chemotactic and mitotic effect on mesenchymal stem cells. Recombinant forms have recently been utilised in periodontal regenerative therapies in the treatment of intrabony and furcation defects (Darby and Morris, 2013). A recent systematic review found that the use of recombinant human platelet–derived growth factor BB (rhPDGF-BB) led to greater clinical attachment level gain of $\approx$ 1 mm compared to an osteoconductive control, β-tricalcium phosphate. Furthermore, the use of rhPDGF-BB led to greater percentage bone fill of $\approx$ 40% compared to the control (Darby and Morris, 2013).

However, there are relatively few clinical studies that have examined the use of PDGF in periodontal regeneration, and hence the effectiveness of PDGF needs to be confirmed in further studies.

P-15

P-15 is a 15-amino-acid peptide that mimics the cell binding part of the α1 chain of Type I collagen, which has been shown to have the capacity to enhance the rate and the extent of attachment and migration of periodontal cells on root surfaces (Lallier et al., 2003). Clinical results indicate that the commercially available combination of P-15 and a bovine-derived hydroxyapatite matrix (ABM) (PEPGEN P-15, Dentsply Friadent, Mannheim, Germany) results in a significant improvement of clinical and radiographic parameters when compared with either open flap debridement (Yukna et al., 1998) or ABM alone (Yukna et al., 2000) in the treatment of intrabony defects. Although these results were shown to be maintained for at least 3 years in a case report (Yukna et al., 2002), the effectiveness of P-15/ABM in promoting periodontal regeneration needs to be confirmed by large-cohort, controlled trials.

Platelet-rich plasma (PRP)

Platelet rich plasma is a platelet concentrate that contains a number of different growth factors, including PDGF, TGF-β, and IGF, which have been shown to exert a positive effect on periodontal wound healing. PRP has the advantage of being able to be prepared chairside, and safety issues are minimal as autologous material is being used. There are no randomised controlled clinical trials evaluating the clinical effect of PRP alone in periodontal regeneration. However, the use of PRP combined with several types of grafts for the treatment of intrabony defects resulted in contradictory results ranging from a significant enhancement of clinical attachment gain (Hanna et al., 2004; Okuda et al., 2005) to no effect (Demir et al., 2007; Yassibag-Berkman et al., 2007). No additional benefit of PRP has been shown when combined with a graft and GTR, compared with the use of only a graft and GTR in intrabony defects (Dori et al., 2007). The discrepancy in clinical outcomes using PRP may be partly due to differences in the methods used to obtain the PRP preparations, which may in turn affect the content of platelets and inflammatory cytokines, as well as lead to contamination of the platelet preparation with leucocytes and erythrocytes (Weibrich et al., 2003). The use of PRP does not result in adverse healing events following surgery, and there are some reports that suggest that PRP may lead to more rapid healing, less postoperative pain, and less membrane exposure (Dori et al., 2007).

Although it has been shown that PRP may exert a positive adjunctive effect when used in combination with graft materials (but not with GTR) for the treatment of intrabony defects, recent systematic reviews suggest that there is limited evidence for the use of platelet-rich plasma or other platelet concentrates as adjuncts in periodontal regeneration (Panda et al., 2014; Del Fabbro, 2011).

Summary of clinical performance of current techniques

Although GTR and EMD have been shown to be effective in regenerating a limited range of periodontal defects, such as three-wall intrabony defects and Class 2 furcations, currently available clinical techniques are generally unpredictable and cannot be utilised in the vast majority of periodontal defects.

The reasons for failure for most regenerative techniques have been outlined by Bartold et al. (2000):

- inability to control the formation of a long junctional epithelium;
- inability to adequately seal the healing site from the oral environment and prevent infection;
- inability to maintain the wound as a closed rather than open system;
- restriction of regeneration to the bone compartment whilst ignoring regenerative processes required for cementogenesis and fibrous attachment;
- inability to define precisely the growth and differentiation factors needed for regeneration;
- the possibility that growth factors may not be sufficiently discriminative in their ability to induce regeneration, and thus the induction of particular transcription factors as an earlier event of cell stimulation may be warranted; and
- infection of the implanted membrane or regenerative material postoperatively.

Periodontal tissue engineering

Tissue engineering involves using techniques for the fabrication of tissues outside the body for implantation into the body to regenerate the lost biological function

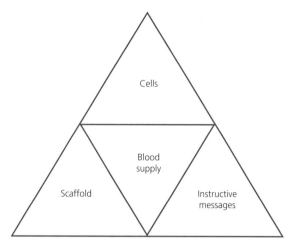

Figure 7.2 Diagrammatic representation of the key components of a tissue-engineered construct: cells, scaffold, instructive messages, and blood supply.

of a given tissue. The requirements for tissue engineering are the presence of adequate numbers of responsive progenitor cells, the appropriate levels and sequencing of regulatory signals, and a suitable carrier or scaffold (Bartold et al., 2000). For successful periodontal regeneration via tissue engineering, the engineered tissues should have sufficient biomechanical strength, architectural properties, and space-maintaining ability. The engineered construct has to maintain space for in-growth of alveolar bone, but it also has to be exclusionary with respect to the epithelial tissues to prevent the formation of a long junctional epithelium. A key requirement is to facilitate the special and temporal coordination of the wound healing process in order to allow formation of new periodontal attachment consisting of periodontal ligament fibres perpendicularly inserted into newly formed cementum on the root surface. A critical but sometimes overlooked prerequisite is the need to ensure a viable blood supply to the newly formed tissues (Figure 7.2).

Cells

A key requirement of cells for use in tissue engineering approaches is that they have sufficient plasticity in order to be guided by the surrounding instructive environment to form the cellular and extracellular components of the required tissues. Undifferentiated progenitor or stem cells are ideal for periodontal tissue engineering applications as they can be manipulated to contribute to the formation of the various soft and hard tissues necessary to regenerate the periodontium. Stem cells are characterised by the ability to differentiate into multiple cell lineages as well as by their self-renewal potential, whereas progenitor cells are descendants of stem cells with a more committed differentiation status and the tendency to be found locally within target tissues.

Progenitor cells in the periodontium and their differentiation

It has been widely hypothesised for many years that periodontal regeneration would be more practically achieved if the properties of progenitor or stem cells could be harnessed. However, for a long time, the origin and ontogeny of these progenitor cells remained largely unknown. A series of experiments carried out in the 1980s began to provide insight into the source and fate of progenitior cells in the periodontium.

Cell kinetic experiments (McCulloch et al., 1987; McCulloch and Melcher, 1983b) showed that periodontal ligament fibroblast populations represent a steady-state renewal system, with the number of new cells generated by mitosis equal to the number of cells lost through apoptosis and migration (McCulloch and Melcher, 1983a; Schellens et al., 1982). This capacity for self-renewal, which is further evidenced by the rapid turnover of the periodontal ligament, supports the notion of progenitor/stem cell populations. Furthermore, a significant number of periodontal cells do not enter the cell cycle (McCulloch and Melcher, 1983c), suggesting that these cells may act in a similar manner to quiescent, self-renewable, and multipotent hematopoietic stem cells (Uchida et al., 1993).

The exact relationship between progenitor cells in regenerating tissues and normally functioning (steady-state) tissues is not clear. Studies performed in normal mouse periodontal ligament (McCulloch, 1985), wounded mouse periodontal ligament (Gould et al., 1980), normal rat gingiva (Pender et al., 1988), and inflamed monkey gingiva (Nemeth et al., 1993) identified a common paravascular location for fibroblast progenitors. These cells exhibited some of the classical cytological features of stem cells, including small size, responsiveness to stimulating factors, and slow cycle time (Gould et al., 1980; McCulloch, 1985; McCulloch and Melcher, 1983a).

Experimental approaches that used cell kinetic (McCulloch et al., 1987) and cell culture methods (Melcher et al., 1986) showed that periodontal ligament cell populations in adult rodents are derived from cells residing in both the periodontal ligament and endosteal spaces, suggesting that considerable mixing of cell populations occurs in periodontal tissues. It has been demonstrated that mesenchymal cells from the dental follicle can differentiate into cementoblasts and form cementum, then subsequently detach from the cementum surface and contribute towards early periodontal fibroblast populations (Cho and Garant, 1989). Other possible sources of osteoblast and cementoblast precursors are the endosteal spaces of alveolar bone from which cells have been observed to adopt a paravascular location in the periodontal ligament of mice (McCulloch et al., 1987).

Collectively, from these early studies, it was apparent that cells with the characteristics of progenitor cells are located in the periodontal ligament, primarily in paravascular sites or in vascular channels of the alveolar bone. It was suggested that these cells may retain their multipotency throughout life, and may periodically divide and differentiate to assure periodontal homeostasis and contribute towards periodontal turnover and remodelling.

The use of PDL cells *in vivo* for periodontal regeneration

In principle, evidence for the viability of using transplanted PDL cells to support periodontal regeneration was first demonstrated in 1998 in an animal study that showed that autologous cultured periodontal cells can support regeneration *in vivo* (Lang et al., 1998). Subsequent studies have confirmed that PDL cells have the ability to facilitate regeneration in animal models. Isaka and colleagues (2001) placed PDL cells in a surgically created defect in an autologous dog model and found that they were capable of the formation of new cementum but had a limited influence on alveolar bone formation.

Similarly, it was shown that seeding PDL cells in autologous blood coagulum under a Teflon membrane promoted regeneration of surgically created furcation and fenestration defects in dogs (Dogan et al., 2002, 2003). Although these studies chiefly examined bone formation, not cementum and hence "true regeneration", this again provided an indication that PDL cells do have a regenerative capacity.

Autologous periodontal ligament–derived cells have also been combined with collagen sponges and resulted in superior regeneration compared to nonseeded scaffolds in surgically created defects in a beagle dog model (Nakahara et al., 2004). The sites treated with the cell-seeded sponges had uniform new cementum formation, whereas the control sites only showed scattered cementum deposits. This suggests that the PDL cell-seeded approach promoted not only bone formation but new cementum and hence regeneration.

More recently, it has been shown that transplanted PDL cells have superior periodontal regenerative properties compared to other cells of periodontal origin, namely gingival fibroblasts and alveolar bone osteoblasts (Dan et al., 2014). In a study utilising a rat defect model, PDL cells showed superior ability to promote cementogenesis and periodontal fibre attachment compared to alveolar bone osteoblasts, while gingival fibroblasts inhibited bone formation (Dan et al., 2014).

The literature therefore supports the principle that cultured PDL cells applied in a scaffold or gel can facilitate periodontal regeneration. However, it must be noted that complete periodontal regeneration is often unobtainable, and adverse outcomes such as ankylosis have been shown to occur. This indicates that although theoretically possible, approaches to regeneration have so far lacked the sophistication to become sufficiently predictable for mainstream clinical practice. It is possible that the key to regeneration lies in the ability to isolate those cells residing within the PDL that possess stem cell properties.

Stem cells

Stem cells are defined by two characteristics: (a) the ability for indefinite self-renewal to give rise to more stem cells; and (b) the ability to differentiate into a variety of specialised daughter cells to perform specific functions. Stem cells can be broadly divided into two broad categories, embryonic stem cells and adult stem cells, and further classified according to their origin and differentiation potential.

Human embryonic stem cells, derived from the inner cell mass of blastocysts, are pluripotent cells capable of differentiating into cells of all three germ layers—ectoderm, mesoderm, and endoderm. Human embryonic stem cell research has, however, been associated with major ethical concerns, which has resulted in increasing focus on adult stem cells. Adult stem cells are found in the majority of fetal and adult tissues and are thought to play roles in long-term tissue maintenance and/or repair by replacing cells that are either injured or lost. They are generally multipotent stem cells that can form a limited number of cell types. Two common examples are hematopoietic and mesenchymal stem cells (MSCs). As the periodontium is mesenchymal in origin, MSCs have been studied in periodontal regeneration research.

Extraoral mesenchymal stem cells and periodontal regeneration

Several preclinical trials have shown that bone marrow–derived MSCs (BMMSCs) have the capacity to promote periodontal regeneration through enhanced generation of cementum, periodontal ligament, alveolar bone, and neovascularisation. The implantation of BMMSCs has been shown to promote cementum and alveolar bone regeneration in furcation defects in dogs (Kawaguchi et al., 2004; Li et al, 2009). Cell labelling showed that the implanted cells directly contributed to the regenerated periodontal tissues, showing that BMMSCs differentiated into cementoblasts, periodontal ligament fibroblasts, and alveolar bone osteoblasts *in vivo* (Hasegawa et al., 2006). Subsequently, a human clinical case report showed that autologous BMMSCs combined with PRP resulted in a reduction in intrabony defect depth and resolution of bleeding (Yamada et al., 2006).

Aside from bone marrow, adipose tissue is another commonly utilised extraoral source of MSCs. Adipose-derived stromal cells mixed with PRP have been shown to promote regeneration of periodontal ligament–like structures along with alveolar bone in rats (Tobita et al., 2008). These observations suggest that adipose-derived stromal cells may be another useful source for future clinical cell-based therapy for periodontal tissue engineering, which may be obtained via relatively noninvasive lipoaspirates that have lower morbidity than bone aspirates. Nevertheless, the difficulty associated with the sourcing of extraoral MSCs for use in the clinical setting has led to the exploration of dental-tissue-derived MSC populations that may be more simply obtained chairside, as well as having superior potential to differentiate into the local periodontal tissues.

Mesenchymal stem cells in dental and periodontal tissues

The first human dental stem cells were isolated from dental pulp tissue of extracted third molar teeth and were characterised relative to BMMSCs (Gronthos et al., 2000). Since then, populations of stem cells have been identified in the pulp tissue of exfoliated deciduous teeth, the apical papilla of human teeth, the dental follicle of human third molar teeth, and the periodontal ligament (Lin et al., 2008). Periodontal ligament stem cells (PDLSCs) have been shown to give rise to adherent clonogenic clusters resembling fibroblasts, and have been shown to be capable of developing into adipocytes, osteoblasts, and cementoblast-like cells *in vitro*, as well as producing cementum- and periodontal ligament–like tissues *in vivo* (Seo et al., 2004). Recent studies have also shown their ability to differentiate into neuronal precursors (Techawattanawisal et al., 2007). PDLSCs also express an array of cementoblast and osteoblast markers as well as the perivascular-associated markers, STRO-1 and CD146 antigens (Trubiani et al., 2005).

A recent systematic review identified a total of 17 studies that have been conducted to assess the regenerative capacity of PDLSCs in a range of periodontal defects in various animal models and one human clinical study (Bright et al., 2014). It was found that 70.5% of studies showed a statistically significant improvement in histological parameters associated with periodontal regeneration, including new bone, cementum, and connective tissue formation with the use of PDLSCs. PDLSCs appear to have a greater capacity to generate dental associated structures in comparison to other MSC-like cells, making them highly amenable for use in periodontal regeneration. The one human clinical study carried out to date (a case series of three patients) (Feng et al., 2010) concluded that the use of autologous PDLSCs in cell-based surgical treatment for periodontitis may be effective in promoting regeneration.

Induced pluripotent stem cells (iPSCs)

Induced pluripotent stem cells are a population of pluripotent stem cells that resemble embryonic stem cells and are generated from somatic cells through the induced expression of key transcription factors such as Oct4, Sox2, C-Myc and Klf4 (Takahashi and Yamanaka, 2006). This generation of iPSCs represented a fundamental shift in understanding of cell differentiation because it demonstrated that cell differentiation can be reversed, meaning that differentiation is not the one-way process it was once believed to be. Interest in iPSCs centres around their close similarity to embryonic stem cells and their capacity to differentiate into all three germ layers *in vitro* (Takahashi and Yamanaka, 2006). The finding that iPSCs are very similar to

embryonic stem cells led to the notion that iPSCs could function as a more easily accessible source of pluripotent stem cells for use in patient therapies, as generation of iPSCs does not require the use of an embryo. It has been suggested that iPSCs could be used to generate patient-specific stem cells for a wide variety of regenerative medicine applications.

Since their discovery, iPSCs have been generated from a wide range of tissues, including those of dental origin. To date iPSCs have been generated from multiple dental tissues, including adult and deciduous teeth pulps, oral mucosa, third molar mesenchymal stromal cells, gingival fibroblasts, and periodontal ligament fibroblasts (Oda et al., 2010; Tamaoki et al., 2010; Yan et al., 2010; Wada et al 2011). iPSCs have been utilised for periodontal regeneration in a mouse periodontal fenestration defect model (Duan et al., 2011). iPSCs, combined with EMD and a silk scaffold and implanted into a fenestration defect, were shown to promote the formation of new cementum, alveolar bone, and normal periodontal ligament (Duan et al., 2011). However, the direct use of iPSCs is associated with an increased risk of teratoma formation, and a safer approach is considered to be the use of cells differentiated from iPSCs. To this end, MSCs differentiated from iPSCs have also been utilised in a rat periodontal defect model, and have been shown to promote periodontal regeneration (Hynes et al., 2013).

Issues with iPSCs and MSCs for periodontal regeneration

Considerable research has been performed to assess the capacity of dental derived MSC-like cell populations to enhance periodontal regeneration, and there are some promising results being obtained. Whilst varying levels of regenerative potential are exhibited by the various MSC-like populations, PDLSCs are by far the most studied cell population and are showing good potential for use in periodontal regeneration; however, a limiting factor to their clinical use is that tooth extraction is required in order to obtain the PDLSCs. Hence, research is ongoing into more easily accessible stem cell populations, one of which is iPSCs. While the early results regarding the use of iPSCs in periodontal regeneration look promising, significantly more work is required in this area. There are also major concerns that need to be addressed regarding the effect genetic manipulation has had on iPSCs and the potential of these cells to form tumours. There are also questions surrounding the ability to control the differentiation of iPSCs once implanted, as iPSCs have the capacity to differentiate into any cell type of the body, and it is necessary to ensure that the cells differentiate into the desired cell types.

Another important consideration in relation to the use of cellular therapy is the need to deliver the cells in the correct spatial and temporal orientation in order to regenerate the complex architecture of the periodontium. To this end, the combination with an appropriate scaffold that will ensure that the correct cell type is delivered and retained within the appropriate part of the defect is important. In this context, the use of a tissue-engineering construct, whereby the appropriate cell type is incorporated into a three-dimensional carrier scaffold, is an important consideration.

Cell sheet technology

A novel technique for harvesting and delivering cells in tissue engineering approaches involves the use of cell sheets (Matsuura et al., 2014). Cell sheet construction involves the use of a temperature-sensitive polymer biomaterial, poly N-isopropylacrylamide (PIPA Am), in the cell culturing process. Once cell confluence is reached, the cells are harvested as an intact cell sheet by decreasing the temperature, which leads to the detachment from the temperature-sensitive substrate. Unlike traditional cell harvesting, which utilises enzymatic approaches to fragment the extracellular matrix in order to release the cells, this cell sheet method allows harvesting of a complete sheet of cellular material with an intact extracellular matrix and cell-cell junctions.

Cell sheet fabrication has been reported from various cell types, including fibroblasts, endothelial cells, hepatocytes, macrophages, and retinal pigmented epithelial cells (Shimizu et al., 2004; Tsuda et al., 2007). Indeed, cell sheet technology has been applied to different tissue engineering applications, including utilising corneal epithelial cell sheets for the preparation of a transplantable cornea and constructing myocardial tissues using multilayered cardiomyocyte cell sheets (Sawa and Miyagawa, 2013; Zavala et al., 2013; Shimizu et al., 2004). Subsequently, cell sheets have been shown to facilitate periodontal regeneration in a number of animal studies using dogs, rats, and mice (Wang et al., 2014). Because of the delicate and fragile nature of the cell sheet, this technology also requires a supportive membrane or scaffold to facilitate its manipulation and implantation into the defect site. Current advances have focused on the use of cell sheets in conjunction with 3D biphasic scaffold engineering technology to promote simultaneous regeneration for different adjacent tissue types (Vaquette et al., 2012). The critical issue of utilising a scaffold that provides appropriate support to cell sheets to ensure predictable harvesting, delivery, and stabilisation within the defect will be addressed later in this chapter.

Regulatory growth factor and differentiation factors

Platelet-derived growth factor (PDGF) and insulin-like growth factor-1 (IGF-1)

Platelet-derived growth factor is a dimeric molecule produced by a variety of cells and tissues, including fibroblasts and osteoblasts (Antoniades et al., 1991; Hauschka et al., 1988). PDGF is mitogenic for various cells of mesenchymal origin, such as glial, smooth muscle, and bone cells, as well as fibroblasts (Antoniades and Owen, 1982; Ross et al., 1986; Stiles, 1983).

In fibroblastic systems, the primary effect of PDGF is that of a mitogen. It initiates cell division by acting as a competence factor, thus making the cell competent for division (Pledger et al., 1977). A progression factor, such as IGF-1 or dexamethasone, is then necessary to induce mitosis (Lynch et al., 1989a). PDGF, however, also acts as a paracrine factor by stimulating certain cells to produce their own progression growth factors (Clemmons and Van Wyk, 1985). Several investigators have demonstrated the potent mitogenic effect of PDGF on gingival and periodontal ligament fibroblasts (Bartold and Raben, 1996; Haase et al., 1998; Oates et al., 1993).

Insulin growth factors I and II are closely related growth factors with biochemical and functional similarities to insulin (Daughaday and Rotwein, 1989; Rall et al., 1987). They are synthesised by multiple tissues, including liver, smooth muscle, and placenta (Caffesse and Quinones, 1993). IGF-I has been shown to be chemotactic for cells derived from the periodontal ligament, and it has strong effects on periodontal ligament mitogenesis and protein synthesis *in vitro* (Haase et al., 1998; Matsuda et al., 1992).

It has been recognised that PDGF and IGF-I might promote periodontal regeneration as they have the potential to potentiate growth of multiple tissues. Consequently, combinations of PDGF and IGF-I have been tested clinically in order to assess their ability to promote periodontal regeneration (Lynch et al., 1989a; Lynch et al., 1991; Lynch et al., 1989b; Rutherford et al., 1992). It was shown that a combination of purified PDGF and recombinant IGF-I can stimulate periodontal regeneration in dogs, including new cementum formation (Lynch et al., 1989b). Subsequently, similar results were obtained with a combination of recombinant PDGF-BB and IGF-I in periodontitis defects in beagle dogs (Lynch et al., 1991) and in ligature-induced periodontitis defects in the cynomolgus monkey (Rutherford et al., 1992). These studies showed that the half-life for release of the growth factors from the carrier was rapid (within 3–4 hours). Since these factors are rapidly cleared or bound, the successful use of a single-dose application suggests that the mechanism for regenerating tissues occurs via stimulation of a cascade of events that result in multiple tissue formation and integration. Subsequently, a number of studies have shown that PDGF, used either with dexamethasone or IGF-I, and with or without guided tissue regeneration with ePTFE membranes, stimulates periodontal regeneration (Cho et al., 1995; Giannobile et al., 1994; Giannobile et al., 1996; Howell et al., 1997; Park et al., 1995; Rutherford et al., 1993).

These studies were the basis of a currently available commercial product that contains PDGF and tricalcium phosphate (GEM 21); the results of clinical trials using this product are discussed earlier in this chapter. However, the less than optimal results obtained by this approach suggest that additional work is required to fully harness the potential of PDGF in periodontal regeneration.

Fibroblast growth factor 2 (FGF-2)

Fibroblast growth factor is a polypeptide that consists of approximately 150–200 amino acid residues. FGF stimulates undifferentiated mesenchymal cells to differentiate and proliferate, and can also induce angiogenesis (Murakami, 2011). The effect of topical application of recombinant human basic fibroblast growth factor (rhFGF-2) on periodontal regeneration in furcation defects has been investigated in beagle dogs (Murakami et al., 2003). Histological analysis showed that sites treated with rhFGF-2 resulted in periodontal regeneration with new cementum, new alveolar bone, and new

Sharpey's fibres with functional new periodontal ligament (Murakami et al., 2003).

However, in a randomised controlled double blind human clinical study, no statistically significant differences were found in clinical attachment level (CAL) gain and alveolar bone gain in FGF-2 treated subjects. There was, however, a significant difference in alveolar bone height between the two groups after 36 weeks, suggesting FGF-2 could have a long-term effect in stimulating bone regeneration in intrabony periodontal defects (Kitamura et al., 2008).

Bone morphogenetic proteins (BMPs)

Bone morphogenetic proteins (BMPs) constitute a large family of regulatory factors that are structurally related members of the TGF-β superfamily (Wozney, 1992). They are characterised by their ability to initiate *de novo* endochondral bone formation by committing undifferentiated pluripotent cells to differentiate into cartilage- and bone-forming cells (Reddi and Cunningham, 1993; Wozney, 1992). BMPs exert multiple effects on bone by acting as mitogens on undifferentiated mesenchymal cells and osteoblast precursors, inducing the expression of the osteoblast phenotype (e.g., increasing alkaline phosphatase [ALP] activity in bone cells) and acting as chemoattractants for mesenchymal cells and monocytes as well as binding to the extracellular matrix (Paralkar et al., 1990).

BMPs are known to stimulate stem cells to differentiate into osteoblasts and chondroblasts. Most of the research in periodontology has focused on three BMPs for their capability to enhance periodontal regeneration: BMP-2, BMP-3, and BMP-7 (Kao et al., 2009). Demineralised freeze-dried bone allograft preparations contain BMPs that enhance periodontal and bone regeneration; however, it has been shown that the concentration in these bone preparations is low. Therefore, currently commercially available BMP products (containing BMP-2 and BMP-7) utilise proteins that are prepared using recombinant DNA technology (Schwartz et al., 1998). These recombinant proteins are then combined with a collagen matrix. In animal studies, recombinant human BMP-2 (rhBMP-2) has been shown to enhance new cementum, alveolar bone, and periodontal ligament formation; however, in this study the authors reported areas of root resorption and ankylosis (Sigurdsson et al., 1995). Compared to rhBMP-2, rhBMP-7 did not show increased ankylosis or root resorption, as demonstrated in a study utilising critical-sized surgically created defects in beagle dogs. (Giannobile et al., 1998). The use of BMPs in periodontal regeneration requires further validation, especially in regards to adverse outcomes including resorption and ankyloses. Another significant consideration is the cost associated with using these recombinant proteins.

Growth/differentiation factor 5 (GDF-5)

Growth/differentiation factor 5 is another member of the TGF-β/BMP superfamily that shares 40%–50% protein sequence homology with BMP-2 and BMP-7 (Hötten et al., 1994). GDF-5 plays critical roles in mesenchymal cell differentiation and in the morphogenesis of skeletal, tendon, and ligament tissues (Dines et al., 2007). A recent systematic review assessed the available literature that utilised GDF-5 for periodontal regeneration (Lee and Wikesjö, 2014). Eleven animal studies utilising a dog model, as well as two human studies, were identified. Several materials, namely, absorbable collagen sponge, β-tricalcium phosphate, and a poly(lactic-co-glycolic) acid were evaluated as candidate carriers for GDF-5 using various doses and healing intervals. Significantly enhanced periodontal regeneration was demonstrated including cementum, periodontal ligament and alveolar bone, with limited, if any, adverse effects. These studies suggest that GDF-5 may be a promising candidate for promoting periodontal regeneration.

Issues associated with the use of growth and differentiation factors

There are several limitations involved in the use of growth factors. There is considerable difficulty with determining exactly what function each growth factor performs and its precise influence on different cell types in a complex *in vivo* environment. Even if the factors can be isolated and function perfectly understood, delivery of these to the appropriate cells in the right concentrations at the ideal time during development/regeneration is a problem constrained by numerous practical considerations. There is also the difficulty common to all periodontal regenerative procedures, which is the inability to obtain primary surgical closure and allow the growth factor to have an influence in a sterile, closed environment. Therefore, it is important to combine growth factors with an appropriate carrier scaffold, as well as responsive cells

(if required), in order to maximise the favourable properties of these bioactive molecules.

Scaffolds

Key scaffold characteristics

The fundamental concept underlying tissue engineering is to combine a scaffold with living cells and/or biologically active molecules to form a "tissue engineering construct", which promotes the repair and/or regeneration of tissues (Bartold et al., 2000; Bartold et al., 2006). The scaffold is expected to perform various functions, including the support of cell colonisation, migration, growth, and differentiation. The design of these scaffolds also needs to consider physico-chemical properties, morphology, and degradation kinetics. The external size and shape of the construct are of importance, particularly if the construct is customised for an individual patient. Most importantly, clinically successful constructs should stimulate and support both the onset and the continuance of tissue in-growth as well as subsequent remodelling and maturation by providing optimal stiffness and external and internal geometrical orientation. Scaffolds must provide sufficient initial mechanical strength and stiffness to substitute for the loss of mechanical function of the diseased, damaged, or missing tissue. Continuous cell and tissue remodelling is important for achieving stable biomechanical conditions and vascularisation at the host site. In addition to these essentials of mechanics and geometry, a suitable construct will (a) possess a three-dimensional and highly porous interconnected pore network with surface properties that are optimised for the attachment, migration, proliferation, and differentiation of cell types of interest and enable flow transport of nutrients and metabolic waste; and (b) be biocompatible and biodegradable with a controllable rate to complement cell/tissue growth and maturation (Hutmacher and Cool, 2007). It is essential to understand and control the scaffold degradation process in order to achieve successful tissue formation, remodelling, and maturation at the defect site.

Initially, it was believed that scaffolds should be degraded as the tissue is growing. Yet, tissue in-growth and maturation differ temporally from tissue to tissue, and simply achieving tissue in-growth does not necessarily equate to tissue maturation and remodelling. Indeed, many scaffold-based strategies have failed in the past as the scaffold degradation was more rapid than tissue remodelling and/or maturation. It is now recognised that the onset of degradation should only occur after the regenerated tissue within the scaffold has remodelled at least once in the natural remodelling cycle. Thus, it is important that the scaffold remain intact as the tissue matures within the scaffold, with bulk degradation occurring later (Woodruff and Hutmacher, 2010).

Scaffolds and carriers for periodontal tissue engineering

There are different scaffold materials that could be used as a carrier for cells in tissue engineering (Figure 7.3). Generally, they could be divided into natural (for example, collagen, gelatin, and chitosan) and synthetic scaffolds (for example, β-tricalcium phosphate, polyglycolic acid, and polycarpolactone), and also could be classified into resorbable and nonresorbable scaffolds (Bartold et al., 2006; Shue et al., 2012).

Three-dimensional electrospun nanofibrous scaffolds are receiving widespread interest in bone and cartilage regeneration, and have also been utilised for periodontal regeneration (Li et al., 2014). Studies have shown good attachment and proliferation of periodontal ligament cells on electrospun gelatin scaffolds (Zhang et al., 2009) and a variety of multilayered electrospun polymeric membranes and scaffolds (Inanc et al., 2009; Bottino et al., 2011; Vaquette et al., 2012).

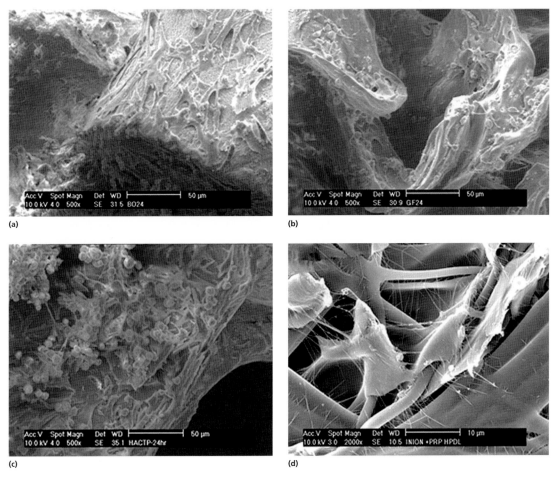

(a)

(b)

(c)

(d)

Figure 7.3 Scanning electron microscope images of periodontal ligament fibroblasts grown on (a) hydroxyapatite-tricalcium phosphate (HA-TCP), (b) polytetrafluoroethlylene (PTFE), (c) demineralised bone xenograft, and (d) gelatin sponge.

Advanced tissue-engineered construct design with multiphasic scaffolds

A multiphasic scaffold can be defined by the variation within the architecture (porosity, pore organisation, etc.) and/or the chemical composition of the resulting construct, which usually recapitulates to some extent the structural organisation and/or the cellular and biochemical composition of the native tissue. Multiphasic scaffolds aimed at imparting biomimetic functionality to tissue-engineered bone and soft tissue grafts have been recognised for some time as having significant potential to enable clinical translation in the field of orthopaedic tissue engineering, and are more recently emerging in the field of periodontal tissue regeneration. Multiphasic scaffolds represent an attractive option for facilitating periodontal regeneration because of the requirement to temporally and spatially control the interaction between multiple soft and hard tissues. Recently, the use of multiphasic scaffolds for periodontal tissue engineering purposes has been employed by several groups.

Carlo-Reis and colleagues (2011) developed a semi-rigid PLGA (polylactide-co-glycolide acid)/CaP (calcium phosphate) bilayered biomaterial construct with a continuous outer barrier membrane obtained by solvent casting and an inner topographically complex and porous component fabricated by solvent casting sugar leaching. The scaffold was tested in Class II furcation defects in dogs and was shown to promote cementum, bone, and periodontal ligament fibre insertion. This bilayered construct approach represents a modification of the traditional "guided tissue regeneration", whereby the construct acts as both a barrier and an enhanced space maintainer. Despite these promising results, the authors noted that the periodontium was not fully regenerated in the most coronal regions of the defect. They hypothesised that the space maintenance properties of the bilayered construct were decreased over time as the scaffold was gradually degraded. Indeed, at 120 days postimplantation, no traces of the polymeric material were found. This study highlights the importance of appropriate material selection and demonstrates that a polymer undergoing a slow *in vivo* degradation might be more suited for periodontal regeneration. The approach proposed by Carlo-Reis and colleagues relies solely on the regenerative performance of the host progenitors residing in the vicinity of the damaged area, and it can be hypothesised that the combination with exogenous progenitor cells could enhance the regenerative process.

Another interesting approach involves the use of polycaprolactone (PCL)-polyglycolic acid constructs for controlling fibre orientation and facilitating morphogenesis of the periodontal tissue complexes (Park et al., 2010, 2012). This approach utilised multicompartmental scaffold architecture using computational scaffold design and manufacturing by 3D printing. When combined with BMP-7 transfected gingival cells, newly formed tissues demonstrated the interfacial generation of parallel- and obliquely oriented fibres that formed human tooth dentin-ligament-bone complexes in an *in vivo* ectopic mouse periodontal regeneration model (Park et al., 2010). Subsequently, biomimetic fibre-guiding scaffolds using similar 3D wax/solvent casting methods combined with BMP-7 transduced PDL cells were tested in an athymic rat periodontal defect model, and resulted in perpendicularly oriented micro-channels that provided guidance for periodontal fibre orientation at the root-ligament interface (Park et al., 2012). The authors advocated the manufacture of individualised multiphasic scaffolds via computational design and 3D printing (Park et al., 2013).

A biphasic tissue-engineered construct has also been utilised, which comprises an elecrospun membrane for the delivery of a periodontal cell sheet attached to a three-dimensional porous scaffold for bone regeneration (Figure 7.4) (Vaquette et al., 2012). The periodontal compartment was composed of a solution electrospun PCL membrane for the purpose of facilitating the delivery of PDL cell sheets and improving the stability and the application of the cell sheets onto the dentine root surface. This study showed that the PCL membrane provided additional anchorage to the cell sheets, which resulted in enhanced adhesion and stability. *In vitro*, it was shown that the bone compartment supported cell growth and mineralisation, and the periodontal component was suitable for supporting multiple PDL cell sheets. When applied onto a dentine block and implanted in a subcutaneous animal model, cementum deposition was seen on the surface of the dentine. This approach demonstrated that a biphasic scaffold combined with cell sheet technology could be beneficial for periodontal regeneration. The concept was further developed by enhancing the osteoconductive nature of the bone compartment by coating with a layer of calcium phosphate, as well as utilising a periodontal compartment possessing a larger pore size that could enhance the integration of PDL tissue with the newly formed alveolar bone (Costa et al., 2014).

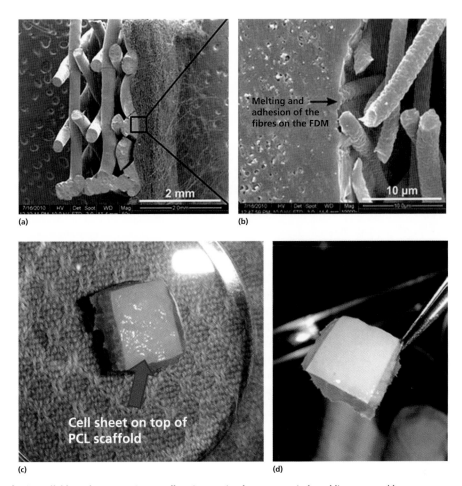

Figure 7.4 Biphasic scaffold (a) demonstrating excellent integration between periodontal ligament and bone compartments (b). Tissue-engineered construct with a periodontal ligament cell sheet placed on periodontal side of biphasic PCL scaffold (c), ready for insertion into periodontal defect (d).

Another approach has been to utilise PCL-HA (90:10 wt%) scaffolds, which were fabricated using three-dimensional printing in three phases: 100-μm microchannels in Phase A designed for cementum/dentine interface, 600-μm microchannels in Phase B designed for the PDL, and 300-μm microchannels in Phase C designed for alveolar bone (Lee et al., 2014). Recombinant human amelogenin, connective tissue growth factor, and bone morphogenetic protein-2 were delivered in Phases A, B, and C, respectively. Upon 4-week *in vitro* incubation with either dental pulp stem/progenitor cells, PDL stem/progenitor cells, or alveolar bone stem/progenitor cells, distinctive tissue phenotypes were formed in each compartment. The strategy used for the regeneration of multiphase periodontal tissues in this study involved the spatiotemporal delivery of multiple proteins. Using this method, it was shown that a single stem/progenitor cell population appeared to differentiate into putative cementum, PDL, and alveolar bone complex by using the scaffold's biophysical properties, combined with spatially released bioactive cues.

Tissue-engineered decellularised matrices and periodontal regeneration

The use of decellularised matrices as a biologic scaffold is gaining increasing attention in regenerative medicine. The rationale of using this approach is to produce three-dimensional scaffolds that mimic natural tissue's composition, microstructure, and biological and mechanical properties. The aim is to enhance the recruitment of host progenitor cells into these scaffolds and induce them to differentiate into the target tissue cell phenotype. Decellularised matrices can be obtained by decellularising native tissues or organs, or by removing the cellular components of tissue-engineered constructs (Hoshiba et al., 2010). In a recent study, it was demonstrated that periodontal cell sheets placed on melt electrospun PCL membranes can be decellularised by bidirectional perfusion with NH_4OH/Triton X-100 and DNase solutions. The decellularised cell sheets demonstrated an intact extracellular matrix, retained growth factors, and had the capacity to support the proliferation of allogenic PDL cells (Farag et al., 2014). Indeed, decellularised matrices have been obtained from various tissues and organs, such as heart valves, blood vessels, small intestinal submucosa (SIS), lung, trachea, skin, nerves, and cornea (reviewed in Hoshiba et al., 2010). It has also been demonstrated that the decellularisation process not only results in preservation of the ECM microstructure, but retention of biologically active components, such as the growth factors, is also achievable (Badylak, 2007). Importantly, tissue-engineered decellularised scaffolds did not elicit an immune response when implanted *in vivo* (Bloch et al., 2011).

Blood supply: Vascularisation and endothelial progenitors

Vascularisation is an important part of any regeneration approach in order to avoid tissue necrosis, and the use of prevascularised tissue engineered scaffolds is receiving increasing attention in regenerative medicine (Baldwin et al., 2014). In the context of periodontal tissue engineering, Nagai and colleagues (2009) used a tissue engineering construct of human PDL fibroblasts (HPDLFs) co-cultured with or without human umbilical vein endothelial cells (HUVECs). The HUVECs were found to form capillary-like structures when co-cultured with the HPDLFs. These cultures demonstrated longer survival, higher ALP activity, and lower osteocalcin production than the HDPLF cultures alone. These findings suggest that the incorporation of endothelial progenitors into tissue-engineered constructs may be beneficial in maintaining adequate vascularisation, which would in turn improve regenerative outcomes.

Gene therapy

One way to overcome the issue of the short half-life of growth factors and ensure a sustained local release is to deliver cells capable of producing the growth factor *in situ* within the periodontal defect. This can be achieved by gene therapy, which involves the genetic manipulation of cells to enhance their ability to produce a given protein, in this case, a growth or differentiation factor. More specifically, this strategy utilises vectors to insert genetic material into cells that are subsequently inserted into the periodontal defect, eliciting transcription of these genes and subsequent growth and differentiation of surrounding host cells, leading to new attachment formation.

Gene delivery of PDGF has been accomplished by the successful transfer of the gene into various periodontal cell types (Jin et al., 2004; Chang et al., 2009; Park et al., 2010; Park et al., 2012). Animal studies have demonstrated that gene delivery of PDGF stimulated more cementoblast activity and improved regeneration compared with a single application of recombinant PDGF (Chang et al., 2009). Although our understanding of the *in vivo* effect of sustained growth factor activity has improved with experimental gene therapy studies, significant safety concerns remain in relation to this technology.

Conclusions

Periodontal regeneration requires the coordinated healing of multiple soft and hard tissues. Current clinically utilised techniques have demonstrated the importance of space maintenance and wound stability for successful regeneration, but the available techniques are not able to achieve predictable regeneration in the vast majority of periodontal defects. Tissue engineering is an attractive approach to periodontal regeneration, as it may permit spatial and temporal control over the periodontal wound healing process. A variety of approaches utilising progenitor cells, bioactive molecules, and carrier scaffolds have shown potential in promoting periodontal regeneration to the extent that they justify testing in human clinical trials. However, successful results are likely to require the use of approaches that utilise a combination of cellular, growth factor, and scaffold properties, based on an understanding of both the complex architecture of the periodontium and the unique challenges associated with surgical intervention involving a nonvascular tooth surface and a nonsterile oral environment. The use of three-dimensional constructs that mimic the anatomy of the periodontium and may also be combined with progenitor/stem cells, growth factors, and/or extracellular molecules, is showing considerable promise in promoting periodontal regeneration that is translatable to the clinical setting.

References

ANTONIADES, H. N., GALANOUPOULOS, T., NEVILLE-GOLDEN, J., KIRITSY, C. P., & LYNCH, S. E. 1991. Injury induces *in vivo* expression of platelet-derived growth factor (PDGF) and PDGF receptor in RNAs in skin epithelial cells and PDGF mRNA in connective tissue fibroblasts. *Proc Natl Acad Sci USA*, 88, 565–9.

ANTONIADES, H. N., & OWEN, A. J. 1982. Growth factors and regulation of cell growth. *Annu Rev Med*, 33, 445–63.

BADYLAK, S. F. 2007. The extracellular matrix as a biologic scaffold material. *Biomaterials*, 28, 3587–93.

BALDWIN, J., ANTILLE, M., BONDA, U., DE-JUAN-PARDO, E. M., KHOSROTEHRANI, K., IVANOVSKI, S., PETCU, E. B., & HUTMACHER, D. W. 2014. In vitro pre-vascularisation of tissue-engineered constructs: a co-culture perspective. *Vasc Cell*, 6, 13.

BARTOLD, P. M., MCCULLOCH, C. A., NARAYANAN, A. S., & PITARU, S. 2000. Tissue engineering: a new paradigm for periodontal regeneration based on molecular and cell biology. *Periodontol 2000*, 24, 253–69.

BARTOLD, P. M., & RABEN, A. 1996. Growth factor modulation of fibroblasts in simulated wound healing. *J Periodontal Res*, 31, 205–16.

BARTOLD, P. M., XIAO, Y., LYNGSTAADAS, S. P., PAINE, M. L., & SNEAD, M. L. 2006. Principles and applications of cell delivery systems for periodontal regeneration. *Periodontol 2000*, 41, 123–35.

BLOCH, O., GOLDE, P., DOHMEN, P. M., POSNER, S., KONERTZ, W., & ERDBRÜGGER, W. 2011. Immune response in patients receiving a bioprosthetic heart valve: lack of response with decellularized valves. *Tissue Eng Part A*, 17, 399–405.

BOTTINO, M. C., THOMAS, V., & JANOWSKI, G. M. 2011. A novel spatially designed and functionally graded electrospun membrane for periodontal regeneration. *Acta Biomater*, 7, 216–24.

BRIGHT, R., HYNES, K., GRONTHOS, S., & BARTOLD, P. M. 2014. Periodontal ligament-derived cells for periodontal regeneration in animal models: a systematic review. *J Periodontal Res*, 50, 160–72.

CAFFESSE, R. G., & QUINONES, C. R. 1993. Polypeptide growth factors and attachment proteins in periodontal wound healing and regeneration. *Periodontol 2000*, 1, 69–79.

CARLO-REIS, E. C., BORGES, A. P. B., ARAÚJO, M. V. F., MENDES, V. C., GUAN, L., & DAVIES, J. E. 2011. Periodontal regeneration using a bilayered PLGA/calcium phosphate construct. *Biomaterials*, 32, 9244–53.

CATON, J., NYMAN, S., & ZANDER, H. 1980. Histometric evaluation of periodontal surgery II. Connective tissue attachment levels after four regenerative procedures. *J Clin Periodontol*, 7, 224–31.

CHANG, P. C., CIRELLI, J. A., JIN, Q., SEOL, Y. J., SUGAI, J. V., D'SILVA, N. J., et al. 2009. Adenovirus encoding human platelet-derived growth factor-B delivered to alveolar bone defects exhibits safety and biodistribution profiles favorable for clinical use. *Hum Gene Ther*, 20, 486–96.

CHO, M. I., & GARANT, P. R. 1989. Radioautographic study of 3H-Mannose utilization during cementoblast differentiation, formation of acellular cementum and development of periodontal ligament principal fibres. *Anat Rec*, 223, 209–22.

CHO, M. I., LIN, W. L., & GENCO, R. J. 1995. Platelet-derived growth factor-modulated guided tissue regenerative therapy. *J Periodontol*, 66, 522–30.

CLEMMONS, D. R., & VAN WYK, J. J. 1985. Evidence for a functional role of endogenously produced somatomedin-like peptides in the regulation of DNA synthesis in cultured human fibroblasts and porcine smooth muscle cells. *J Clin Invest*, 75, 1914–18.

COSTA, P. F., VAQUETTE, C., ZHANG, Q., REIS, R. L., IVANOVSKI, S., & HUTMACHER, D. W. 2014. Advanced tissue engineering scaffold design for regeneration of the complex hierarchical periodontal structure. *J Clin Periodontol*, 41, 283–94.

DAN, H., VAQUETTE, C., FISHER, A., HAMLET, S. M., XIAO, Y., HUTMACHER, D. W., et al. 2014. The influence of cellular source on periodontal regeneration using calcium phosphate coated polycaprolactone scaffold supported cell sheets. *Biomaterials*, 35, 113–22.

DARBY, I. B., & MORRIS, K. H. 2013. A systematic review of the use of growth factors in human periodontal regeneration. *J Periodontol*, 84, 465–76.

DAUGHADAY, W. H., & ROTWEIN, P. 1989. Insulin-like growth factors I and II. Peptide, messenger ribonucleic acid and gene structures, serum, and tissue concentrations. *Endocr Rev*, 10, 68–91.

DEL FABBRO, M., BORTOLIN, M., TASCHIERI, S., & WEINSTEIN, R. 2011. Is platelet concentrate advantageous for the surgical treatment of periodontal diseases? A systematic review and meta-analysis. *J Periodontol*, 82, 1100–11.

DEMIR, B., SENGUN, D., & BERBEROGLU, A. 2007. Clinical evaluation of platelet-rich plasma and bioactive glass in the treatment of intra-bony defects. *J Clin Periodontol*, 34, 709–15.

DINES, J. S., WEBER, L., RAZZANO, P., PRAJAPATI, R., TIMMER, M., BOWMAN, S. et al., 2007. The effect of growth differentiation factor-5-coated sutures on tendon repair in a rat model. *J Shoulder Elbow Surg*, 16(5 Suppl), S215–21.

DOGAN, A., OZDEMIR, A., KUBAR, A., & OYGUR, T. 2002. Assessment of periodontal healing by seeding of fibroblast-like cells derived from regenerated periodontal ligament in artificial furcation defects in a dog: a pilot study. *Tissue Eng*, 8, 273–82.

DOGAN, A., OZDEMIR, A., KUBAR, A., & OYGUR, T. 2003. Healing of artificial fenestration defects by seeding of fibroblast-like cells derived from regenerated periodontal ligament in a dog: a preliminary study. *Tissue Eng*, 9, 1189–96.

DORI, F., HUSZAR, T., NIKOLIDAKIS, D., ARWEILER, N. B., GERA, I., & SCULEAN, A. 2007. Effect of platelet-rich plasma on the healing of intrabony defects treated with an anorganic bovine bone mineral and expanded polytetrafluoroethylene membranes. *J Periodontol*, 78, 983–90.

DRAGOO, M. R., & KALDAHL, W. B. 1983. Clinical and histological evaluation of alloplasts and allografts in regenerative periodontal surgery in humans. *Int J Periodontics Restorative Dent*, 3, 8–29.

DUAN, X., TU, Q., ZHANG, J., YE, J., SOMMER, C., MOSTOSLAVSKY, G., KAPLAN, D., YANG, P., & CHEN, J. 2011. Application of induced pluripotent stem (iPS) cells in periodontal tissue regeneration. *J Cell Physiol*, 226, 150–7.

ESPOSITO, M., GRUSOVIN, M. G., PAPANIKOLAOU, N., COULTHARD, P., & WORTHINGTON, H. V. 2005. Enamel matrix derivative (Emdogain) for periodontal tissue regeneration in intrabony defects. *Cochrane Database Syst Rev*, CD003875.

FARAG, A., VAQUETTE, C., THEODOROPOULOS, C., HAMLET, S. M., HUTMACHER, D. W., & IVANOVSKI, S. 2014. Decellularized periodontal ligament cell sheets with recellularization potential. *J Dent Res*, 93, 1313–9.

FENG, F., AKIYAMA, K., LIU, Y., YAMAZA, T., WANG, T. M., CHEN, J. H., et al., 2010. Utility of PDL progenitors for in vivo tissue regeneration: a report of 3 cases. *Oral Dis*, 16, 20–8.

GIANNOBILE, W. V., FINKELMAN, R. D., & LYNCH, S. E. 1994. Comparison of canine and non-human primate animal models for periodontal regenerative therapy: results following a single administration of PDGF/IGF-I. *J Periodontol*, 65, 1158–68.

GIANNOBILE, W. V., HERNANDEZ, R. A., FINKELMAN, R. D., RYAN, S., KIRITSY, C. P., D'ANDREA, M., & LYNCH, S. E. 1996. Comparative effects of platelet-derived growth factor-BB and insulin- like growth factor-I, individually and in combination, on periodontal regeneration in *Macaca fascicularis*. *J Periodont Res*, 31, 301–12.

GIANNOBILE, W. V., RYAN, S., SHIH, M. S., SU, D. L., KAPLAN, P. L., & CHAN, T. C. 1998. Recombinant human osteogenic protein-1 (OP-1) stimulates periodontal wound healing in class III furcation defects. *J Periodontol*, 69, 129–37.

GIANNOBILE, W. V., & SOMERMAN, M. J. 2003. Growth and amelogenin-like factors in periodontal wound healing: a systematic review. *Ann Periodontol*, 8, 193–204.

GOTTLOW, J., NYMAN, S., LINDHE, J., KARRING. T., & WENNSTROM, J. 1986. New attachment formation in the human periodontium by guided tissue regeneration. *J Clin Periodontol*, 13, 604–16.

GOULD, T. R. L., MELCHER, A. H., & BRUNETTE, D. M. 1980. Migrations and division of progenitor cell populations in periodontal ligament after wounding. *J Periodont Res*, 15, 20–42.

GRONTHOS, S., MANKANI, M., BRAHIM, J., ROBEY, P. G., & SHI, S. 2000. Postnatal human dental pulp stem cells (DPSCs) in vitro and in vivo. *Proc Natl Acad Sci USA*, 97, 13625–30.

HAASE, H. R., CLARKSON, R. W., WATERS, M. J., & BARTOLD, P. M. 1998. Growth factor modulation of mitogenic responses and proteoglycan synthesis by human periodontal fibroblasts. *J Cell Physiol*, 174, 353–61.

HAMMARSTROM, L. 1997. Enamel matrix, cementum development and regeneration. *J Clin Periodontol*, 24, 658–68.

HAMMARSTROM, L., HEIJL, L., & GESTRELIUS, S. 1997. Periodontal regeneration in a buccal dehiscence model in monkeys after application of enamel matrix proteins. *J Clin Periodontol*, 24, 669–77.

HANNA, R., TREJO, P. M., & WELTMAN, R. L. 2004. Treatment of intrabony defects with bovine-derived xenograft alone and in combination with platelet-rich plasma: a randomized clinical trial. *J Periodontol*, 75, 1668–77.

HASEGAWA, N., KAWAGUCHI, H., HIRACHI, A., TAKEDA, K., MIZUNO, N., NISHIMURA, M., et al. 2006. Behavior of transplanted bone marrow-derived mesenchymal stem cells in periodontal defects. *J Periodontol*, 77, 1003–7.

HAUSCHKA, P. V., CHEN, T. L., & MAVRAKOS, A. E. 1988. Polypeptide growth factors in bone matrix. *Ciba Found Symp*, 136, 207–25.

HEDEN, G., & WENNSTROM, J. L. 2006. Five-year follow-up of regenerative periodontal therapy with enamel matrix derivative at sites with angular bone defects. *J Periodontol*, 77, 295–301.

HEIJL, L. 1997. Periodontal regeneration with enamel matrix derivative in one human experimental defect: a case report. *J Clin Periodontol*, 24, 693–96.

HIATT, W. H., SCHALLHORN, R. G., & AARONIAN, A. J. 1978. The induction of new bone and cementum formation. IV. Microscopic examination of the periodontium following human bone and marrow allograft, autograft and nongraft periodontal regenerative procedures. *J Periodontol*, 49, 495–512.

HOSHIBA, T., LU, H., KAWAZOE, N., & CHEN, G. 2010. Decellularized matrices for tissue engineering. *Expert Opin Biol Ther*, 10, 1717–28.

HÖTTEN, G., NEIDHARDT, H., JACOBOWSKY, B., & POHL, J. 1994. Cloning and expression of recombinant human growth/differentiation factor 5. *Biochem Biophys Res Commun*, 204, 646–52.

HOWELL, T. H., FIORELLINI, J. P., PAQUETTE, D. W., OFFENBACHER, S., GIANNOBILE, W. V., & LYNCH, S. E. 1997. A phase I/II clinical trial to evaluate a combination of recombinant human platelet-derived growth factor-BB and recombinant human insulin- like growth factor-I in patients with periodontal disease. *J Periodontol*, 68, 1186–93.

HUTMACHER, D. W., & COOL, S. 2007. Concepts of scaffold-based tissue engineering: the rationale to use solid free-form fabrication techniques. *J Cell Mol Med*, 1, 654–69.

HYNES, K., MENICANIN, D., HAN, J,. MARINO, V., MROZIK, K., GRONTHOS, S., & BARTOLD, P. M. 2013. Mesenchymal stem cells from iPS cells facilitate periodontal regeneration. *J Dent Res*, 92, 833–9.

INANC, B., ARSLAN, Y., SEKER, S., ELCIN, A., & ELCIN, Y. 2009. Periodontal ligament cellular structures engineered with electrospun poly(DL-lactide-coglycolide) nanofibrous membrane scaffolds. *J Biomed Mater Res A*, 90, 186–95.

ISAKA, J., OHAZAMA, A., KOBAYASHI, M., NAGASHIMA, C., TAKIGUCHI, T., KAWASAKI, H., TACHIKAWA, T., & HASEGAWA, K. 2001. Participation of periodontal ligament cells with regeneration of alveolar bone. *J Periodontol*, 72, 314–23.

JEPSEN, S. R., EBERHARD, J. R., HERRERA, D., & NEEDLEMAN, I. 2002. A systematic review of guided tissue regeneration for periodontal furcation defects. What is the effect of guided tissue regeneration compared with surgical debridement in the treatment of furcation defects? *J Clin Periodontol*, 3, 103–16.

JIN, Q., ANUSAKSATHIEN, O., WEBB, S. A., PRINTZ, M. A., & GIANNOBILE, W. V. 2004. Engineering of tooth-supporting structures by delivery of PDGF gene therapy vectors. *Mol Ther*, 9, 519–26.

KAO, R. T., MURAKAMI, S., & BEIRNE, O. R. 2009. The use of biologic mediators and tissue engineering in dentistry. *Periodontol 2000*, 50, 127–53.

KARRING, T., NYMAN, S., & LINDHE, J. 1980. Healing follow-ing implantation of periodontitis affected teeth into bone tissue. *J Clin Periodontol*, 7, 96–105.

KAWAGUCHI, H., HIRACHI, A., HASEGAWA, N., IWATA, T., HAMAGUCHI, H., SHIBA, H. et al., 2004. Enhancement of periodontal tissue regeneration by transplantation of bone marrow mesenchymal stem cells. *J Periodontol*, 75, 1281–7.

KITAMURA, M., NAKASHIMA, K., KOWASHI, Y., FUJII, T., SHIMAUCHI, H., SASANO, T., et al. 2008. Periodontal tissue regeneration using fibroblast growth factor-2: randomized controlled phase II clinical trial. *PLoS One*, 3, e2611.

LALLIER, T. E., PALAIOLOGOU, A. A., YUKNA, R. A., & LAYMAN, D. L. 2003. The putative collagen-binding peptide P-15 promotes fibroblast attachment to root shavings but not hydroxyapatite. *J Periodontol*, 74, 458–67.

LANG, H., SCHULER, N., & NOLDEN, R. 1998. Attachment formation following replantation of cultured cells into periodontal defects: a study in minipigs. *J Dent Res*, 77, 393–405.

LEE, C. H., HAJIBANDEH, J., SUZUKI, T., FAN, A., SHANG, P., & MAO, J. J. 2014. Three-dimensional printed multiphase scaffolds for regeneration of periodontium complex. *Tissue Eng Part A*, 20, 1342–51.

LEE, J., & WIKESJÖ, U. M. 2014. Growth/differentiation factor-5: pre-clinical and clinical evaluations of periodontal regeneration and alveolar augmentation: review. *J Clin Periodontol*, 41, 797–805.

LI, G., ZHANG, T., LI, M., FU, N., FU, Y., BA, K., et al. 2014. Electrospun fibers for dental and craniofacial applications. *Curr Stem Cell Res Ther*, 9, 187–95.

LI, H., YAN, F., LEI, L., LI, Y., & XIAO, Y. 2009. Application of autologous cryopreserved bone marrow mesenchymal stem cells for periodontal regeneration in dogs. *Cells Tissues Organs*, 190, 94–101.

LIN, N. H., GRONTHOS, S., & BARTOLD, P. M. 2008. Stem cells and periodontal regeneration. *Aust Dent J*, 53, 108–21.

LYNCH, S. E., COLVIN, R. B., & ANTONIADES, H. N. 1989a. Growth factors in wound healing. Single and synergistic effects on partial thickness porcine skin wounds. *J Clin Invest*, 84, 640–6.

LYNCH, S. E., DE CASTILLA, G. R., WILLIAMS, R. C., KIRITSY, C. P., HOWELL, T. H., et al. 1991. The effects of short-term application of a combination of platelet- derived and insulin-like growth factors on periodontal wound healing. *J Periodontol*, 62, 458–67.

LYNCH, S. E., WILLIAMS, R. C., POLSON, A. M., HOWELL, T. H., REDDY, M. S., ZAPPA, U. E., & ANTONIADES, H. N. 1989b. A combination of platelet-derived and insulin-like growth factors enhances periodontal regeneration. *J Clin Periodontol*, 16, 545–48.

MARIOTTI, A. 2003. Efficacy of chemical root surface modifiers in the treatment of periodontal disease: a systematic review. *Ann Periodontol*, 8, 205–26.

MATSUDA, N., LIN, W. L., KUMAR, N. M., CHO, M. I., & GENCO, R. J. 1992. Mitogenic, chemotactic, and synthetic responses of rat periodontal ligament fibroblastic cells to polypeptide growth factors *in vitro*. *J Periodontol*, 63, 515–25.

MATSUURA, K., UTOH, R., NAGASE, K., & OKANO, T. 2014. Cell sheet approach for tissue engineering and regenerative medicine. *J Control Release*, 190, 228–39.

MELCHER, A. H. 1976. On the repair potential of periodontal tissues. *J Periodontol*, 47, 256–60.

MELCHER, A. H., CHEONG, T., COX, J., NEMETH, E., & SHIGA, A. 1986. Synthesis of cementum-like tissue *in vitro* by cells cultured from bone: a light and electron microscopic study. *J Periodontal Res*, 21, 592–612.

MCCULLOCH, C. A. G. 1985. Progenitor cell populations in the periodontal ligament of mice. *Anat Rec*, 211, 258–62.

MCCULLOCH, C. A. G., & MELCHER, A. H. 1983a. Cell density and cell generation in the periodontal ligament of mice. *Am J Anat*, 167, 43–58.

MCCULLOCH, C. A. G, & MELCHER, A. H. 1983b. Cell migration in the periodontal ligament of mice. *J Periodontal Res*, 18, 339–52.

MCCULLOCH, C. A. G., & MELCHER, A. H. 1983c. Continuous labelling of the periodontal ligament of mice. *J Periodontal Res*, 18, 231–41.

MCCULLOCH, C. A. G., NEMETH, E., LOWENBURG, B., & MELCHER, A. H. 1987. Paravascular cells in endosteal spaces of alveolar bone contribute to periodontal ligament cell populations. *Anat Rec*, 219, 2233–42.

MURAKAMI, S. 2011. Periodontal tissue regeneration by signaling molecule(s): what role does basic fibroblast growth factor (FGF-2) have in periodontal therapy? *Periodontol 2000*, 56, 188–208.

MURAKAMI, S., TAKAYAMA, S., KITAMURA, M., SHIMABUKURO, Y., YANAGI, K., IKEZAWA, K., et al. 2003. Recombinant human basic fibroblast growth factor (bFGF) stimulates periodontal regeneration in class II furcation defects created in beagle dogs. *J Periodontal Res*, 38, 97–103.

NAGAI, N., HIRAKAWA, A., OTANI, N., & MUNEKATA, M. 2009. Development of tissue-engineered human periodontal ligament constructs with intrinsic angiogenic potential. *Cells Tissues Organs*, 190, 303–12.

NAKAHARA, T., NAKAMURA, T., KOBAYASHI, E., KUREMOTO, K., MATSUNO, T., TABATA, Y. et al. 2004. In situ tissue engineering of periodontal tissues by seeding with periodontal ligament-derived cells. *Tiss Eng*, 10, 537–44.

NEEDLEMAN, I. G., WORTHINGTON, H. V., GIEDRYS-LEEPER, E., & TUCKER, R. J. 2006. Guided tissue regeneration for periodontal infra-bony defects. *Cochrane Database Syst Rev*, 19(2), CD001724.

NEMETH, E., KULKARNIE, G., & MCCULLOCH, C. A. G. 1993. Disturbances of gingival fibroblast population homeostasis due to experimentally induced inflammation in the cynomolgus monkey (*Macaca fascicularis*): potential mechanism for disease progression. *J Periodontal Res*, 28, 180–90.

NYMAN, S., GOTTLOW, J., KARRING, T., & LINDHE, J. 1982. The regenerative potential of the periodontal ligament: an experimental study in the monkey. *J Clin Periodontol*, 9, 257–65.

NYMAN, S., KARRING, T., LINDHE, J., & PLANTEN, S. 1980. Healing following implantation of periodontitis affected roots into gingival connective tissue. *J Clin Periodontol*, 7, 394–401.

OATES, T. W., ROUSE, C. A., & COCHRAN, D. L. 1993. Mitogenic effects of growth factors on human periodontal ligament cells *in vitro*. *J Periodontol*, 64, 142–8.

ODA, Y., YOSHIMURA, Y., OHNISHI, H., TADOKORO, M., KATSUBE, Y., SASAO, M., et al. 2010. Induction of pluripotent stem cells from human third molar mesenchymal stromal cells. *J Biol Chem*, 285, 29270–8.

OKUDA, K., TAI, H., TANABE, K., SUZUKI, H., SATO, T., KAWASE, T., et al. 2005. Platelet-rich plasma combined with a porous hydroxyapatite graft for the treatment of intrabony periodontal defects in humans: a comparative controlled clinical study. *J Periodontol*, 76, 890–8.

PANDA, S., DORAISWAMY, J., MALAIAPPAN, S., VARGHESE, S. S., & DEL FABBRO, M. 2014. Additive effect of autologous platelet concentrates in treatment of intrabony defects: a systematic review and meta-analysis. *J Investig Clin Dent*, doi: 10.1111/jicd.12117.

PARALKAR, V. M., NANDEDKAR, K. N., POINTER, R. H., KLEINMAN, H. K, & REDDI, A. H. 1990. Interaction of osteogenin, a heparin binding bone morphogenetic protein, and demineralized bone matrix in calverial defects of adult primates. *J Biol Chem*, 265, 17281–4.

PARK, C. H., RIOS, H. F., JIN, Q., BLAND, M. E., FLANAGAN, C. L., HOLLISTER, S. J., et al. 2010. Biomimetic hybrid scaffolds for engineering human tooth-ligament interfaces. *Biomaterials*, 31, 5945–52.

PARK, C. H., RIOS, H. F., JIN, Q., SUGAI, J. V., PADIAL-MOLINA, M., TAUT, A. D., et al. 2012. Tissue engineering bone-ligament complexes using fiber-guiding scaffolds. *Biomaterials*, 33, 137–45.

PARK, C. H., RIOS, H. F., TAUT, A. D., PADIAL-MOLINA, M., FLANAGAN, C. L., PILIPCHUK, S. P., et al. 2013. Image-based, fiber guiding scaffolds: a platform for regenerating tissue interfaces. *Tissue Eng Part C Methods*, 20, 533–42.

PARK, J. B., MATSUURA, M., HAN, K. Y., NORDERYD, O., LIN, W. L., GENCO, R. J., & CHO, M. I. 1995. Periodontal regeneration in class III furcation defects of beagle dogs using guided tissue regenerative therapy with platelet-derived growth factor. *J Periodontol*, 66, 462–77.

PENDER, N., HEANEY, T. G., PYCOCK, D., & WEST, C. R. 1988. Progenitor connective tissue cell populations in the gingival papillae of the rat. *J Periodontal Res*, 23, 175–81.

PLEDGER, W. J., STILES, C. D., ANTONIADES, H. N., & SCHER, D. 1977. Induction of DNA synthesis in BALB/c-3T3 cells by serum components: reevaluation of the commitment process. *Proc Natl Acad Sci USA*, 74, 4481–5.

PRITCHARD, J. 1957. Regeneration of bone following periodontal therapy: report of cases. *Oral Surg Oral Med Oral Pathol*, 10, 247–52.

RALL, L. B., SCOTT, J. J., & BELL, G. I. 1987. Human insulin-like growth factor I and II messenger RNA: isolation and complimentary DNA analysis of expression. *Methods Enzymol*, 146, 239–48.

REDDI, A. H., & CUNNINGHAM, N. S. 1993. Initiation and promotion of bone differentiation by bone morphogenetic proteins. *J Bone Miner Res*, 8(Suppl 2), S499–502.

REYNOLDS, M. A., AICHELMANN-REIDY, M. E., BRANCH-MAYS, G. L., & GUNSOLLEY, J. C. 2003. The efficacy of bone replacement grafts in the treatment of periodontal osseous defects: a systematic review. *Ann Periodontol*, 8, 227–65.

ROSS, R., RAINES, E. W., & BOWEN-POPE, D. F. 1986. The biology of platelet derived growth factor. *Cell*, 46, 155–69.

RUTHERFORD, R. B., NIEKRASH, C. E., KENNEDY, J. E., & CHARETTE, M. F. 1992. Platelet-derived and insulin-like growth factors stimulate regeneration of periodontal attachment in monkeys. *J Periodont Res*, 27, 285–90.

RUTHERFORD, R. B., RYAN, M. E., KENNEDY, J. E., TUCKER, M. M., & CHARETTE, M. F. 1993. Platelet-derived growth factor and dexamethasone combined with a collagen matrix induce regeneration of the periodontium in monkeys. *J Clin Periodontol*, 20, 537–44.

SAWA, Y., & MIYAGAWA, S. 2013. Present and future perspectives on cell sheet-based myocardial regeneration therapy. *Biomed Res Int*, 2013, 583912.

SCHELLENS, J. P. M., EVERTS, V., & BEERTSEN, W. 1982. Quantitative analysis of connective tissue resorption in the supra-alveolar region of the mouse incisor ligament. *J Periodontal Res*, 17, 407–22.

SCHWARTZ, Z., SOMERS, A., MELLONIG, J. T., CARNES, D. L. JR, WOZNEY, J. M., DEAN, D. D., et al. 1998. Addition of human recombinant bone morphogenetic protein-2 to inactive commercial human demineralized freeze-dried bone allograft makes an effective composite bone inductive implant material. *J Periodontol*, 69, 1337–45.

SCULEAN, A., DONOS, N., BLAES, A., LAUERMANN, M., REICH, E., & BRECX, M. 1999. Comparison of enamel matrix proteins and bioabsorbable membranes in the treatment of intrabony periodontal defects: a split-mouth study. *J Periodontol*, 70, 255–62.

SEO, B. M., MIURA, M., GRONTHOS, S., BARTOLD, P. M., BATOULI, S., BRAHIM, J., et al. 2004. Investigation of multipotent postnatal stem cells from human periodontal ligament. *Lancet*, 364, 149–55.

SHIMIZU, T., YAMATO, M., KIKUCHI, A., & OKANO, T. 2004. Two-dimensional manipulation of cardiac myocyte sheets utilizing temperature-responsive culture dishes augments the pulsatile amplitude. *Tissue Engineering*, 7, 141–51.

SHUE, L., YUFENG, Z., & MONY, U. 2012. Biomaterials for periodontal regeneration: a review of ceramics and polymers. *Biomatter*, 2, 271–7.

SIGURDSSON, T. J., LEE, M. B., KUBOTA, K., TUREK, T. J., WOZNEY, J. M., & WIKESJÖ, U. M. 1995. Periodontal repair in dogs: recombinant human bone morphogenetic protein-2 significantly enhances periodontal regeneration. *J Periodontol*, 66, 131–8.

STILES, C. D. 1983. The molecular biology of platelet-derived growth factor. *Cell*, 33, 653–9.

TAKAHASHI, K., & YAMANAKA, S. 2006. Induction of pluripotent stem cells from mouse embryonic and adult fibroblast cultures by defined factors. *Cell*, 126, 663–76.

TAMAOKI, N., TAKAHASHI, K., TANAKA, T., ICHISAKA, T., AOKI, H., TAKEDA-KAWAGUCHI, T., et al. 2010. Dental pulp cells for induced pluripotent stem cell banking. *J Dent Res*, 89, 773–8.

TECHAWATTANAWISAL, W., NAKAHAMA, K., KOMAKI, M., ABE, M., TAKAGI, Y., & MORITA, I. 2007. Isolation of multipotent stem cells from adult rat periodontal ligament by neurosphere-forming culture system. *Biochem Biophys Res Commun*, 357, 917–23.

TOBITA, M., UYSAL, A.C., OGAWA, R., HYAKUSOKU, H., & MIZUNO, H. 2008. Periodontal tissue regeneration with adipose-derived stem cells. *Tissue Eng Part A*, 14, 945–53.

TROMBELLI, L., & FARINA, R. 2008. Clinical outcomes with bioactive agents alone or in combination with grafting or guided tissue regeneration. *J Clin Periodontol*, 35, 117–35.

TRUBIANI, O., DI PRIMIO, R., TRAINI, T., PIZZICANNELLA, J., SCARANO, A., PIATTELLI, A., & CAPUTI, S. 2005. Morphological and cytofluorimetric analysis of adult mesenchymal stem cells expanded ex vivo from periodontal ligament. *Int J Immunopathol Pharmacol*, 18, 213–21.

TSUDA, Y., SHIMIZU, T., YAMATO, M., KIKUCHI, A., SASAGAWA, T., SEKIYA, S., KOBAYASHI, J., CHEN, G., & OKANO, T. 2007. Cellular control of tissue architectures using a three-dimensional tissue fabrication technique. *Biomaterials*, 28, 4939–46. Epub 2007 Aug 20.

UCHIDA, N., FLEMING, W. H., ALPERN, E. J., & WEISSMAN, I. L. 1993. Heterogeneity of hematopoietic stem cells. *Curr Opin Immunol*, 5, 177–84.

VAQUETTE, C., FAN, W., XIAO, Y., HAMLET, S., HUTMACHER, D. W., IVANOVSKI, S. 2012. A biphasic scaffold design combined with cell sheet technology for simultaneous regeneration of alveolar bone/periodontal ligament complex. *Biomaterials*, 33, 5560–73.

WADA, N., WANG, B., LIN, N. H., LASLETT, A. L., GRONTHOS, S., & BARTOLD, P. M. 2011. Induced pluripotent stem cell lines derived from human gingival fibroblasts and periodontal ligament fibroblasts. *J Periodont Res*, 46, 438–47.

WANG, J., ZHANG, R., SHEN, Y., XU, C., QI, S., LU, L., WANG, R., & XU, Y. 2014. Recent advances in cell sheet technology for periodontal regeneration. *Curr Stem Cell Res Ther*, 9, 162–73.

WEIBRICH, G., KLEIS, W. K., HAFNER, G., HITZLER, W. E., & WAGNER, W. 2003. Comparison of platelet, leukocyte, and growth factor levels in point-of-care platelet-enriched plasma, prepared using a modified Curasan kit, with preparations received from a local blood bank. *Clin Oral Implants Res*, 14, 357–62.

WOODRUFF, M. A., & HUTMACHER, D. W. 2010. The return of a forgotten polymer: polycaprolactone in the 21st century. *Progress in Polymer Science*, 35, 1217–56.

WOZNEY, J. M. 1992. The bone morphogenetic protein and osteogenesis. *Mol Rep Dev*, 32, 160–7.

YAMADA, Y., UEDA, M., HIBI, H., & BABA, S. 2006. A novel approach to periodontal tissue regeneration with mesenchymal stem cells and platelet-rich plasma using tissue engineering technology: a clinical case report. *Int J Periodontics Restorative Dent*, 26, 363–9.

YAN, X., QIN, H., QU, C., TUAN, R. S., SHI, S., & HUANG, G. T. 2010. iPS cells reprogrammed from human mesenchymal-like stem/progenitor cells of dental tissue origin. *Stem Cells Dev*, 19, 469–80.

YASSIBAG-BERKMAN, Z., TUNCER, O., SUBASIOGLU, T., & KANTARCI, A. 2007. Combined use of platelet-rich plasma and bone grafting with or without guided tissue regeneration in the treatment of anterior interproximal defects. *J Periodontol*, 78, 801–9.

YUKNA, R., SALINAS, T. J., & CARR, R. F. 2002. Periodontal regeneration following use of ABM/P-15: a case report. *Int J Periodontics Restorative Dent*, 22, 146–55.

YUKNA, R. A., CALLAN, D. P., KRAUSER, J. T., EVANS, G. H., AICHELMANN-REIDY, M. E., MOORE, K., et al. 1998. Multi-center clinical evaluation of combination anorganic bovine-derived hydroxyapatite matrix (ABM)/cell binding peptide (P-15) as a bone replacement graft material in human periodontal osseous defects: 6-month results. *J Periodontol*, 69, 655–63.

YUKNA, R. A., KRAUSER, J. T., CALLAN, D. P., EVANS, G. H., CRUZ, R., & MARTIN, M. 2000. Multi-center clinical comparison of combination anorganic bovine-derived hydroxyapatite matrix (ABM)/cell binding peptide (P-15) and ABM in human periodontal osseous defects. 6-month results. *J Periodontol*. 71, 1671–9.

ZAVALA, J., LÓPEZ JAIME, G. R., RODRÍGUEZ BARRIENTOS, C. A., & VALDEZ-GARCIA, J. 2013. Corneal endothelium: developmental strategies for regeneration. *Eye (Lond)*, 27, 579–88.

ZHANG, S., HUANG, Y., YANG, X., MEI, F., MA, Q., & CHEN G. 2009. Gelatin nanofibrous membrane fabricated by electrospinning of aqueous gelatine solution for guided tissue regeneration. *J Biomed Mater Res A*, 90, 671–9.

CHAPTER 8

Clinical strategies for dental and periodontal disease management: A way forward

Anibal Diogenes, Vanessa Chrepa, and Nikita B. Ruparel

School of Dentistry, University of Texas Health Science Center, San Antonio, TX, USA

Dentistry dates back to ancient civilizations. Archeological findings suggest that rudimentary dental extractions, bone trephinations to drain abscesses and splinting of loose teeth with gold wires and various forms of dental adornments were practiced by ancient Chinese and Egyptians as early as 6,000 BC (Xu and MacEntee, 1994; Marion 1996; Shimizu et al., 2013). Other remarkable findings include use of various forms of medicaments to treat dental pain, and evidence of dental implants in ancient Turkey and Egypt (el-Ansary, 1989; Atilla, 1993; Irish, 2004). Since these primordial times, the evolution of dentistry is largely marked by the development of dental materials and techniques that aim to address replacing lost or diseased tissues with nonbiologic materials. Thus, prosthetic replacement of missing dental tissues has prevailed in dentistry since early examples of dental treatments in ancient civilizations (Lucas and Maes, 2013; McFadden et al., 2013; Unterholzner, 2013).

In contrast, the goal of regenerative dentistry is to induce biologic replacement of dental tissues and their supporting structures. The potential for regenerative dentistry is in large part due to advancements in biologic therapies that apply principles of tissue engineering with the spatial and temporal assembly of stem cells, growth factors, and scaffolds to achieve the functional regeneration. Tissue engineering is defined as an interdisciplinary field that applies the principles of engineering and life sciences toward the development of biological substitutes that restore, maintain, or improve tissue or organ function. This is accomplished by the concerted interplay between stem cells, scaffolds, and growth factors, known as the tissue engineering triad (Langer and Vacanti, 1993). However, it is important to keep in mind that the outcome of the interplay among this triad is greatly modified by environmental factors such as the presence of microbes or their antigens (Figure 8.1). This is particularly important for regenerative endodontics and periodontics, which aim to restore the physiology and function of previously infected tissues with residual presence of microbial antigens.

Cao and colleagues (1997) captured worldwide attention when they published a study reporting the development of engineered human ears grown on the dorsum of athymic mice. Later, a groundbreaking clinical case report announced the successful engineering of a functional human mandible on a patient with a subtotal mandibulectomy due to oral cancer, who was unable to have solid meals and had severe functional and esthetics issues for more than 8 years (Warnke et al., 2004). A titanium mesh scaffold filled with bone mineral block was molded to fit the defect through computer-aided design (CAD). The titanium/mineral bone scaffold was injected with bone morphogenic protein 7 (BMP-7) and the patient's own bone marrow–derived mesenchymal stem cells. The engineered construct was then implanted into the patient's right latissimus dorsi muscle (Warnke et al., 2004). In this case report, the patient was used as his own bioreactor for 7 weeks, after which the construct was harvested and transplanted onto the mandibular defect. The blood vessels that had developed within the construct were anastomosed on the external

Tissue Engineering and Regeneration in Dentistry: Current Strategies, First Edition. Edited by Rachel J. Waddington and Alastair J. Sloan.

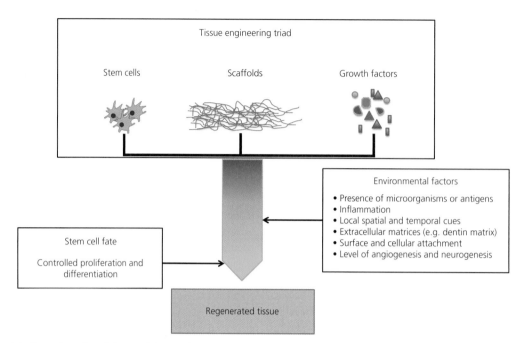

Figure 8.1 Illustration of modulation of the "triad of tissue engineering" by environmental factors, affecting the downstream stem cell fate and regenerated tissue.

carotid artery and cephalic veins. Skeletal scintilography with a 600 MBq Tc99m-oxydronate tracer revealed that the engineered mandible had metabolically active bone with evident remodeling and mineralisation processes. Importantly, this patient was able to have his first solid meal in over 9 years.

Another remarkable clinical report of tissue engineering in dentistry was published in 2009 (d'Aquino et al., 2009). Dental pulp stem cells (DPSCs) were isolated from extracted maxillary third molars and expanded *in vitro*. Later, these autologous DPSCs were combined with collagen sponge and implanted into the extraction sockets of impacted mandibular molars. The regeneration of the osseous defects was assessed by both radiographic and histological methods. There was radiographic evidence of approximately 60% more bone formed on the sites that received the DPSCs in the scaffold as compared with a site that received scaffold only (control). Importantly, the bone formed in the sites that received the DPSCs was better organised and dense compared with the control site. This study was a pioneer in the use of autologous DPSCs in cell-based therapies in dentistry (d'Aquino et al., 2009). Also, it is noteworthy that the unsorted dental pulp cells used in this study enhanced bone formation without evidence of ectopic

dentin formation. This observation highlights the importance of the environment growth factors and attachment molecules to dictate the fate of mesenchymal stem cells.

The last decade has been marked with significant increased knowledge of the biology of the pulp and periradicular tissues, including the role of stem cells, scaffolds, and growth factors. The realisation of the intrinsic regenerative potential of the pulp and periradicular tissues has created a paradigm shift in treatment approaches, addressing many unmet needs such as the arrest of dental development in immature teeth with necrotic pulp. Importantly, these new treatment modalities propelled further advances that have been quickly incorporated into chairside therapies. This chapter focuses on describing regenerative clinical advances in both endodontics and periodontics.

Clinical strategies in regenerative endodontics

Regenerative endodontics is a new field within the specialty of endodontics that focuses on promoting the physiological and functional regeneration of the damaged pulp-dentin complex. There has been much attention to the fast-evolving field of regenerative endodontics since the first contemporary case report published in 2001: the successful treatment of a permanent immature tooth with the use of a double antibiotic paste medicament (ciprofloxacin and metronidazole) and intracanal bleeding from the apical tissues (Iwaya et al., 2001). As a result, there have been significant advances in stem cell biology, microbiology, and biomaterials. Indeed, regenerative endodontics research and development has evolved into a multidisciplinary effort. It is noteworthy that the foundations of regenerative endodontics date back to more than a century ago with the first attempts of vital pulp therapy to maintain the physiologic function of an injured pulp (Dammaschke, 2008). Phillip Pfaff in 1756 performed the first reported pulp capping procedure. He concluded that the exposed injured pulp had the potential of repair if the tissue was further irritated with a caustic agent or heated instruments to promote the cauterisation of the pulp stumps (Francke, 1971; Gelbier, 2010). It was not until 1920 that Datwyler introduced zinc eugenol–based cement as a direct pulp capping agent (Grossman, 1976). Subsequently, Herman introduced calcium hydroxide in 1921 as a biocompatible agent to be used in both vital and nonvital therapies (Dammaschke, 2008). Importantly, both agents are still important adjuvants in the modern endodontic armamentarium.

Vital pulp therapies

Therapies such as direct pulp capping procedures and pulpotomies have become primarily restricted to deciduous or immature teeth with open apices due to their alleged poor predictabililty when applied to mature teeth (Barthel et al., 2000). However, Cvek (1978) reported that pulp vitality could be maintained in 96% of teeth with pulp exposures due to complicated crown fractures following a partial pulpotomy and direct pulp capping with calcium hydroxide. In this pioneer work, Cvek demonstrated that the pulp, when confirmed vital by testing and direct clinical visualisation, had an intrinsic capacity of repair and regeneration as calcific barriers were often observed under the capping material. He also demonstrated that this desirable outcome was not limited to immature teeth since 53% of teeth treated in this study were fully formed mature teeth. In the last

decade, knowledge gained on the participation of stem cells and progenitor cells within the dental pulp on the process of tertiary reparative dentinogenesis has dramatically changed the therapeutic potential of vital pulp therapies. Thus, it has created a paradigm shift with clinical techniques and materials designed to optimise stem cell fate towards a reparative cell type, often called odontoblast-like cells.

Although calcium hydroxide has been considered the gold standard for direct pulp capping procedures, newer materials designed to have better biocompatibility and inductive effects on stem cells such as mineral trioxide aggregate (MTA) and tricalcium silicate cements (e.g., Biodentine) have increased the success and predictability of these procedures. It is now appreciated that desired clinical outcomes rely heavily on the many effects of these materials on the local environment, reducing inflammation while promoting the recruitment, proliferation, and differentiation of undifferentiated MSCs into odontoblast-like cells. Elegant *ex vivo* models have been used to demonstrate that both MTA and Biodentine when used as direct capping materials promote greater reparative tertiary dentinogenesis as compared with calcium hydroxide due to both direct (calcium-mediated increase in proliferation and recruitment) and indirect effects (e.g., release of transforming growth factor β-1 from dentin) (Tecles et al., 2008; Laurent et al., 2012). These materials have been shown to promote unprecedented regeneration in the injured dental pulp and have quickly transitioned to clinical practice.

A recent randomised clinical trial using a practice-based research network evaluated the clinical outcomes of direct pulp capping procedures performed with either calcium hydroxide or MTA (Hilton et al., 2013). In this large study, the use of MTA resulted in significantly greater clinical success (81.3%) compared with the calcium hydroxide group (68.5%) (Hilton et al., 2013). These results confirmed a previous clinical study that reported an 80.5% success with the use of MTA as compare to 59% when calcium hydroxide was used (Mente et al., 2014). It is important to emphasise that desirable clinical outcomes such as resolution of the disease process and lack of symptoms is directly influenced by the biocompatibility of these materials and their effects on local stem cells and growth factors. Indeed, an interesting study reported the histologic evaluation of human dental pulp capped with MTA or calcium hydroxide following extraction of the treated teeth for orthodontic reasons (Accorinte Mde et al., 2008). Similar desirable histological findings were found in an independent study evaluating the histological outcome of pulp capping procedures in patients using MTA or Biodentine. These findings, including presence of a dentinal bridge without tubular defects lined with odontoblast-like cells and minimal inflammation, were found in another histological study in treated human teeth (Nowicka et al., 2013). Therefore, the greater clinical success rates achieved with contemporary biomaterials in pulp capping procedures appear directly related to the ability of these materials to "facilitate" stem cell–mediated pulp regeneration with the formation of tertiary dentin and reestablishment of normal pulp physiology.

Successful outcomes have recently been reported for vital pulp therapy in mature teeth diagnosed with reversible pulpitis using contemporary endodontic techniques and materials (Simon et al., 2013). There are still many barriers to be overcome in order that vital pulp therapies become the first line of treatment for both mature and immature teeth. One of the major challenges to be overcome is the development of meaningful inflammation markers that could be used chairside to determine the extent of pulpal inflammation while correlating the results to the prognosis of a regenerative procedure. Currently, clinicians rely on responses to cold stimulus, history of spontaneous pain, and degree of pulpal hemorrhage to determine whether pulpal inflammation should be deemed reversible or irreversible. This remains a very subjective determination that has limited the application of capping procedures in teeth with a diagnosis of irreversible pulpitis. It has been recently reported that a contemporary pulpotomy was capable of "reversing" the irreversible pulpitis status of a secondary mandibular molar in a 19-year-old patient (Chueh and Chiang, 2010). The tooth was extracted for orthodontic reasons 10 months after the procedure and examined histologically. A vital pulp was observed with normal appearance with presence of a mineralised barrier in intimate contact with the coronal MTA capping material (Figure 8.2) (Chueh and Chiang, 2010).

Despite these significant advances and promising results, vital pulp therapy has not yet become the first treatment alternative for mature teeth with vital pulps requiring endodontic treatment. This is an important area that requires further translational research to better explore the inherent regenerative potential of the dental pulp, allowing the maintenance of a complex tissue with sensorial and immunological functions not easily recapitulated by our current regenerative approaches.

Nonvital pulp therapies

Regenerative endodontic procedures

The occurrence of pulpal necrosis in the permanent immature tooth often represents a challenging clinical situation because the thin and often short roots increase the risk of subsequent fracture, resulting in difficulties in debriding and sealing a large canal space. Although apexification procedures allow for healing of apical periodontitis, they fail to promote continued root development and reestablishment of a functional, competent pulp-like tissue. Unfortunately, alternative procedures, such as implants, are often contraindicated because of the still-growing craniofacial skeleton in these young patients. Therefore, immature teeth with pulpal necrosis present unique challenges not previously addressed by apexification procedures.

Regenerative endodontic procedures (REPs) include, but are not limited to, procedures first described in the literature as revascularisation procedures (Banchs and Trope, 2004) (Figure 8.3). These procedures first emerged from the observation that the pulp of replanted immature teeth could revascularise and regain vitality (Kling et al., 1986; Cvek et al., 1990; Andreasen et al., 1995). Indeed, *revascularisation* is a term used for the reestablishment of the vascularity of an ischemic tissue, such as the dental pulp of an avulsed tooth. There was an initial focus on the role of the blood clot in promoting wound healing that started in the early 1960s (Nyggard-Ostby, 1961), and it remained prevalent until 2011 with the demonstration that revascularisation procedures delivered a substantial number of undifferentiated MSCs into root canals (Lovelace et al., 2011). Nonetheless, the seminal work of Nyggard-Ostby laid the foundation for contemporary regenerative endodontic procedures (Nyggard-Ostby, 1961; Nygaard-Ostby and Hjortdal, 1971).

The first of the contemporary case reports demonstrated that a necrotic pulp with chronic apical abscess is suitable for healing using REP. Clinical success was seen as complete resolution of pre-operative sinus tract and symptoms. Unique to conventional endodontic procedures was that these cases also demonstrated thickening

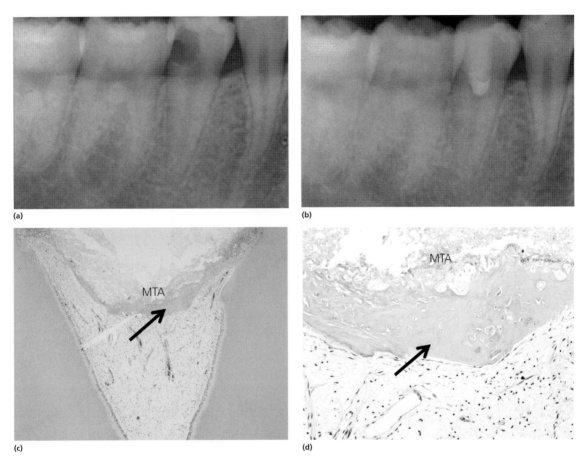

Figure 8.2 Radiographs and micrograph of tooth #29 treated with a partial pulpotomy and direct pulp capping using MTA. (a) Preoperative radiograph showing a large distal proximal carious lesion. (b) Recall radiograph taken 10 months after the pulpotomy showing absence of pathosis; in addition, the patient was asymptomatic. (c and d) Histologic examination of tooth #29 after extraction for orthodontic reasons reveals absence of inflammation and a thick reparative dentinal bridge as seen in both 10X (c) and 50X (d) magnification. (Modified from Chueh and Chiang, 2010. Reproduced with permission from Operative Dentistry, Inc.)

and elongation of the root as well as apical closure (Diogenes et al., 2013). Moreover, treated teeth were vital to testing. These reports demonstrated that adequate disinfection using chemical means without any mechanical instrumentation can satisfactorily heal chronic infections. Combination irrigation and a multiple-visit approach using intracanal antimicrobials successfully healed sinus tracts in both cases prior to completion of treatment.

Following these cases, to date, we now have more than 200 published cases demonstrating successful clinical outcomes using regenerative endodontic therapies. Additionally, a wide range of etiologies such as trauma (complicated and uncomplicated crown fractures, avulsions, luxation injuries including intrusive luxation), developmental defects (dens evaginatus and invaginatus), and caries have also been reported (Diogenes et al., 2013). This points to an encouraging trend that despite what the cause of pulp trauma may be, the current procedures aid in restoring the environment suitable for a positive effect. In addition to the varied etiologies, there exists a wide variety of clinical procedures and protocols being performed, which indicates the lack of a standardised treatment protocol (Kontakiotis et al., 2014; Kontakiotis et al., 2015). Despite this, a closer look at the contemporary procedures reveals certain common features. A representative protocol is given in Textbox 8.1. The rest of this

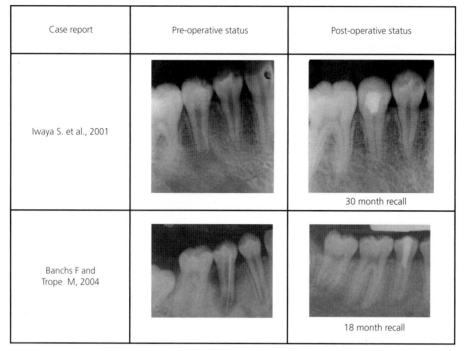

Case report	Pre-operative status	Post-operative status
Iwaya S. et al., 2001		30 month recall
Banchs F and Trope M, 2004		18 month recall

Figure 8.3 Two case reports showing successful clinical outcomes using REPs. Both cases reported immature permanent premolar teeth diagnosed with pulp necrosis. Large radiolucent areas are seen surrounding the apex and roots of both teeth, suggesting advanced apical periodontitis in the preoperative radiographs. Teeth were treated with revascularisation procedures, resulting in complete resolution of signs and symptoms of disease. Complete radiographic healing of apical periodontitis is seen in the postoperative radiographs. (Modified from Iwaya et al., 2001, and Banchs and Trope, 2004. Reproduced with permission from Wiley and Elsevier.)

Textbox 8.1 A recommended clinical protocol for regenerative endodontics.

First treatment visit for regenerative endodontics

1. Informed consent, including explanation of risks and alternative treatments or no treatment.
2. After ascertaining adequate local anesthesia, dental dam isolation is obtained.
3. The root canal systems are accessed and working length is determined (radiograph of a file loosely positioned at 1 mm from root end).
4. The root canal systems are slowly irrigated first with 1.5% NaOCl (20 mL/canal, 5 min) and then irrigated with saline (20 mL/canal, 5 min), with irrigating needle positioned about 1 mm from root end.
5. Canals are dried with paper points.
6. Calcium hydroxide, or DAP or TAP (0.1–1 mg/mL) is delivered to canal system.
7. Access is temporarily restored.

Final (second) treatment visit for regenerative endodontics

1. A clinical exam is first performed to ensure that there is no moderate to severe sensitivity to palpation and percussion. If such sensitivity is observed, or a sinus tract or swelling is noted, then the treatment provided at the first visit is repeated.
2. After ascertaining adequate local anesthesia with 3% mepivacaine (no epinephrine), dental dam isolation is obtained.
3. The root canal systems are accessed; the intracanal medicament is removed by irrigating with saline (20 mL) followed by 17% EDTA (10 mL/canal, 5 min).
4. The canals are dried with paper points.
5. Bleeding is induced by rotating a precurved K-file size #25 at 2 mm past the apical foramen with the goal of having the entire canal filled with blood to the level of the cementoenamel junction.
6. Once a blood clot has formed, a premeasured piece of Collaplug (Zimmer Dental Inc., Warsaw, IN) is carefully placed on top of the blood clot to serve as an internal matrix for the placement of approximately 3 mm of white MTA (Dentsply, Tulsa, OK) or Biodentine (Septodont, France).
7. A 3–4 mm layer of glass ionomer (e.g., Fuji IX, GC America, Alsip, IL) is flowed gently over the MTA.
8. A bonded reinforced composite resin restoration is placed over the glass ionomer.
9. The case needs to be followed up at 3 months, 6 months, and yearly after that for a total of 4 years.

chapter will focus on each of these to better understand the biological principles behind REPs.

Inclusion criteria

Our knowledge of treating immature necrotic teeth with REPs has emerged over years through therapies such as apexogenesis. Previous work by Andreason and Cvek on avulsed teeth treated with apexogenesis demonstrated that a minimum of 1.1 mm of apical opening is required for teeth to successfully regain vitality and undergo root development via apexogenesis (Cvek, 1974; Andreasen et al., 1995). Apart from this criterion, patient's age and the stage of root development also play a key role in predicting outcomes. Barring one case report (Kim et al., 2010), almost all other reports published have been on young patients with an age range of 6–20 years (Kontakiotis et al., 2015). This points to an important characteristic that despite the large evidence of successful cases, REPs at this time are largely limited to a subset of the population. This may in part be due to the number and cellular properties of stem cells present in young versus adult patients. Numerous studies have demonstrated that there is a decrease in the number as well as a decrease in the proliferative and differentiation capacity of mesenchymal stem cells (MSCs) in the older population (Yu et al., 2011). This has been attributed to changes in cell-cycle regulation, signaling mechanisms, cell damage over time, and systemic changes (Piccin and Morshead 2010). These features directly translate to a suboptimal regenerative potential and can therefore lead to an unpredictable clinical outcome in aged individuals. Nevertheless, it cannot be excluded that findings from the present studies can be extrapolated to the adult population and therefore a larger group of patients, as the number or the regenerative potential of adult dental stem cells has not been evaluated.

Evoked bleeding

Since the inception of regenerative endodontics, bleeding evoked inside the canal system has been a common step during the second appointment (Diogenes et al., 2013). However, prior to 2011, it was believed that the blood clot promoted by this step mediated the healing by inducing angiogenesis similar to a blood clot in an extraction socket following exodontia. It is well appreciated that angiogenesis is a requirement for tissue regeneration; however, the focus on this alone fundamentally ignores the role of the stem cells, local growth

factors, and scaffolds. Importantly, random healing or repair does not explain the continued root development and gain in vitality, suggesting the functional reinnervation of the tissue, as reported in 60% of the case reports (Diogenes et al., 2013).

A study by Lovelace and colleagues in 2011 demonstrated that evoked bleeding in immature teeth from young patients not only brings in vascular components but also allows for ingress of mesenchymal stem cells that were not seen circulating in the patient's systemic blood (Lovelace et al., 2011). The amount of these cell types was 600–700-fold greater than systemic blood. Interestingly, the first speculated mention of the presence of perivascular mesenchymal components was also from Nygaard-Ostby's work (Ostby, 1961). However, further research in the field of tissue engineering and dentistry reveals many sources of stem cells, especially ones located in the periapical region (Diogenes et al., 2013). Stem cells of the apical papilla (SCAP), inflammatory periapical progenitor cells, periodontal ligament stem cells, and bone marrow stem cells appear to be the most likely sources of periapical stem cells when lacerating apical tissues. Of these, SCAPs have been shown to be a rich source of stem cells with superior population doubling capacity, proliferation rate, telomerase activity, and cell migration ability (Sonoyama et al., 2008). Collectively, these findings point to an important concept that regeneration of pulp tissue is a stem cell–based process and may be governed by the multipotency of mesenchymal stem cells and their acquired phenotype such as connective tissue, endothelium, dentin, cementum, and bone.

The ability of stem cells to proliferate and differentiate into the desired phenotypes is dependent on signaling from bioactive molecules such as growth factors and their three-dimensional carrier, a biodegradable scaffold. The combination of adequate numbers of stem cells, appropriate growth factors, and a suitable scaffold form the basis of tissue engineering (Murray et al., 2007). Tissue engineering in endodontics is defined as "biologically based procedures designed to replace damaged structures, including dentin and root structures, as well as cells of the pulp-dentin complex" (Murray et al., 2007). In order to achieve the goals of these procedures, several strategies have been proposed for optimizing differentiation of DPSCs and SCAPs into desired phenotypes (Diogenes et al., 2013). These include increasing bioavailability of growth factors already present within the root canal system; dentin has been shown to harbor a wide range of growth factors, namely, transforming growth factor beta (TGF-β), basic fibroblast growth factor, vascular endothelial growth factor, bone morphogenetic proteins (BMPs), and others (Smith et al., 2012). *In vitro* studies have shown that dentin conditioning with either calcium hydroxide treatment, MTA, or 17% ethylenediamine tetraacetic acid (EDTA) allows for solubilisation of some of the dentin-matrix components (Graham et al., 2006; Tomson et al., 2007; Casagrande et al., 2010; Galler et al., 2015). Additionally, platelet-rich plasma extracted from a patient's own blood has been used greatly due to its use as an autologous scaffold as well as a rich source of growth factors (Torabinejad and Kiger, 1980; Torabinejad and Turman, 2011; Chen et al., 2012; Sachdeva et al., 2014; Torabinejad et al., 2014). The results of the clinical case reports are equivocal at this point. However, this may be due to the lack of standardised protocols being used. Other options include exogenous introduction of growth factors as used by several *in vivo* animal studies (Huang et al., 2010; Iohara et al., 2011; Kodonas et al., 2012) and one prospective clinical trial (Nagy et al., 2014).

The third component of tissue engineering includes a bioactive substance that can carry stem cells and growth factors and act as a template for tissue regeneration (Galler et al., 2011a). Ideal characteristics of a scaffold have been described by many and include the following: biocompatibility; biodegradability; strong mechanical properties to withstand handling; and conducive architecture to allow for adequate loading of cells and penetration of their nutrients and growth factors and facilitate proliferation, adhesion, and migration of stem cells (Galler et al., 2011a). Several groups are now attempting to develop an ideal scaffolding material. These include natural polymers, synthetic polymers, hydrogels, and bioceramics (Galler et al., 2011a). Injectable scaffolds are an attractive strategy when dealing with a small region such as a root canal system. To this end, *in vitro* and *in vivo* animal models have demonstrated that creating a suitable and conducive environment for stem cells by providing the necessary scaffold such as poly(lactic) acid and poly(glycolic) acid in combination with chemotactic and growth factors can lead to desirable outcomes not just clinically but also histologically (Huang et al., 2010; Iohara et al., 2011; Kodonas et al., 2012). Other strategies include optimizing the release profiles of growth factors

embedded in scaffolds. Biodegradable polymeric chitosan nanoparticles have been studied as a potential delivery means of large proteins using temporal controlled release of growth factors, thereby facilitating bioavailability and efficacy of a regenerative phenomenon (Shrestha et al., 2014). In addition, photodynamically activated chitosan nanoparticles have been shown to inactivate bacterial endotoxins, thereby participating not only in the regenerative process but also in the disinfection process of the root canal system. Collectively, optimum results for tissue engineering will require the active participation of stem cells, scaffold, and bioactive molecules.

Disinfection

Thorough debridement of the root canal system is critical to any endodontic treatment. Similar to wound healing, the presence of bacteria and their toxins can sustain a proinflammatory environment, which can greatly hinder the regenerative potential of stem cells. Regenerative endodontic procedures rely heavily on chemical disinfection and debridement since most published cases reported none to minimal mechanical instrumentation to preserve the already thin fragile dentinal walls (Diogenes et al., 2013; Diogenes et al., 2014). Because disinfection in necrotic cases may present with established biofilms, it is conceivable that the canal system is required to be first disinfected maximally before attempting regeneration. The role of passive ultrasonic activation and other nonabrasive methods of debridement has never been evaluated for these procedures, but they may represent an important method of optimizing disinfection while maintaining the integrity of the weak dentinal walls. Thus, chemical disinfection, like other endodontic procedures, involves usage of a combination of irrigants and intracanal medicaments.

Irrigation at first and second appointments has been accomplished, in published cases, with a range of irrigants, namely, 2.5% or 5.25% sodium hyperchlorite (NaOCl), 3% hydrogen peroxide (H_2O_2), saline, 2% chlorhexidine, 17% EDTA, 4% formaldehyde, and others (Nygaard-Ostby and Hjortdal, 1971; Iwaya et al., 2001; Banchs and Trope, 2004; Kontakiotis et al., 2015). Whilst all combinations of irrigation protocols have shown successful clinical outcomes, recent studies evaluating the effect of various irrigants on the survival and differentiation of stem cells demonstrate that higher concentrations of NaOCl are detrimental to the survival and differentiation of stem cells (Casagrande et al., 2010; Galler et al., 2011b; Trevino et al., 2011; Martin et al., 2012). However, when 17% EDTA is used post-NaOCl rinse, these effects are almost completely reversed (Galler et al., 2011b; Trevino et al., 2011; Martin et al., 2012). Moreover, dentin discs irrigated with 5.25% NaOCl plus 17% EDTA demonstrate pulp-like tissue formation as well as expression of dentin sialoprotein on the dentin walls, whereas discs irrigated with 5.25% NaOCl alone result in clastic activity (Galler et al., 2011b). EDTA also promotes stem cell adhesion and maintains their morphology compared with other irrigant protocols as shown by an *in vitro* study (Ring et al., 2008). Above all, EDTA has been shown to release growth factors such as TGF-β embedded in dentin, which have been shown to promote differentiation of stem cells into odontoblast-like cell types (Casagrande et al., 2010). These findings indicate that a final rinse with EDTA at the second appointment would not only maintain stem cell viability but could also make available the necessary growth factors required by stem cells to differentiate into appropriate phenotypes.

Similar to irrigation protocols, the use of intracanal medicaments can also have a beneficial or detrimental effect of stem cells. Two instances when medicaments can come in contact with stem cells are the following: (a) extrusion of material into periapical tissues at first appointment and (b) direct contact from dentin walls due to inadequate removal of them at second appointment. The most widely used intracanal medicament is the triple antibiotic paste (TAP) followed by calcium hydroxide (Ca[OH]$_2$), formocresol, double antibiotic paste (DAP), and others (Iwaya et al., 2001; Banchs and Trope 2004; Diogenes et al., 2013). Recent studies have demonstrated that concentrations greater than 0.1 mg/mL of TAP, DAP, DAP with Cefaclor, and Augmentin cause severe death of SCAPs (Ruparel et al., 2012; Althumairy et al., 2014). Interestingly, Ca(OH)$_2$ has been seen as beneficial to stem cells in that it not only supports their survival but also promotes proliferation (Ruparel et al., 2012). These studies indicate that concentrations that are bactericidal as well as nondetrimental to stem cells must be used in order to satisfy the disinfection as well as regenerative potential of REPs. Following the above-mentioned studies, recent studies have evaluated the antibactericidal effects of diluted TAP and DAP on *Enterococcus faecalis* and *Porphyromonas gingivalis* biofilms (Sabrah et al., 2013; Sabrah et al., 2015). Data from these studies demonstrate that concentrations ranging from 0.1 mg/mL to 0.3 mg/mL are significantly bactericidal against the tested biofilms and in turn provide strong and encouraging evidence for the use of "balanced" disinfection that is not only efficacious against bacterial biofilms but also innocuous to the regeneration process. Overall, studies concerning irrigation as well as intracanal medicaments demonstrate a cautious use of materials that come in contact with stem cells to create a conducive environment for the regenerative phenomenon.

Expected outcomes and challenges

The goals of REPs are many. These include (a) resolution of pathosis (signs and symptoms of apical periodontitis), (b) gain in root width and root length at the apex as well as at the cemento-enamel junction (CEJ), and (c) regaining lost vasculature and innervation and histological regeneration in terms of true pulp-like and dentin-like tissue formation. Two retrospective and one prospective study demonstrate that in addition to resolution for periapical pathosis, regenerative endodontic procedures allow for significant gain in root length as well as width compared with conventional MTA apexification therapy (Figure 8.4) (Bose et al., 2009; Jeeruphan et al., 2012; Nagy et al., 2014). Another prospective study of 16 cases demonstrated similar findings in that 90.3% of the treated teeth showed complete resolution of signs and symptoms, 19.4% showed complete apical closure, 2.7% to 25.3% had change in root length, and 1.9% to 72.6% gained root dentin thickness (Kahler et al., 2014). It is noteworthy to state that the study employed teeth with different etiologies leading to pulp necrosis, such as dens evaginatus, uncomplicated crown fracture, subluxation, and avulsion (Kahler et al., 2014), demonstrating that the success of REPs is not dependent on a specific etiology and patients with varied etiologies can benefit from this therapy. Moreover, an analysis of the published case reports also indicates that approximately 60% of successful cases also regain vitality responses in the treated tooth (Iwaya et al., 2001; Banchs and Trope, 2004; Petrino, 2007; Reynolds et al., 2009; Ding et al., 2010; Thomson and Kahler, 2010; Cehreli et al., 2011; Iwaya et al., 2011; Cehreli et al., 2012; Miller et al., 2012; Shivashankar et al., 2012). Collectively, REPs to date have generated significant evidence as a viable treatment option for immature teeth with pulp necrosis.

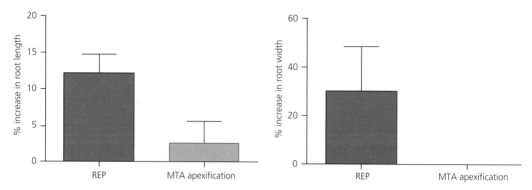

Figure 8.4 Composite representation of two retrospective and one prospective study showing percentage change in root width and root length between regenerative endodontic procedures and MTA apexification procedures. (Modified from Bose et al., 2009; Jeeruphan et al., 2012; and Nagy et al., 2014).

There is considerable discussion on the expected histologic nature of the formed tissue in order to call these procedures "regenerative" in the strict sense of the word. Histological success, however, is limited. Only one case report thus far demonstrates pulp-like and dentin-like tissue deposition in the canal space (Shimizu et al., 2012). Other studies report fibrous connective tissue, cementum, and bonelike hard tissue depositions (Fouad and Nosrat, 2013; Martin et al., 2013; Shimizu et al., 2013; Becerra et al., 2014; Lin et al., 2014). However, a closer look at the etiology of all published cases with histology reveal that the majority of cases have pulp necrosis with either acute apical abscess or chronic apical abscess as their periapical diagnosis (Martin et al., 2013; Nosrat et al., 2013; Shimizu et al., 2013; Lin et al., 2014). This indicates the presence of an established biofilm in the canal system. Since disinfection is key to a successful regenerative outcome, inadequate removal of the biofilm can hinder an optimal regenerative outcome either clinically, histologically, or both.

Other challenges using REP as a treatment modality include (a) staining from TAP and MTA (Nosrat et al., 2013; Kahler et al., 2014), (b) inadequate bleeding into the canal system, and (c) lack of cervical thickness, which may be the most fracture-prone site of the tooth. Staining from TAP has largely been overcome by the use of DAP, which excludes the use of minocycline, the tetracycline class of drug primarily responsible for the yellow to dark brown stain. Discoloration of the crown and cervical region has been minimised with the use a bonding system prior to placement of MTA (Petrino, 2007). Other options include internal bleaching post-MTA placement or full-coverage crown or veneers, if indicated. The use of local anesthetics not containing epinephrine (for example, 3% mepivicaine) has been advocated as the local anesthetic for use during the second appointment to prevent any vaso-constriction due to presence of epinephrine (Diogenes et al., 2013). Last, gain of dentin thickness at the CEJ is hugely missing in most published case reports. This is because of the placement of MTA or a biocompatible barrier below or at the CEJ to avoid crown staining. However, a handful of studies have used Collaplug as a matrix over the formed blood clot to allow for placement of MTA in the pulp chamber thereby (Petrino, 2007; Jeeruphan et al., 2012). Therefore, published case reports have provided important information on clinical findings, inciting researchers to find solutions for the presented challenges and limitations. This has allowed for the development of techniques and approaches, and therefore accelerated evolution of this young field in endodontics.

Future approaches

The field of regenerative endodontics is rapidly evolving due to a constant cross-talk between translational preclinical and clinical studies. This desirable bridging between basic sciences and clinical practice allows for a more timely transfer of technology to helping patients. There are still many challenges to be overcome, including the progressive recruitment of stem cells into the canal system (cell homing) and perhaps the use of autologous transplantation of stem cells (cell-based therapies). It is important to emphasise that both strategies have successfully been employed in preclinical studies, resulting in the regeneration of a pulp-like tissue that closely resembled the native pulp.

It is well appreciated that nearly all cells in the human body are located within 0.1 mm from the nearest blood vessel in order to maintain adequate supply of nutrients and oxygen (Helmlinger et al., 1997; Nie et al., 2010). Conversely, current regenerative endodontic procedures deliver a substantial number of MSCs to root canals devoid of blood supply (Lovelace et al., 2011). However, MSCs likely to be involved in endodontics regeneration, such as SCAPs, are known to be present in a niche that is poorly vascularised (Diogenes et al., 2013), and they respond to hypoxia by releasing proangiogenic and neurogenic factors (Vanacker et al., 2014). Nonetheless, the successful survival of cells placed in the most coronal part of the root canal remains dependent on the kinetics of angiogenesis and the ability of these cells to resist hypoxia. A case report showing the histology of a revascularisation procedure performed 3.5 weeks earlier demonstrated the presence of a well-vascularised pulp-like tissue (Shimizu et al., 2012). Therefore, there is evidence that blood vessels can be recruited into root canals in less than 1 month after the procedure. Unfortunately, the kinetics of angiogenesis in regenerative endodontics is largely unknown, and likely modulated by several factors including etiology, duration and virulence of infection, and host biology. In order to overcome this issue, future procedures will likely depend on a progressive recruitment of apical stem cells into the canal system, containing a suitable scaffold and signaling molecules directing stem cell migration, proliferation, and differentiation concomitantly with angiogenesis. This cell homing approach is being intensively studied in preclinical studies.

Another approach that has been shown to promote pulpal regeneration in animal models is the transplantation of autologous stem cells (Iohara et al., 2011; Iohara et al., 2013). In this approach, autologous stem cells are expanded, selected, and transplanted into the apical region of disinfected teeth, while the middle and coronal thirds of the canal are filled with an injectable hydrogel containing chemotactic factors (Nakashima and Iohara, 2014). The advantages of such an approach include the opportunity to enrich and deliver a large number of cells to initiate the repair process at the apical region of teeth. Also, these cells would proliferate and migrate apically, allowing time for the supportive blood vessels to form into the formed tissue. Unfortunately, this approach is challenged by several factors. The source of these stem cells remains a major issue to be overcome. It is conceivable that patients with pulpal necrosis also have the need for third molar extractions, making dental pulp stem cells available for culturing, although adipose-derived MSCs and bone marrow MSCs have also been shown to be conducive with pulpal regeneration (Figure 8.5). Inducible pluripotent stem cells (iPSCs, reviewed in Chapter 2) may also represent an alternative cell type for this treatment modality. However, regulation of proliferation and differentiation of iPSCs is difficult due to pluripotency potential, directly hindering their use in patients (Okita et al., 2007). Regardless of the cell type to be used, MSCs need to be cultured in a good manufacturing practice facility, under strict regulations to minimise chances of contamination and risk to the recipient. The high cost of these facilities and the lack of continuum with the dental clinic where the patient is being treated create additional barriers for the use of this technology in a daily endodontic practice.

Overall, the current work in the field of regenerative endodontics has broadened our understanding of the biological principles of tissue engineering. This in turn has led to a change in concepts and clinical procedures, as well as in the mindsets of practitioners in adopting this unique treatment strategy as a viable option for immature teeth with pulp necrosis.

Clinical techniques for periodontal regeneration

Periodontitis is among the most prevalent inflammatory diseases affecting almost half of the U.S. adult population and, if left untreated, is the leading cause of tooth loss in adulthood (Eke et al., 2012). In established periodontal disease, the periodontium, which is composed of the bone, the periodontal ligament (PDL), and the cementum, progressively degenerates, leading to compromised tooth function and eventually tooth loss. Periodontal regenerative therapy has been developed under the premise of regenerating the lost periodontal structures, given that the inflammation is controlled (Figure 8.6). True periodontal regeneration is defined as regeneration of tooth supporting tissues, including new alveolar bone, new functionally oriented PDL, and new cementum over a previously diseased root surface (Bowers et al., 1989).

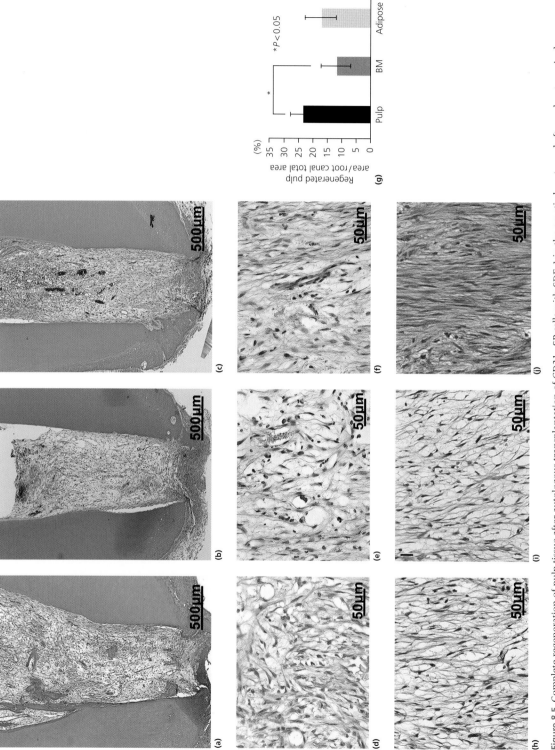

Figure 8.5 Complete regeneration of pulp tissue after autologous transplantation of CD31– SP cells with SDF-1 in the emptied root canal after pulpectomy in dogs. (a, d, and h) Pulp CD31– SP cell transplantation. (b, e, and i) Bone marrow CD31– SP cell transplantation. (c, f, and j) Adipose CD31– SP cell transplantation. (a–g) 14 days. (h–j) 28 days after transplantation. (j) Enhanced matrix formation. (g) Ratio of regenerated area to root canal area. Data are expressed as means ± SD. (From Nakashima and Iohara, 2014. Reproduced with permission from Elsevier.)

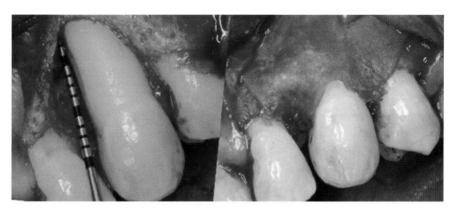

Figure 8.6 Intraoral clinical view following flap elevation showing significant bone loss due to periodontal disease. In this case, a resorbable collagen membrane in combination with a calcium phosphosilicate (bioglass) bone substitute was utilised for periodontal regeneration to enhance the long-term prognosis of this maxillary canine. (Clinical case courtesy of Dr. George Kotsakis, University of Washington, Seattle, WA.)

Numerous periodontal regeneration techniques have been developed and evaluated with overall successful clinical outcomes (Nabers and O'Leary, 1965; Anderegg et al., 1991; Blumenthal, 1993; Heijl et al., 1997; McClain and Schallhorn, 2000; Scheyer et al., 2002; Nevins et al., 2005). These treatment modalities may incorporate the use of bone grafting materials, barrier membranes, and growth factors/matrix proteins as well as their combination to achieve true regeneration of the periodontium. Guided tissue regeneration and osseous grafting are the most extensively evaluated techniques that also have histological documentation (Dragoo and Sullivan, 1973; Nyman et al., 1982; Bowers et al., 1989; Bowers et al., 1989; Bowers et al., 1989). Histological evaluation of the regeneration outcome is crucial to confirm the presence of truly regenerated tissue; however, ethical limitations often impede harvesting periodontal tissues from humans to provide evidence for true periodontal regeneration. The majority of the published evidence on periodontal regeneration deals with clinical outcomes such as clinical attachment level (CAL), pocket depth (PD) reduction, and bone fill (BF) as surrogate endpoints for treatment. Despite the lack of histological support, these criteria are clinically important and have been shown to be associated with tooth survival (Kao et al., 2014).

Historically, attempts for periodontal regeneration have been reported since the 1950s (Prichard, 1957). Autogenous grafts were initially investigated for regenerating bone in human periodontal defects (Schaffer, 1958; Nabers and O'Leary, 1965; Schallhorn, 1968; Dragoo and Sullivan, 1973). Schallhorn and coworkers were among the first to show clinical reattachment in periodontal bone defects after the implantation of autogenous iliac bone. Histological analysis in these defects revealed a true reattachment with osteogenesis, cementogenesis, and new PDL formation (Schallhorn, 1968; Dragoo and Sullivan, 1973). Subsequently, Bowers et al. (1989) performed a three-part human study and compared regeneration of intrabony defects in submerged or nonsubmerged environments with or without the use of decalcified freeze-dried bone allograft (DFDBA). Histological results showed that grafted areas had significantly greater periodontal regeneration than nongrafted areas (Bowers et al., 1989). Moreover, regeneration of the periodontal apparatus was far greater in submerged sites when compared with nonsubmerged sites, which indicated that secluded defects that were protected from the microbial challenge of the oral environment were advantageous in terms of regeneration (Bowers et al., 1989). Collectively, landmark human studies have provided substantial histological evidence confirming beyond any doubt that true periodontal regeneration is feasible under clinical conditions following appropriate surgical technique and careful selection of biomaterials (Cortellini and Bowers, 1995). The following section will focus on current periodontal regenerative techniques and biomaterials.

Osseous grafts

Bone grafts are widely used as a therapeutic strategy to enhance periodontal regeneration. Bone grafts are categorised as autografts (bone graft derived from patient's own body), allografts (bone originated from human donors), xenografts (bone matrix originating from different species), or alloplasts/synthetic grafts (bone substitutes composed by synthetic materials) (Reynolds et al., 2003; Hanes 2007; Kotsakis et al., 2014). Bone grafts possess osteogenic, osteoinductive, and/or osteoconductive properties based on their source and the processing that they undergo. An osteogenic graft contains mesenchymal stem cells encapsulated in its matrix. These cells when grafted in the graft-host site undergo osteoblastic differentiation. Osteoinductive grafts have the capacity to recruit stem cells from surrounding tissues and induce their differentiation into osteoblastic lineages. Lastly, osteoconductive materials act as scaffolds that allow stem cell survival, proliferation, and osteoblastic differentiation (Chen and Jin, 2010).

Autogenous bone grafts are indicated for bone regeneration procedures as they demonstrate all three osteogenic, osteoconductive, and osteoinductive properties (Cypher and Grossman, 1996). Cancellous or mixed cortico-cancellous bone is preferred over cortical bone in contained defects since the presence of vascular supply allows for greater cell survival (Khan et al., 2005). Intraoral and extraoral sites have been used as donor sites with similarly successful outcomes (Nabers and O'Leary, 1965; Hiatt and Schallhorn, 1973; Froum et al., 1976). Intraoral cancellous bone is usually obtained from the maxillary tuberosity, the ramus, or the chin. For extraoral harvesting, either the iliac crest or the tibia are most often employed. Studies have shown a mean bone fill varying from 1.2 mm to 3.4 mm with the use of intraoral bone grafts (Hiatt and Schallhorn, 1973; Renvert et al., 1985). Autogenous iliac cancellous bone has also shown good results in terms of bone fill in various bony defects (Nabers and O'Leary, 1965; Schallhorn, 1968). Nevertheless, morbidity associated with obtaining autografts from the iliac bone as well as the possibility of root resorption associated with fresh iliac grafts have detrimentally impaired its clinical use (Dragoo and Sullivan, 1973). Human histological data from osseous grafting procedures using autografts appear controversial. Histological evaluation of intraoral autogenous grafts has shown evidence of periodontal regeneration and new connective tissue attachment in some studies while others have reported formation of long junctional epithelium (Nabers and O'Leary, 1965; Hiatt et al., 1978; Listgarten and Rosenberg, 1979). Bone grafting with autografts without the simultaneous use of barrier membranes may not predictably lead to true periodontal regeneration (Chen and Jin, 2010).

Various clinical and preclinical studies have evaluated the bone regeneration ability of allogenic bone grafts in periodontal defects as substitutes to autogenous bone. Allografts consist, among others, of freeze-dried bone allografts (FDBA) and DFDBA. Their advantages are their wide availability as well as the fact that they are available without the need for an additional surgical site as compared with autografts (Giannoudis et al., 2005). Their drawbacks include a decreased osteoconductive and osteoinductive potential as compared with autografts, due to their processing, and a very small but not inexistent risk of immunological reactions associated with their use (Giannoudis et al., 2005). DFDBA and FDBA have been shown to lead to similar clinical outcomes with respect to BF, CAL, and PD (Mellonig, 1984; Rummelhart et al., 1989). Results from a recent systematic review showed that the addition of DFDBA following periodontal flap surgery led to significantly greater BF than did open flap debridement (OFD) procedures (Reynolds et al., 2003). A clinical study evaluated the use of mineralised bone allograft for the treatment of periodontal osseous defects in 12 patients. After 6 months, the surgical sites were reentered and PD, CAL, and BF measurements were obtained. Mineralised bone allograft led to significant differences in PD, CAL, and BF measurements as compared with baseline (Browning et al., 2009). Collectively, allografts have shown great clinical potential for regeneration of periodontal defects.

Histologically, controlled human studies have shown new attachment and true periodontal regeneration with the use of allografts in intrabony defects versus conventional root cleaning and flap adaptation (Bowers et al., 1989). DFDBA-grafted areas resulted in significantly greater regeneration than did nongrafted areas (Bowers et al., 1989). A systematic review concluded that the use of DFDBA in intrabony defects led to formation of a new attachment apparatus whilst OFD led to long junctional epithelium formation, which is considered periodontal repair (Bowers et al., 1989). A comparative histological and histochemical analysis of bone regeneration processes with the use of FDBA and DFDBA demonstrated that FDBA had a better osteoconductive potential (Piattelli et al., 1996). Moreover, according to this study, there was no osteo-inductive potential with either one of the allografts tested (Piattelli et al., 1996). However, a series of pre-clinical studies have shown an osteoinductive potential of DFDBA when implanted in intramuscular sites (Committee on Research, Science, and Therapy of the American Academy of Periodontology, 2001). This effect has been showed to vary largely with donor age and with tissue bank preparation (Schwartz et al., 1996; Schwartz et al., 1998).

Xenografts and alloplastic grafts have also been uti-lised as bone substitutes for use around periodontal defects. However, limited evidence from human studies exists to support their use alone for periodontal regen-eration (Older, 1967; Pietruska, 2001). These grafts only possess osteoconductive properties and act as scaffolds that allow revascularisation, cell migration, and osteo-blastic differentiation (Spector, 1994). Xenografts used in periodontal regeneration are usually of bovine origin. Alloplasts can be ceramics, composites, polymers, or silica-based materials (Giannoudis et al., 2005). Clinical studies that used bovine hydroxyapatite combined with collagen membrane showed clinical improvement in PD and CAL (Camelo et al., 2001; Paolantonio et al., 2001). Moreover, similar clinical outcomes to DFDBA have been demonstrated with the use of bioactive glass in intrabony defects (Lovelace et al., 1998). Histological evidence also supports true periodontal regeneration with the use of xenografts in periodontal defects (Reynolds et al., 2003).

In summary, osseous grafts significantly improve clinical periodontal outcomes when implanted in periodontal osseous defects as compared with no-graft controls. However, among bone substitutes, strong his-tological evidence for regeneration exists for allografts. The use of autografts has been limited in clinical practice due to the reduced benefit to hazard ratio as compared with allografts.

Guided tissue regeneration (GTR)

Guided tissue regeneration is a distinctly different approach that aims to regenerate a new periodontal apparatus on a previously diseased root surface. This technique relies on the use of a biocompatible membrane to allow for selective population of the root

surface by mesenchymal stem cells. According to GTR principles, this membrane acts as a barrier to delay epithelial migration in the healing site. During wound healing, epithelial cells are the first to migrate in the site of injury, which leads to long-junctional epithelial formation. GTR membranes allow selective cellular repopulation of the healing site from the surrounding tissues and thus lead to formation of new cementum, bone, and periodontal ligament (Phillips and Palou, 1992).

GTR techniques deploy either resorbable or nonre-sorbable materials as membranes. Nonresorbable mem-branes have been used in early studies with great success (Becker et al., 1988; Gottlow et al., 1992). However, an important limitation to their use is the necessity of a second surgical procedure for membrane removal that may contribute to additional patient discomfort as well as possible postsurgical infection (Nowzari et al., 1995). Resorbable membranes overcome these limitations and at the same time yield equally favorable outcomes in periodontal regeneration (Chung et al., 1990; Blumenthal, 1993). *In vitro* studies have compared resorbable and nonresorbable membranes and their biological effect on fibroblasts and osteoblast-like cells (Alpar et al., 2000; Kasaj et al., 2008). Resorbable membranes have been shown to demonstrate superior cytocompatibility and to allow for increased cell growth and adhesion as compared with nonresorbable mem-branes (Alpar et al., 2000; Kasaj et al., 2008). Yet clinical studies have consistently reported similar results bet-ween the two types of membranes when used to achieve periodontal regeneration (Caffesse et al., 1997; Windisch et al., 1999; Wadhawan et al., 2012). Both membrane types resulted in significant improvement in PD and CAL measurements at various time points and were found equally effective (Caffesse et al., 1997; Windisch et al., 1999; Wadhawan et al., 2012). Collectively, resorbable and nonresorbable membranes both dem-onstrate similar clinical outcomes, although resorb-able membranes may lead to improved patient-related outcomes.

Various studies have reported successful clinical out-comes with GTR techniques mainly for the treatment of furcation and intrabony defects (McClain and Schallhorn, 2000; Aichelmann-Reidy and Reynolds, 2008). A systematic review and meta-analysis assessed the efficacy of GTR in the treatment of intrabony defects compared to OFD in terms of clinical and patient-oriented outcomes (Needleman et al., 2005). This study found a 1.22 mm mean difference in CAL and a 1.21 mm mean difference in PD reduction favoring GTR procedures as compared with OFD. The same study also reported a statistically significant difference in gingival recession between the different techniques, with OFD exhibiting more recession. Patient-centered outcomes such as surgical complications and esthetic assessment were very limited or completely absent in the studies reviewed and no conclusion could be made (Needleman et al., 2005). Another systematic review and meta-analysis assessed the efficacy of GTR in the treatment of intrabony and furcation defects (Murphy and Gunsolley, 2003). In terms of intrabony defects, GTR procedures resulted in significantly improved CAL and PD outcomes. With regard to furcation defects, GTR led to more favorable outcomes in terms of vertical probing attachment level, vertical PD, and horizontal open probing attachment as compared with OFD (Murphy and Gunsolley, 2003). Both studies reported a significant amount of heterogeneity among the included studies, particularly in terms of defect configuration. Although a high level of evidence supports the use of GTR for well-contained defects, their application in defects with multiple missing bony walls remains equivocal. Limited data have shown the potential of successful periodontal regeneration and consequent tooth survival, even in cases of extreme bone loss (Cortellini et al., 2011). Further controlled studies are warranted to delineate the indications and limitations of GTR.

Human histology has demonstrated that regeneration of new cementum, bone, and PDL can occur following GTR procedures (Nyman, Lindhe et al., 1982; Stahl et al., 1990; Cortellini et al., 1993). A case report on histological findings after GTR treatment for buccal recession reported 3.66 mm of new connective tissue attachment. This tissue was associated with newly formed cementum and bone growth (Cortellini et al., 1993). GTR techniques in intrabony lesions have shown periodontal regeneration as early as 5 weeks after surgery (Stahl et al., 1990). Another case report revealed new cementum formation and connective tissue attachment 6 months after GTR procedure on a previously diseased root surface (Nyman et al., 1982). Nonetheless, in contemporary periodontics GTR is often combined with bone substitutes to support the barrier membrane and to increase the predictability of achieving clinical success, as will be discussed later in this chapter. There is histological evidence of true periodontal regeneration in humans after GTR procedures, but the available information for the various combination approaches is scarce. Hence, further research is necessary to verify how efficacious these results are and to investigate the effect of various bone substitutes utilised in GTR to yield periodontal regeneration.

Growth factors/matrix proteins

An increasing body of periodontal regeneration research investigates the effect of growth factors and biomimetic molecules in the treatment of periodontal defects. Growth factors have an important role in regulating the proliferation, migration, and differentiation of a variety of cell types. Several factors and matrix proteins such as BMP-2, BMP-7, BMP-12, TGF-β1, platelet-derived growth factor (PDGF), basic fibroblast growth factors, insulin-like growth factor ([IGF]-I), and enamel matrix derivative (EMD) have been investigated to facilitate periodontal regeneration (Heijl et al., 1997; Howell et al., 1997; Mohammed et al., 1998; Tatakis et al., 2000; van den Bergh et al., 2000; Wikesjo et al., 2004; Chen et al., 2006). Importantly, factors such as rhPDGF-BB and EMD have been found to be clinically as effective as bone grafting and GTR procedures (Parashis et al., 2004; Kao et al., 2014).

Delivery systems have been developed for the application of these growth factors (King, 2001; Chen et al., 2007). The use of scaffolds with time-delayed release of biomolecules decreases their degradation and absorption while providing temporal sustained release of their supportive effect on regeneration (King, 2001; Chen et al., 2007). Reported delivery systems include collagen sponges and membranes or gels, gelatin, and synthetic matrices (Nevins et al., 2005; Lee et al., 2008).

Recombinant human (rh) PDGF and rhIGF-I have been clinically evaluated in patients with periodontal disease (Howell et al., 1997; Nevins et al., 2005). A study tested different doses of rhPDGF-BB and rhIGF-I combined in periodontal osseous defects in terms of regeneration outcomes and patient's safety. The study implemented a low dose of 50 μg/mL and a high dose of 150 μg/mL of the growth factors. OFD or OFD with vehicle were used as controls and surgical reentry was performed at 6 and 9 months postsurgery. Results indicated that none of the patients developed any local or systemic problems and that the local application of rhPDGF-BB and rhIGF-I to periodontal lesions is safe.

Moreover, the high dose combination led to a 42.3% bone fill that was found to be statistically significant more than controls (Howell et al., 1997). A more recent multicenter randomised control trial confirmed the regenerative efficacy and safety of rhPDGF-BB in periodontal osseous defects. The study utilised rhPDGF-BB in different concentrations mixed with a synthetic beta-tricalcium phosphate (β-TCP) matrix and β-TCP alone as active control. Treatment with rhPDGF-BB significantly increased the bone fill, the rate of CAL gain, and reduced gingival recession compared to control (Nevins et al., 2005). The clinical use of rhPDGF-BB has been consistently shown in human studies to be safe for clinical use and to result to equally favorable clinical outcomes as GTR techniques.

EMD consists of a group of enamel matrix proteins and is an FDA-approved drug for dental use. A number of clinical studies have utilised EMD for periodontal regeneration with promising results while others showed no additional clinical benefits (Heijl et al., 1997; Scheyer et al., 2002; Francetti et al., 2005). A randomised control trial utilised EMD for the treatment of intrabony lesions and concluded that it led to significantly increased CAL gain, bone fill, and significantly decreased PD compared to vehicle placebo control (Heijl et al., 1997). In a recent systematic review the effect of growth and amelogenin-like factors, used in periodontal osseous defects was evaluated (Giannobile and Somerman, 2003). The study concluded that EMD could be safely used in periodontal defects and is expected to lead to successful clinical outcomes. Longitudinal clinical evaluations have shown that results of periodontal regeneration with EMD are sustainable over 10 years either when EMD is utilised alone or in combination with bone substitutes (Sculean et al., 2008).

In summary, several growth factors and matrix proteins have been tested for periodontal regeneration of osseous defects. However, it is clear that additional clinical and histological data are needed to provide more insight regarding the regenerative potential of these molecules.

Combination therapy

Combination of different periodontal regeneration therapies has been shown to enhance clinical outcomes (Anderegg et al., 1991; Harris, 1997; Murphy and Gunsolley, 2003; Reynolds et al., 2003). One of the most common therapies is combination of osseous grafting with guided tissue regeneration (Figure 8.7). It is believed that the enhanced effect is bidirectional. On one hand, the bone graft may enhance the response to membrane-only therapy due to its osteoinductive properties and by providing structural support (McClain and Schallhorn 2000). On the other hand, the barrier membrane provides better support to the osseous graft and excludes epithelial growth, thus enhancing the clinical results. Results from a systematic review indicated that bone grafts combined with GTR improved clinical outcomes compared with graft alone (Reynolds et al., 2003). Interestingly though, when compared with GTR treatment, combination therapy enhanced clinical results only for furcation (boneless) and not for intrabony defects (Murphy and Gunsolley, 2003). Bioactive molecules have also been evaluated in combination with other regeneration techniques. The use of rhPDGF-BB or EMD combined with osseous graft has been shown to have an enhanced effect compared with the use of the bioactive agent alone. However, EMD combined with a graft appears to have no additional effect compared with the graft-alone treatment. Moreover, available evidence suggests that EMD combined with GTR does not enhance the clinical outcome as compared with EMD or GTR alone. Collectively, combination therapy seems to overall enhance the effect of individual treatments for periodontal regeneration and, especially in furcation defects, may be considered as the treatment of choice.

Concluding remarks

There have been considerable advances in the field of regenerative endodontics and periodontics. Translational science in tissue engineering has dictated a paradigm shift in treatment alternatives for conditions with previously unmet needs, such as loss of dental development of immature teeth with pulpal necrosis and repair of large periodontal defects. These procedures have become permanent treatment alternatives recognised by the American Dental Association as treatment options in both periodontics and endodontics. However, there are still many challenges to be overcome to use these technologies in a wider range of conditions whilst improving the predictability of desirable outcomes. Further research evaluating the interplay of stem cells, growth factors, and scaffolds, along with

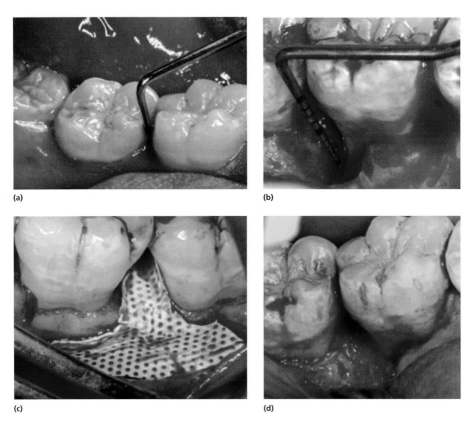

(a)   (b)

(c)   (d)

Figure 8.7 Series of intraoral clinical photographs showing (a) 12 mm probing depth in the distal region of the lower left 1st mandibular molar; (b) combination of a two-wall intrabony defect with a three-wall component at the base of the defect; (c) placement of a nonresorbable barrier membrane through the buccal aspect to provide space maintenance for regeneration in combination with a bone substitute; and (d) 6-month reentry surgical procedure. Note the newly formed tissue covering approximately 65% of the original defect volume. (Clinical case courtesy of University of Washington, Seattle, WA.)

their modulation by local environmental factors, will likely pave the road for the future generation of regenerative procedures.

References

ACCORINTE MDE, L., HOLLAND, R., REIS, A., BORTOLUZZI, M. C., MURATA, S. S., DEZAN, E. JR., SOUZA, V., & ALESSANDRO, L. D. 2008. Evaluation of mineral trioxide aggregate and calcium hydroxide cement as pulp-capping agents in human teeth. *J Endod*, 34, 1–6.

AICHELMANN-REIDY, M. E., & REYNOLDS, M. A. 2008. Predictability of clinical outcomes following regenerative therapy in intrabony defects. *J Periodontol*, 79, 387–93.

ALPAR, B., LEYHAUSEN, G., GUNAY, H., & GEURTSEN, G. 2000. Compatibility of resorbable and nonresorbable guided tissue regeneration membranes in cultures of primary human periodontal ligament fibroblasts and human osteoblast-like cells. *Clin Oral Investig*, 4, 219–25.

ALTHUMAIRY, R. I., TEIXEIRA, F. B., & DIOGENES, A. 2014. Effect of dentin conditioning with intracanal medicaments on survival of stem cells of apical papilla. *J Endod*, 40, 521–5.

ANDEREGG, C. R., MARTIN, S. J., GRAY, J. L., MELLONIG, J. T., & GHER, M. E. 1991. Clinical evaluation of the use of decalcified freeze-dried bone allograft with guided tissue regeneration in the treatment of molar furcation invasions. *J Periodontol*, 62, 264–8.

ANDREASEN, J. O., BORUM, M. K., JACOBSEN, H. L., & ANDREASEN, F. M. 1995. Replantation of 400 avulsed permanent incisors. 2. Factors related to pulpal healing. *Endod Dent Traumatol*, 11, 59–68.

ATILLA, G. 1993. A rare find in Anatolia: a tooth implant (mid-sixth century B.C.). *J Oral Implantol*, 19, 54–7.

BANCHS, F., & TROPE, M. 2004. Revascularization of immature permanent teeth with apical periodontitis: new treatment protocol? *J Endod*, 30, 196–200.

BARTHEL, C. R., ROSENKRANZ, B., LEUENBERG, A., & ROULET, J. F. 2000. Pulp capping of carious exposures: treatment outcome after 5 and 10 years: a retrospective study. *J Endod*, 26, 525–8.

BECERRA, P., RICUCCI, D. LOGHIN, S., GIBBS, J. L., & LIN, L. M. 2014. Histologic study of a human immature permanent premolar with chronic apical abscess after revascularization/revitalization. *J Endod*, 40, 133–9.

BECKER, W., BECKER, B. E., BERG, L., PRICHARD, J., CAFFESSE, R., & ROSENBERG, E. 1988. New attachment after treatment with root isolation procedures: report for treated Class III and Class II furcations and vertical osseous defects. *Int J Periodontics Restorative Dent*, 8, 8–23.

BLUMENTHAL, N. M. 1993. A clinical comparison of collagen membranes with e-PTFE membranes in the treatment of human mandibular buccal class II furcation defects. *J Periodontol*, 64, 925–33.

BOSE, R., NUMMIKOSKI, P., & HARGREAVES, K. 2009. A retrospective evaluation of radiographic outcomes in immature teeth with necrotic root canal systems treated with regenerative endodontic procedures. *J Endod*, 35, 1343–9.

BOWERS, G. M., CHADROFF, B. CARNEVALE, R., MELLONIG, J., CORIO, R., EMERSON, J., STEVENS, M., & ROMBERG, E. 1989. Histologic evaluation of new attachment apparatus formation in humans: Part I. *J Periodontol*, 60, 664–74.

BROWNING, E. S., MEALEY, B. L., & MELLONIG, J. T. 2009. Evaluation of a mineralized cancellous bone allograft for the treatment of periodontal osseous defects: 6-month surgical reentry. *Int J Periodontics Restorative Dent*, 29, 41–7.

CAFFESSE, R. G., MOTA, L. F., QUINONES, C. R., & MORRISON, E. C. 1997. Clinical comparison of resorbable and non-resorbable barriers for guided periodontal tissue regeneration. *J Clin Periodontol*, 24, 747–52.

CAMELO, M., NEVINS, M. L., LYNCH, S. E., SCHENK, R. K., SIMION, M., & NEVINS, M. 2001. Periodontal regeneration with an autogenous bone-Bio-Oss composite graft and a Bio-Gide membrane. *Int J Periodont Restor Dent*, 21, 109–19.

CAO, Y., VACANTI, J. P., PAIGE, K. T., UPTON, J., & VACANTI, C. A. 1997. Transplantation of chondrocytes utilizing a polymer-cell construct to produce tissue-engineered cartilage in the shape of a human ear. *Plast Reconstr Surg*, 100, 297–302; discussion 303–4.

CASAGRANDE, L., DEMARCO, F. F., ZHANG, Z., ARAUJO, F. B., SHI, S., & NOR, J. E. 2010. Dentin-derived BMP-2 and odontoblast differentiation. *J Dent Res*, 89, 603–8.

CEHRELI, Z. C., ISBITIREN, B., SARA, S., & ERBAS, G. 2011. Regenerative endodontic treatment (revascularization) of immature necrotic molars medicated with calcium hydroxide: a case series. *J Endod*, 37, 1327–30.

CEHRELI, Z. C., SARA, S., & AKSOY, B. 2012. Revascularization of immature permanent incisors after severe extrusive luxation injury. *J Can Dent Assoc*, 78, c4.

CHEN, F. M., & JIN, Y. 2010. Periodontal tissue engineering and regeneration: current approaches and expanding opportunities. *Tissue Eng Part B Rev*, 16, 219–55.

CHEN, F. M., ZHAO, Y. M., WU, H., DENG, Z. H., WANG, Q. T., ZHOU, W., et al., 2006. Enhancement of periodontal tissue regeneration by locally controlled delivery of insulin-like growth factor-I from dextran-co-gelatin microspheres. *J Control Release*, 114, 209–22.

CHEN, M. Y., CHEN, K. L., CHEN, C. A., TAYEBATY, F., ROSENBERG, P. A., & LIN, L. M. 2012. Responses of immature permanent teeth with infected necrotic pulp tissue and apical periodontitis/abscess to revascularization procedures. *Int Endod J*, 45, 294–305.

CHEN, R. R., SILVA, E. A., YUEN, W. W. BROCK, A. A., FISCHBACH, C., LIN, A. S., GULDBERG, R. E., & MOONEY, D. J. 2007. Integrated approach to designing growth factor delivery systems. *FASEB J*, 21, 3896–903.

CHUEH, L. H., & CHIANG, C. P. 2010. Histology of Irreversible pulpitis premolars treated with mineral trioxide aggregate pulpotomy. *Oper Dent*, 35, 370–4.

CHUNG, K. M., SALKIN, L. M., STEIN, M. D., & FREEDMAN, A. L. 1990. Clinical evaluation of a biodegradable collagen membrane in guided tissue regeneration. *J Periodontol*, 61, 732–6.

COMMITTEE ON RESEARCH, SCIENCE, AND THERAPY OF THE AMERICAN ACADEMY OF PERIODONTOLOGY. 2001. Tissue banking of bone allografts used in periodontal regeneration. *J Periodontol*, 72, 834–8.

CORTELLINI, P., & BOWERS, G. M. 1995. Periodontal regeneration of intrabony defects: an evidence-based treatment approach. *Int J Periodont Restor Dent*, 15, 128–45.

CORTELLINI, P., CLAUSER, C., & PRATO, G. P. 1993. Histologic assessment of new attachment following the treatment of a human buccal recession by means of a guided tissue regeneration procedure. *J Periodontol*, 64, 387–91.

CORTELLINI, P., STALPERS, G., MOLLO, A., & TONETTI, M. S. 2011. Periodontal regeneration versus extraction and prosthetic replacement of teeth severely compromised by attachment loss to the apex: 5-year results of an ongoing randomized clinical trial. *J Clin Periodontol*, 38, 915–24.

CVEK, M. 1974. Treatment of non-vital permanent incisors with calcium hydroxide. IV. Periodontal healing and closure of the root canal in the coronal fragment of teeth with intra-alveolar fracture and vital apical fragment. A follow-up. *Odontol Revy*, 5, 239–46.

CVEK, M. 1978. A clinical report on partial pulpotomy and capping with calcium hydroxide in permanent incisors with complicated crown fracture. *J Endod*, 4, 232–7.

CVEK, M., CLEATON-JONES, P., AUSTIN, J., LOWNIE, J., KLING, M., & FATTI, P. 1990. Pulp revascularization in reimplanted immature monkey incisors: predictability and the effect of antibiotic systemic prophylaxis. *Endod Dent Traumatol*, 6, 157–69.

CYPHER, T. J., & GROSSMAN, J. P. 1996. Biological principles of bone graft healing. *J Foot Ankle Surg*, 35, 413–7.

D'AQUINO, R., DE ROSA, A., LANZA, V., TIRINO, V., LAINO, L., GRAZIANO, A., DESIDERIO, V. LAINO, G., & PAPACCIO, G. 2009. Human mandible bone defect repair by the grafting of dental pulp stem/progenitor cells and collagen sponge biocomplexes. *Eur Cell Mater*, 18, 75–83.

DAMMASCHKE, T. 2008. The history of direct pulp capping. *J Hist Dent*, 56, 9–23.

DING, G., LIU, Y., AN, Y., ZHANG, C., SHI, S., WANG, W., & WANG, S. 2010. Suppression of T cell proliferation by root apical papilla stem cells in vitro. *Cells Tissues Organs*, 191, 357–64.

DIOGENES, A., M. HENRY, A. TEIXEIRA, F. B., & HARGREAVES, K. M. 2013. An update on clinical regenerative endodontics. *Endodontic Topics*, 28, 2–23.

DIOGENES, A. R., RUPAREL, N. B., TEIXEIRA, F. B., & HARGREAVES, K. M. 2014. Translational science in disinfection for regenerative endodontics. *J Endod*, 40, S52–7.

DRAGOO, M. R., & SULLIVAN, H. C. 1973. A clinical and histological evaluation of autogenous iliac bone grafts in humans. I. Wound healing 2 to 8 months. *J Periodontol*, 44, 599–613.

EKE, P. I., DYE, B. A., WEI, L., THORNTON-EVANS, G. O., & GENCO, R. J. 2012. CDC Periodontal Disease Surveillance workgroup: James Beck. Prevalence of periodontitis in adults in the United States: 2009 and 2010. *J Dent Res*, 91, 914–20.

EL-ANSARY, M. M. 1989. History of pain relief by ancient Egyptians. *Middle East J Anaesthesiol*, 10, 99–105.

FOUAD, A. F., & NOSRAT, A. 2013. Pulp regeneration in previously infected root canal space. *Endodontic Topics*, 28, 24–37.

FRANCETTI, L., TROMBELLI, L., LOMBARDO, G.,. GUIDA, L., CAFIERO, C., ROCCUZZO, M., CARUSI, G., & DEL FABBRO, M. 2005. Evaluation of efficacy of enamel matrix derivative in the treatment of intrabony defects: a 24-month multicenter study. *Int J Periodon Restor Dent*, 25, 461–73.

FRANCKE, O. C. 1971."Capping of the living pulp: from Philip Pfaff to John Wessler. *Bull Hist Dent*, 19, 17–23.

FROUM, S. J., ORTIZ, M., WITKIN, R. T., THALER, R., SCOPP, I. W., & STAHL, S. S. 1976. Osseous autografts. III. Comparison of osseous coagulum-bone blend implants with open curetage. *J Periodontol*, 47, 287–94.

GALLER, K. M., BUCHALLA, W., HILLER, K. A., FEDERLIN, M., EIDT, A., SCHIEFERSTEINER, M., & SCHMALZ, G. 2015. Influence of root canal disinfectants on growth factor release from dentin. *J Endod*, 41, 363–8.

GALLER, K. M., D'SOUZA, R. N., HARTGERINK, J. D., & SCHMALZ, G. 2011a. Scaffolds for dental pulp tissue engineering. *Adv Dent Res*, 23, 333–9.

GALLER, K. M., D'SOUZA, R. N., FEDERLIN, M., CAVENDER, A. C., HARTGERINK, J. D., HECKER, S., & SCHMALZ, G. 2011b.Dentin conditioning codetermines cell fate in regenerative endodontics. *J Endod*, 37, 1536–41.

GELBIER, M. J. 2010. Pulp capping and pulpotomy: 1750–2008. *Dent Hist*, 52, 58–69.

GIANNOBILE, W. V., & SOMERMAN, M. J. 2003. Growth and amelogenin-like factors in periodontal wound healing. A systematic review. *Ann Periodontol*, 8, 193–204.

GIANNOUDIS, P. V., DINOPOULOS, H., & TSIRIDIS, E. 2005. Bone substitutes: an update. *Injury*, 36, S20–7.

GOTTLOW, J., NYMAN, S., & KARRING, T. 1992. Maintenance of new attachment gained through guided tissue regeneration. *J Clin Periodontol*, 19, 315–7.

GRAHAM, L., COOPER, P. R., CASSIDY, N., NOR, J. E., SLOAN, A. J., & SMITH, A. J. 2006. The effect of calcium hydroxide on solubilisation of bio-active dentine matrix components. *Biomaterials*, 27, 2865–73.

GROSSMAN, L. I. 1976. Endodontics 1776–1976: a bicentennial history against the background of general dentistry. *J Am Dent Assoc*, 93, 78–87.

HANES, P. J. 2007. Bone replacement grafts for the treatment of periodontal intrabony defects. *Oral Maxillofac Surg Clin North Am*, 19, 499–512, vi.

HARRIS, R. J. 1997. A clinical evaluation of guided tissue regeneration with a bioabsorbable matrix membrane combined with an allograft bone graft. A series of case reports. *J Periodontol*, 68, 598–607.

HEIJL, L., HEDEN, G., SVARDSTROM, G., & OSTGREN, A. 1997. Enamel matrix derivative (EMDOGAIN) in the treatment of intrabony periodontal defects. *J Clin Periodontol*, 24, 705–14.

HELMLINGER, G., YUAN, F., DELLIAN, M., & JAIN, R. K. 1997. Interstitial pH and pO2 gradients in solid tumors in vivo: high-resolution measurements reveal a lack of correlation. *Nat Med*, 3, 177–82.

HIATT, W. H., & SCHALLHORN, R. G. 1973. Intraoral transplants of cancellous bone and marrow in periodontal lesions. *J Periodontol*, 44, 194–208.

HIATT, W. H., SCHALLHORN, R. G., & AARONIAN, A. J. 1978. The induction of new bone and cementum formation. IV. Microscopic examination of the periodontium following human bone and marrow allograft, autograft and nongraft periodontal regenerative procedures. *J Periodontol*, 49, 495–512.

HILTON, T. J., FERRACANE, J. L., & MANCL, L.; Northwest Practice-based Research Collaborative in Evidence-based Dentistry (NWP). 2013. Comparison of CaOH with MTA for direct pulp capping: a PBRN randomized clinical trial. *J Dent Res*, 92, 16S–22S.

HOWELL, T. H., FIORELLINI, J. P., PAQUETTE, D. W., OFFENBACHER, S. GIANNOBILE, W. V., & LYNCH, S. E. 1997. A phase I/II clinical trial to evaluate a combination of recombinant human platelet-derived growth factor-BB and recombinant human insulin-like growth factor-I in patients with periodontal disease. *J Periodontol*, 68, 1186–93.

HUANG, G. T., YAMAZA, T., SHEA, L. D., DJOUAD, F., KUHN, N. Z., TUAN, R. S., & SHI, S. 2010. Stem/progenitor cell-mediated de novo regeneration of dental pulp with newly deposited continuous layer of dentin in an in vivo model. *Tissue Eng Part A*, 16, 605–15.

IOHARA, K., IMABAYASHI, K., ISHIZAKA, R., WATANABE, A. NABEKURA, J. ITO, M. MATSUSHITA, K. NAKAMURA, H, & NAKASHIMA, M. 2011. Complete pulp regeneration after pulpectomy by transplantation of CD105+ stem cells with stromal cell-derived factor-1. *Tissue Eng Part A*, 17, 1911–20.

IOHARA, K., MURAKAMI, M., TAKEUCHI, N., OSAKO, Y., ITO, M., ISHIZAKA, R., UTUNOMIYA, S., NAKAMURA, H., MATSUSHITA, K., & NAKASHIMA, M. 2013. A novel combinatorial therapy with pulp stem cells and granulocyte colony-stimulating factor for total pulp regeneration. *Stem Cells Transl Med*, 2, 521–33.

IRISH, J. D. 2004. A 5,500 year old artificial human tooth from Egypt: a historical note. *Int J Oral Maxillofac Implants*, 19, 645–7.

IWAYA, S.-I., IKAWA, M., & KUBOTA, M. 2001. Revascularization of an immature permanent tooth with apical periodontitis and sinus tract. *Dental Traumatology*, 17, 185–7.

IWAYA, S., IKAWA, M., & KUBOTA, M. 2011. Revascularization of an immature permanent tooth with periradicular abscess after luxation. *Dent Traumatol*, 27, 55–8.

JEERUPHAN, T., JANTARAT, J., YANPISET, K., SUWANNAPAN, L., KHEWSAWAI, P., & HARGREAVES, K. M. 2012. Mahidol study 1: comparison of radiographic and survival outcomes of immature teeth treated with either regenerative endodontic or apexification methods: a retrospective study. *J Endod*, 38, 1330–6.

KAHLER, B., MISTRY, S,. MOULE, A., RINGSMUTH, A. K., CASE, P., THOMSON, A., & HOLCOMBE, T. 2014. Revascularization outcomes: a prospective analysis of 16 consecutive cases. *J Endod*, 40, 333–8.

KAO, R. T., NARES, S., & REYNOLDS, M. A. 2014. Periodontal regeneration of intrabony defects: a systematic review. *J Periodontol*, 86, S77–104.

KASAJ, A., REICHERT, C., GOTZ, H., ROHRIG, B., SMEETS, R., & WILLERSHAUSEN, B. 2008. In vitro evaluation of various bioabsorbable and nonresorbable barrier membranes for guided tissue regeneration. *Head Face Med*, 4, 22.

KHAN, S. N., CAMMISA, F. P. JR., SANDHU, H. S., DIWAN, A. D., GIRARDI, F. P., & LANE, J. M. 2005. The biology of bone grafting. *J Am Acad Orthop Surg*, 13, 77–86.

KIM, J.-H., KIM, Y., SHIN, S.-J., PARK, J.-W., & JUNG, I.-Y. 2010. tooth discoloration of immature permanent incisor associated with triple antibiotic therapy: a case report. *Journal of Endodontics*, 36, 1086–91.

KING, G. N. 2001. The importance of drug delivery to optimize the effects of bone morphogenetic proteins during periodontal regeneration. *Curr Pharm Biotechnol*, 2, 131–42.

KLING, M., CVEK, M., & MEJARE, I. 1986. Rate and predictability of pulp revascularization in therapeutically reimplanted permanent incisors. *Endod Dent Traumatol*, 2, 83–9.

KODONAS, K., GOGOS, C., PAPADIMITRIOU, S., KOUZI-KOLIAKOU, K., & TZIAFAS, D. 2012. Experimental formation of dentin-like structure in the root canal implant model using cryopreserved swine dental pulp progenitor cells. *J Endod*, 38, 913–9.

KONTAKIOTIS, E. G., FILIPPATOS, C. G., TZANETAKIS, G. N., & AGRAFIOTI, A. 2015. Regenerative endodontic therapy: a data analysis of clinical protocols. *J Endod*, 41, 146–54.

KOTSAKIS, G. A., SALAMA, M., CHREPA, V., HINRICHS, J. E., & GAILLARD, P. 2014. A randomized, blinded, controlled clinical study of particulate anorganic bovine bone mineral and calcium phosphosilicate putty bone substitutes for socket preservation. *Int J Oral Maxillofac Implants*, 29, 141–51.

LANGER, R., & VACANTI, J. P. 1993. Tissue engineering. *Science*, 260, 920–6.

LAURENT, P., CAMPS, J., & ABOUT, I. 2012. Biodentine induces TGF-beta1 release from human pulp cells and early dental pulp mineralization. *Int Endod J*, 45, 439–48.

LEE, J., CUDDIHY, M. J., & KOTOV, N. A. 2008. Three-dimensional cell culture matrices: state of the art. *Tissue Eng Part B Rev*, 14, 61–86.

LIN, L. M., SHIMIZU, E., GIBBS, J. L., LOGHIN, S., & RICUCCI, D. 2014. Histologic and histobacteriologic observations of failed revascularization/revitalization therapy: a case report. *J Endod*, 40, 291–5.

LISTGARTEN, M. A., & ROSENBERG, M. M. 1979. Histological study of repair following new attachment procedures in human periodontal lesions. *J Periodontol*, 50, 333–44.

LOVELACE, T. B., MELLONIG, J. T., MEFFERT, R. M., JONES, A. A., NUMMIKOSKI, P. V., & COCHRAN, D. L. 1998. Clinical evaluation of bioactive glass in the treatment of periodontal osseous defects in humans. *J Periodontol*, 69, 1027–35.

LOVELACE, T. W., HENRY, M. A., HARGREAVES, K. M., & DIOGENES, A. 2011. Evaluation of the delivery of mesenchymal stem cells into the root canal space of necrotic immature teeth after clinical regenerative endodontic procedure. *J Endod*, 37, 133–8.

LUCAS, K., & MAES, M. 2013. Role of the toll-like receptor (TLR) radical cycle in chronic inflammation: possible treatments targeting the TLR4 pathway. *Mol Neurobiol*, 48, 190–204.

MARION, L. R. 1996. Dentistry of ancient Egypt. *J Hist Dent*, 44, 15–7.

MARTIN, D. E., HENRY, M. A., ALMEIDA, J. F. A., TEIXEIRA, F. B., HARGREAVES, K. M., & DIOGENES, A. R. 2012. Effect of sodium hypochlorite on the odontoblastic phenotype differentiation of SCAP in cultured organotype human roots. *J Endod*, 38, e26.

MARTIN, G., RICUCCI, D., GIBBS, J. L., & LIN, L. M. 2013. Histological findings of revascularized/revitalized immature permanent molar with apical periodontitis using platelet-rich plasma. *J Endod*, 39, 138–44.

MCCLAIN, P. K., & SCHALLHORN, R. G. 2000. Focus on furcation defects: guided tissue regeneration in combination with bone grafting. *Periodontol 2000*, 22, 190–212.

MCFADDEN, J. P., PUANGPET, P., BASKETTER, D. A., DEARMAN, R. J., & KIMBER, I. 2013. Why does allergic contact dermatitis exist? *Br J Dermatol*, 168, 692–9.

MELLONIG, J. T. 1984. Decalcified freeze-dried bone allograft as an implant material in human periodontal defects. *Int J Periodont Restor Dent*, 4, 40–55.

MENTE, J., HUFNAGEL, S., LEO, M., MICHEL, A., GEHRIG, H., PANAGIDIS, D., SAURE, D., & PFEFFERLE, T. 2014.

Treatment outcome of mineral trioxide aggregate or calcium hydroxide direct pulp capping: long-term results. *J Endod*, 40, 1746–51.

MILLER, E. K., LEE, J. Y., TAWIL, P. Z., TEIXEIRA, F. B., & VANN, W. F. JR. 2012. Emerging therapies for the management of traumatized immature permanent incisors. *Pediatr Dent*, 34, 66–9.

MOHAMMED, S., PACK, A. R., & KARDOS, D T. B. 1998. The effect of transforming growth factor beta one (TGF-beta 1) on wound healing, with or without barrier membranes, in a Class II furcation defect in sheep. *J Periodontal Res*, 33, 335–44.

MURPHY, K. G., & GUNSOLLEY, J. C. 2003. Guided tissue regeneration for the treatment of periodontal intrabony and furcation defects. A systematic review. *Ann Periodontol*, 8, 266–302.

MURRAY, P. E., GARCIA-GODOY, F., & HARGREAVES, K. M. 2007. Regenerative endodontics: a review of current status and a call for action. *J Endod*, 33, 377–90.

NABERS, C. L., & O'LEARY, T. J. 1965. Autogenous bone transplants in the treatment of osseous defects. *J Periodontol*, 36, 5–14.

NAGY, M. M., TAWFIK, H. E., HASHEM, A. A., & ABU-SEIDA, A. M. 2014. Regenerative potential of immature permanent teeth with necrotic pulps after different regenerative protocols. *J Endod*, 40, 192–8.

NAKASHIMA, M., & IOHARA, K. 2014. Mobilized dental pulp stem cells for pulp regeneration: initiation of clinical trial. *J Endod*, 40, S26–32.

NEEDLEMAN, TUCKER, I., R., GIEDRYS-LEEPER, E., & WORTHINGTON, H. 2005. Guided tissue regeneration for periodontal intrabony defects: a Cochrane Systematic Review. *Periodontol 2000*, 37, 106–23.

NEVINS, M., GIANNOBILE, W. V., MCGUIRE, M. K. KAO, R. T., MELLONIG, J. T. HINRICHS, J. E., et al. 2005. Platelet-derived growth factor stimulates bone fill and rate of attachment level gain: results of a large multicenter randomized controlled trial. *J Periodontol*, 76, 2205–15.

NIE, K., MOLNAR, Z., & SZELE, F. G. 2010. Proliferation but not migration is associated with blood vessels during development of the rostral migratory stream. *Dev Neurosci*, 32, 163–72.

NOSRAT, A., LI, K. L., VIR, K., HICKS, M. L., & FOUAD, A. F. 2013. Is pulp regeneration necessary for root maturation? *J Endod*, 39, 1291–5.

NOWICKA, A., LIPSKI, M., PARAFINIUK, M., SPORNIAK-TUTAK, K., LICHOTA, D., KOSIERKIEWICZ, A., KACZMAREK, W., & BUCZKOWSKA-RADLINSKA, J. 2013. Response of human dental pulp capped with biodentine and mineral trioxide aggregate. *J Endod*, 39, 743–7.

NOWZARI, H., MATIAN, F., & SLOTS, J. 1995. Periodontal pathogens on polytetrafluoroethylene membrane for guided tissue regeneration inhibit healing. *J Clin Periodontol*, 22, 469–74.

NYGGARD-OSTBY, B. 1961. The role of the blood clot in endodontic therapy: an experimental histological study. *Acta Odontol Scand*, 79, 333–49.

NYGAARD-OSTBY, B., & HJORTDAL, O. 1971. Tissue formation in the root canal following pulp removal. *Scand J Dent Res*, 79, 333–49.

NYMAN, S., LINDHE, J., KARRING, T., & RYLANDER, H. 1982. New attachment following surgical treatment of human periodontal disease. *J Clin Periodontol* 9(4): 290–6.

OKITA, K., ICHISAKA, T., & YAMANAKA, S. 2007. Generation of germline-competent induced pluripotent stem cells. *Nature*, 448, 313–7.

OLDER, L. B. 1967. The use of heterogenous bovine bone implants in the treatment of periodontal pockets. An experimental study in humans. *J Periodontol*, 38, 539–49.

OSTBY, B. N. 1961. The role of the blood clot in endodontic therapy. An experimental histologic study. *Acta Odontol Scand*, 19, 324–53.

PAOLANTONIO, M., SCARANO, A., DI PLACIDO, G., TUMINI, V., D'ARCHIVIO, D., & PIATTELLI A. 2001. Periodontal healing in humans using anorganic bovine bone and bovine peritoneum-derived collagen membrane: a clinical and histologic case report. *Int J Periodontics Restorative Dent*, 21, 505–15.

PARASHIS, A., ANDRONIKAKI-FALDAMI, A., & TSIKLAKIS, K. 2004. Clinical and radiographic comparison of three regenerative procedures in the treatment of intrabony defects. *Int J Periodont Restor Dent*, 24, 81–90.

PETRINO, J. A. 2007. Revascularization of necrotic pulp of immature teeth with apical periodontitis. *Northwest Dent*, 86, 33–5.

PHILLIPS, J. D., & PALOU, M. E. 1992. A review of the guided tissue regeneration concept. *Gen Dent*, 40, 118–23.

PIATTELLI, A., SCARANO, A., CORIGLIANO, M., & PIATTELLI M. 1996. Comparison of bone regeneration with the use of mineralized and demineralized freeze-dried bone allografts: a histological and histochemical study in man. *Biomaterials*, 17, 1127–31.

PICCIN, D., & MORSHEAD, C. M. 2010. Potential and pitfalls of stem cell therapy in old age. *Dis Model Mech*, 3, 421–5.

PIETRUSKA, M. D. 2001. A comparative study on the use of Bio-Oss and enamel matrix derivative (Emdogain) in the treatment of periodontal bone defects. *Eur J Oral Sci*, 109, 178–81.

PRICHARD, J. 1957. Regeneration of bone following periodontal therapy: report of cases. *Oral Surg Oral Med Oral Pathol*, 10, 247–52.

RENVERT, S., GARRETT, S., SHALLHORN, R. G., & EGELBERG, J. 1985. Healing after treatment of periodontal intraosseous defects. III. Effect of osseous grafting and citric acid conditioning. *J Clin Periodontol*, 12, 441–55.

REYNOLDS, K., JOHNSON, J. D., & COHENCA, D N. 2009. Pulp revascularization of necrotic bilateral bicuspids using a modified novel technique to eliminate potential coronal discolouration: a case report. *Int Endod J*, 42, 84–92.

REYNOLDS, M. A., AICHELMANN-REIDY, M. E., BRANCH-MAYS, G. L., & GUNSOLLEY, J. C. 2003. The efficacy of bone replacement grafts in the treatment of periodontal osseous defects. A systematic review. *Ann Periodontol*, 8, 227–65.

RING, K. C., MURRAY, P. E., NAMEROW, K. N., KUTTLER, S., & GARCIA-GODOY, F. 2008. The comparison of the effect of endodontic irrigation on cell adherence to root canal dentin. *J Endod*, 34, 1474–9.

RUMMELHART, J. M., MELLONIG, J. T., GRAY, V., & TOWLE, D H. J. 1989. A comparison of freeze-dried bone allograft and demineralized freeze-dried bone allograft in human periodontal osseous defects. *J Periodontol*, 60, 655–63.

RUPAREL, N. B., TEIXEIRA, F. B., FERRAZ, C. C., & DIOGENES, A. 2012. Direct effect of intracanal medicaments on survival of stem cells of the apical papilla. *J Endod*, 38, 1372–5.

SABRAH, A. H., YASSEN, G. H., & GREGORY, R. L. 2013. Effectiveness of antibiotic medicaments against biofilm formation of *Enterococcus faecalis* and *Porphyromonas gingivalis*. *J Endod*, 39, 1385–9.

SABRAH, A. H., YASSEN, G. H., LIU, W. C., GOEBEL, W. S., GREGORY, R. L., & PLATT, J. A. 2015. The effect of diluted triple and double antibiotic pastes on dental pulp stem cells and established *Enterococcus faecalis* biofilm. *Clin Oral Investig*, e-pub ahead of print.

SACHDEVA, G. S., SACHDEVA, L. T., GOEL, M., & BALA S. 2014. Regenerative endodontic treatment of an immature tooth with a necrotic pulp and apical periodontitis using platelet-rich plasma (PRP) and mineral trioxide aggregate (MTA): a case report. *Int Endod J*, 48, 902–10.

SCHAFFER, E. 1958. Cartilage grafts in human periodontal pockets. *J Periodontol*, 9, 176.

SCHALLHORN, R. G. 1968. The use of autogenous hip marrow biopsy implants for bony crater defects. *J Periodontol*, 39, 145–7.

SCHEYER, E. T., VELASQUEZ-PLATA, D., BRUNSVOLD, M. A., LASHO, D. J., & MELLONIG, J. T. 2002. A clinical comparison of a bovine-derived xenograft used alone and in combination with enamel matrix derivative for the treatment of periodontal osseous defects in humans. *J Periodontol*, 73, 423–32.

SCHWARTZ, Z., MELLONIG, J. T., CARNES, D. L. JR., DE LA FONTAINE, J., COCHRAN, D. L., DEAN, D. D., & BOYAN, B. D. 1996. Ability of commercial demineralized freeze-dried bone allograft to induce new bone formation. *J Periodontol*, 67, 918–26.

SCHWARTZ, Z., SOMERS, A., MELLONIG, J. T., CARNES, D. L. JR., DEAN, D. D., COCHRAN D. L., & BOYAN, B. D. 1998. Ability of commercial demineralized freeze-dried bone allograft to induce new bone formation is dependent on donor age but not gender. *J Periodontol*, 69, 470–8.

SCULEAN, A., KISS, A., MILIAUSKAITE, A., SCHWARZ, F., ARWEILER, N. B., & HANNIG, M. 2008. Ten-year results following treatment of intra-bony defects with enamel matrix proteins and guided tissue regeneration. *J Clin Periodontol*, 35, 817–24.

SHIMIZU, E., JONG, G., PARTRIDGE, N., ROSENBERG, P. A., & LIN L. M. 2012. Histologic observation of a human immature permanent tooth with irreversible pulpitis after revascularization/regeneration procedure. *J Endod*, 38, 1293–7.

SHIMIZU, E., RICUCCI, D., ALBERT, J., ALOBAID, A. S., GIBBS, J. L., HUANG, G. T. LIN, L. M. 2013. Clinical, radiographic, and histological observation of a human immature permanent tooth with chronic apical abscess after revitalization treatment. *J Endod*, 39, 1078–83.

SHIVASHANKAR, V. Y., JOHNS, D. A., VIDYANATH, S., & KUMAR, M. R. 2012. Platelet rich fibrin in the revitalization of tooth with necrotic pulp and open apex. *J Conserv Dent*, 15, 395–8.

SHRESTHA, S., DIOGENES, A., & KISHEN, A. 2014. Temporal-controlled release of bovine serum albumin from chitosan nanoparticles: effect on the regulation of alkaline phosphatase activity in stem cells from apical papilla. *J Endod*, 40, 1349–54.

SIMON, S., PERARD, M., ZANINI, M., SMITH, A. J., CHARPENTIER, E., DJOLE, S. X., & LUMLEY, P. J. 2013. Should pulp chamber pulpotomy be seen as a permanent treatment? Some preliminary thoughts. *Int Endod J*, 46, 79–87.

SMITH, A. J., SCHEVEN, B. A., TAKAHASHI, Y., FERRACANE, J. L., SHELTON, R. M., & COOPER, P. R. 2012. Dentine as a bioactive extracellular matrix. *Arch Oral Biol*, 57, 109–21.

SONOYAMA, W., LIU, Y., YAMAZA, T., TUAN, R. S., WANG, S., SHI, S., & HUANG, G. T. 2008. Characterization of the apical papilla and its residing stem cells from human immature permanent teeth: a pilot study. *J Endod*, 34, 166–71.

SPECTOR, M. 1994. Anorganic bovine bone and ceramic analogs of bone mineral as implants to facilitate bone regeneration. *Clin Plast Surg*, 21, 437–44.

STAHL, S. S., FROUM, S., & TARNOW, D. 1990. Human histologic responses to guided tissue regenerative techniques in intrabony lesions. Case reports on 9 sites. *J Clin Periodontol*, 17, 191–8.

TATAKIS, D. N., WIKESJO, U. M., RAZI, S. S., SIGURDSSON, T. J., LEE, M. B., NGUYEN, T., ONGPIPATTANAKUL, B., & HARDWICK, R. 2000. Periodontal repair in dogs: effect of transforming growth factor-beta 1 on alveolar bone and cementum regeneration. *J Clin Periodontol*, 27, 698–704.

TECLES, O., LAURENT, P., AUBUT, V., & ABOUT, I. 2008. Human tooth culture: a study model for reparative dentinogenesis and direct pulp capping materials biocompatibility. *J Biomed Mater Res B Appl Biomater*, 85, 180–7.

THOMSON, A., & KAHLER, B. 2010. Regenerative endodontics: biologically-based treatment for immature permanent teeth: a case report and review of the literature. *Aust Dent J*, 55, 446–52.

TOMSON, P. L., GROVER, L. M., LUMLEY, P. J., SLOAN, A. J. SMITH, A. J., & COOPER, P. R. 2007. Dissolution of bioactive dentine matrix components by mineral trioxide aggregate. *J Dent*, 35, 636–42.

TORABINEJAD, M., FARAS, H., CORR, R., WRIGHT, K. R., & SHABAHANG, S. 2014. Histologic examinations of teeth treated with 2 scaffolds: a pilot animal investigation. *J Endod*, 40, 515–20.

TORABINEJAD, M., & KIGER, R. D. 1980. Experimentally induced alterations in periapical tissues of the cat. *J Dent Res*, 59, 87–96.

TORABINEJAD, M., & TURMAN, M. 2011. Revitalization of tooth with necrotic pulp and open apex by using platelet-rich plasma: a case report. *J Endod*, 37, 265–8.

TREVINO, E. G., PATWARDHAN, A. N., HENRY, M. A., PERRY, G., DYBDAL-HARGREAVES, N., HARGREAVES, K. M., & DIOGENES, A. 2011. Effect of irrigants on the survival of human stem cells of the apical papilla in a platelet-rich plasma scaffold in human root tips. *J Endod*, 37, 1109–15.

UNTERHOLZNER, L. 2013.The interferon response to intracellular DNA: why so many receptors? *Immunobiology*, 218, 1312–21.

VAN DEN BERGH, J. P., TEN BRUGGENKATE, C. M., GROENEVELD, H. H., BURGER, E. H., & TUINZING, D. B. 2000. Recombinant human bone morphogenetic protein-7 in maxillary sinus floor elevation surgery in 3 patients compared to autogenous bone grafts. *A clinical pilot study. J Clin Periodontol*, 27, 627–36.

VANACKER, J., VISWANATH, A., DE BERDT, P., EVERARD, A., CANI, P. D., BOUZIN, C., FERON, O., DIOGENES, A., LEPRINCE, J. G., & DES RIEUX, A. 2014. Hypoxia modulates the differentiation potential of stem cells of the apical papilla. *J Endod*, 40, 1410–8.

WADHAWAN, A., GOWDA, T. M., & MEHTA, D. S. 2012. Gore-tex(R) versus resolut adapt(R) GTR membranes with perioglas(R) in periodontal regeneration. *Contemp Clin Dent*, 3, 406–11.

WARNKE, P. H., SPRINGER, I. N., WILTFANG, J., ACIL, Y., EUFINGER, H., WEHMOLLER, M., et al. 2004. Growth and transplantation of a custom vascularised bone graft in a man. *Lancet*, 364, 766–70.

WIKESJO, U. M., SORENSEN, R. G. KINOSHITA, A., JIAN LI, X., & WOZNEY, J. M. 2004. Periodontal repair in dogs: effect of recombinant human bone morphogenetic protein-12 (rhBMP-12) on regeneration of alveolar bone and periodontal attachment. *J Clin Periodontol*, 31, 662–70.

WINDISCH, P., SCULEAN, A., & GERA, I. 1999. GTR with three different types of membranes in the treatment of intrabony periodontal defects: three-year results in sixty consecutive cases. *J Long Term Eff Med Implants*, 9, 235–46.

XU, Y., & MACENTEE, M. I. 1994. The roots of dentistry in ancient China. *J Can Dent Assoc*, 60, 613–6.

YU, J. M., WU, X., GIMBLE, J. M., GUAN, X., FREITAS, M. A., & BUNNELL, B. A. 2011. Age-related changes in mesenchymal stem cells derived from rhesus macaque bone marrow. *Aging Cell*, 10, 66–79.

Index

Note: Page references in *italics* refer to Figures and Protocols; those in **bold** refer to Tables

Tissue Engineering and Regeneration in Dentistry: Current Strategies, First Edition. Edited by Rachel J. Waddington and Alastair J. Sloan.
© 2017 John Wiley & Sons, Ltd. Published 2017 by John Wiley & Sons, Ltd.